D0328752

Infantile Spasms and West Syndrome

EDITED BY

OLIVIER DULAC
HARRY T. CHUGANI
BERNARDO DALLA BERNARDINA

W. B. SAUNDERS COMPANY LTD

London · Philadelphia · Toronto · Sydney · Tokyo

W. B. Saunders Company Ltd 24–28 Oval Road
London NW1 7DX

The Curtis Center
Independence Square West
Philadelphia, PA 19106–3399, USA

Harcourt Brace & Company
55 Horner Avenue
Toronto, Ontario M8Z 4X6, Canada

Harcourt Brace & Company, Australia
30–52 Smidmore Street
Marrickville, NSW 2204, Australia

Harcourt Brace & Company Japan
Ichibancho Central Building, 22–1 Ichibancho
Chiyoda-ku, Tokyo, 102, Japan

© 1994 W. B. Saunders Company Ltd

This book is printed on acid-free paper

All rights reserved. No part of this publication
may be reproduced, stored in a retrieval system
or transmitted, in any form or by any means,
electronic, mechanical, photocopying or otherwise,
without the prior permission of W. B. Saunders Company Ltd,
24–28 Oval Road, London NW1 7DX, England

A catalogue record for this book is available from the British Library.

ISBN   0-7020-1777-9

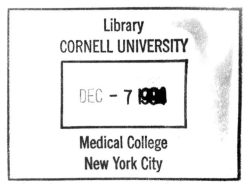

Library
CORNELL UNIVERSITY

DEC - 7 1994

Medical College
New York City

Editorial and Production Services by Fisher Duncan
10 Barley Mow Passage, London W4 4PH

Typeset by Paston Press Ltd, Loddon, Norfolk
Printed in Great Britain by the Cambridge University Press

Contents

III Morphology and Imaging

H. T. CHUGANI

IV Etiology

O. DULAC

V Treatment

H. T. CHUGANI

Acknowledgements

The work in Chapter 3 (S. L. Moshé *et al.*) was supported by NIH Grant NS-20253 and NRSA training grant NS-07183 from the NINDS and a training grant MH-15788 from the NIMH. Dr A. Tempel is thanked for her contributions in the receptor autoradiography studies and Ms Diane Smith for her technical expertise.

Chapter 4: the author gratefully acknowledges Dr Federico Vigevano for several helpful suggestions and for providing four figures.

Chapter 9: work in Dr Vinters' laboratory was supported by United States PHS Grants NS 26312 and 28383. H.V.V. appreciates ongoing discussions with Dr Robin Fisher and Dr Michael DeRosa, and the technical expertise of Diana Lenard Secor, Vadims Poukens, Alex Brooks, Laurel Reed and Yan Cheng.

Chapter 11: the authors would like to thank Dr C. Raynaud for his collaboration.

The editors would like to thank M. C. Henry for technical assistance.

Contributors

Catherine Billard, MD Service de Neurochirurgie, Hôpital de Clocheville, Blvd Béranger, 37044 Tours, France

LL Brown, Albert Einstein College of Medicine, 1330 Morris Park Avenue, Bronx, New York, NY 10461, USA

Catherine Chiron, MD Service Hospitalier F. Joliot, 4 place General Leclerc, 91406 Orsay, France

Harry T. Chugani, Professor of Pediatrics, Neurology and Radiology, Director Positron Emission Tomography Center, Children's Hospital of Michigan, Wayne State University School of Medicine, Detroit, MI 48210-2196, USA

Paolo Curatolo, MD Professor of Pediatric Neurology and Psychiatry, Via dei Sabelli, 108-00185 Rome, Italy

Rafaella Cusmai, MD Ospedale del Bambino Gesus, Servizio di Neurofisiopatologie, Piazza S. Onofrio n. 4, Rome, Italy

Bernardo Dalla Bernardina, Professor of Neuropsychiatry, Policlinico Borgo Rome, 37134 Verona, Italy

Claus Diebler, MD Neuroradiology Department, Hôpital Foch, 40 rue Worth, Suresnes 92150, France

Fritz Dreifuss, MD University of Virginia Medical Center, Dept of Neurology, Charlottesville, Virginia VA 22908, USA

Olivier Dulac, Professor of Pediatric Neurology, Hôpital St Vincent de Paul, 82 ave. Denfert-Rochereau, 75674 Paris Cedex 14, France

Jose Feingold, MD INSERM, Chateau de Longchamp, Bois de Boulogne, Paris 16e, France

Natalio Fejerman, MD Neurologo de Ninos, VIDT 2052, 2 C, 1425 Buenos Aires, Argentina

Lucia Fusco, MD Ospedale del Bambino Gesus, Servizio di Neurofisiopatologie, Piazza S. Onofrio n. 4, Rome, Italy

DS Garant, MD Department of Neurology, Albert Einstein College of Medicine, Bronx, New York, NY 10461, USA

Tiziana Granata, MD C Besta Neurological Institute, Milan, Italy

Daniel L Hurst, MD Texas Tech University Health Sciences Center, Department of Medical & Surgical Neurology, School of Medicine, Lubbock, Texas TX 79430, USA

Paul Hwang, MD EEG & Clinical Neurophysiology Laboratory, Division of Neurology, University of Toronto, 555 University Avenue, Toronto, Ontario M5G 1X8, Canada

Isabelle Jambaqué, MD Service de Neuropediatrie, INSERM U29, Hôpital St Vincent de Paul, 82 ave. Denfert-Rochereau, 75674 Paris Cedex 14, France

Solomon Moshé, MD Albert Einstein College of Medicine, Laboratory of Developmental Epilepsy, Rose F Kennedy Center, Room 316, 1410 Pelham Parkway South, Bronx, New York, NY 10461, USA

Jacques Motte, MD American Memorial Hospital, Reims 51092, France

Jean-Marc Pinard, MD Service de Neuropediatrie, Hôpital St Vincent de Paul, 82 ave. Denfert-Rochereau, 75674 Paris Cedex 14, France

Perrine Plouin, MD Laboratoire Electroencephalographie, INSERM U29, Hôpital St Vincent de Paul, 82 ave. Denfert-Rocherau, 75674 Paris Cedex 14, France

Stefano Ricci, MD Ospedale del Bambino Gesus, Servizio di Neurofisiopatologia, Piazza S. Onofrio n. 4, 00165 Rome, Italy

Raili Riikonen, MD Children's Castel Hospital, Dept of Child Neurology, Lastenlinnantic 11, University of Helsinki, Helsinki SF-00290, Finland

Olivier Robain, MD INSERM U29, Hôpital St Vincent de Paul, 82 ave. Denfert-Rochereau, 75674 Paris Cedex 14, France

J Roger, Centre St Paul, 300 Blvd Sainte Marguerite, Marseilles 13000, France

D Alan Shewmon, MD UCLA Medical School, Department of Pediatrics & Division of Neurology, 10833 Le Comte Avenue, Los Angeles, CA 90024-1752, USA

O Carter Snead III, MD Chief, Division of Neurology, Children's Hospital of Los Angeles & UCLA, 4650 Sunset Blvd, Los Angeles CA90027, USA

EF Sperber, MD Depts of Neurology and Neuroscience, Laboratory of Developmental Epilepsy, Albert Einstein College of Medicine, Bronx, New York, NY 10461, USA

Louis Vallee, MD Hôpital B, CHRU Lille, 59037 Lille Cedex, France

Francesco Viani, MD Regina Elena Hospital, Milan, Italy

Frederico Vigevano, MD Servizio di Neurofisiopatologia, Ospedale del Bambino Gesus, Piazza S. Onofrio n. 4, 00165 Rome, Italy

Harry V Vinters, MD Associate Professor of Pathology and Laboratory Medicine, Chief, Section of Neuropathology, UCLA School of Medicine, 10833 Le Comte Avenue, Los Angeles, CA 90024-1752, USA

Kazuyoshi Watanabe, MD Department of Pediatrics, Nagoya University School of Medicine, 65 Tsuruma-Cho, Showa-Ku, Nagoya, Japan

SG Xu, MD Department of Neurology, Albert Einstein College of Medicine, Bronx, New York, NY 10461, USA

Foreword

The past 10 years have witnessed increasing interest in defining the specific epileptic syndromes, fine-tuning the diagnostic criteria for their delineation in order to predict the etiological influence and identify genetic factors as many of the syndromes have found a place on the human genome. The starting point for the definition of an epileptic syndrome is the accurate identification and definition of the seizure type which is usually the presenting symptom of the condition. Many of the syndromes have yielded to advances in antiepileptic drug therapy or, occasionally, to advances in imaging technology and surgical technique. The last decade has also seen a proliferation of books concerning the epileptic syndromes, the surgical treatment of the epilepsies and the development of new antiepileptic drugs possessing specific modes of action based on improved knowledge of the pathophysiology of the epilepsies. Despite these many advances some of the early childhood epileptic encephalopathies have not been successfully assuaged. One of the outstanding examples has been West syndrome, recognized through its presenting symptom, the infantile spasms, a condition which has to a large degree continued to defy etiologic speculation and therapeutic intervention.

This book represents a collation of advances in diagnostic capability through intensive monitoring, magnetic resonance imaging and positron emission tomography, as well as improvement in knowledge in biochemistry of the inborn errors of metabolism and molecular genetics, as in the case of tuberous sclerosis, neurofibromatosis and various other brain dysplastic disorders. While definitive pharmacological management of infantile spasms remains elusive, still depending largely on steroids, refinement in administration as well as the development of new antiepileptic drugs has resulted in an improved repertoire of medicaments largely devised in response to increase in knowledge about seizure mechanisms. One of the key areas described in this book is the identification of brain dysplasias as an etiology of infantile spasms and as potentially surgically remediable lesions.

The sesqui-centennial of the first description of West syndrome in 1841 illustrates in a microcosm the history of neurological science in this era in its exponential evolution. It is thus a fitting international contribution to the literature of the Decade of the Brain.

FRITZ E. DREIFUSS MB, FRCP, FRACP

Overview

O. DULAC, H.T. CHUGANI, B. DALLA BERNARDINA

Epileptic spasms (ES), when associated with the electroencephalogram (EEG) pattern called "hypsarrhythmia", constitute the best example of an age-related epilepsy syndrome and a unique model for the study of the interaction between epilepsy and brain maturation. Since the major monographs addressing this disorder in the late 1960s, there have been major advances in nosology, diagnostic tools, etiology and treatment, although a number of issues remain controversial.

The syndrome has been called either West syndrome (WS) or infantile spasms (IS). However, spasms are no more than a special type of epileptic seizure. Although in infancy they are usually associated with diffuse paroxysmal interictal EEG activity and therefore part of IS as a syndrome, they may also occur long after infancy has ended. In addition, hypsarrhythmia has a restrictive meaning of generalized nonfocal paroxysmal activity. West syndrome combines ES and hypsarrhythmia, and is thus a subgroup of IS. Therefore, the terms "IS" and "WS" are preferred as epilepsy syndromes, whereas the term "ES" should apply to the type of seizures, whatever the age at which they occur.

Epidemiological data show that IS involves 1 in every 2000–4000 infants. It occurs throughout the world, but although it is likely that the relative frequency for each etiology varies according to socio-economic conditions and genetic background, this issue has not yet been addressed.

The majority of cases of IS are symptomatic. The nonsymptomatic cases are called "cryptogenic" or "idiopathic", although these labels have different meanings. In particular, the existence of an "idiopathic" form which, on the current understanding of the term, implies the absence of any underlying brain lesion, is still not generally accepted.

There have been major advances in the diagnosis of the various disorders associated with IS. Both the clinical and EEG characteristics may be somewhat modified by the underlying pathology. Pharmacological modifications of the interictal EEG, continuous ambulatory EEG monitoring and EEG video-telemetry have demonstrated the previously overlooked high frequency of various lateralizing features such as asymmetry of the interictal tracing, focal

1

discharges (which may occasionally be combined with, or drive, a cluster of spasms), and focal events such as eye deviation during the spasms, all of which provide diagnostic and prognostic information, since they indicate some kind of focal or multifocal cortical damage. Tracings are different in patients with malformations and those with inborn errors of metabolism. Indeed, the interictal EEG may be so characteristic that it provides a major clue to the etiological diagnosis. On the other hand, the electroclinical characteristics of clusters of spasms may be a major clue to the diagnosis of the "idiopathic" form.

Video-polygraphy EEG analysis of the ictal event has shown that the EEG counterpart of spasms is a generalized high-amplitude slow wave. Video EEG and ambulatory EEG monitoring have revealed the previously overlooked high frequency of partial seizures which, combined with ES, help to demonstrate focal cortical involvement. Repeat wake and sleep EEG recordings may be necessary to identify newly recognized conditions, such as benign nonepileptic infantile spasms and ES without diffuse interictal paroxysms, otherwise called "periodic spasms", that are less clearly age-related and do not come under the heading of IS.

One of the major breakthroughs in the diagnosis of disorders producing IS resulted from advances in brain imaging. Structural imaging with computed tomography and in particular magnetic resonance imaging (MRI), have revealed developmental abnormalities such as cortical dysplasia and other types of cerebral dysgenesis. Functional imaging with positron emission tomography and single photon emission tomography, on the other hand, have both disclosed focal abnormalities that have even been overlooked by MRI. In addition, they contribute to the understanding of the basic mechanisms involved in the generation of IS.

Progress in biochemistry has increased the number of inborn errors of metabolism associated with IS. Neuropathological studies have improved our understanding of the major role played by focal cortical malformations in this generalized seizure disorder. Diffuse cortical abnormalities that fail to undergo normal maturation are a major component of chronicity, and this implies that maturation of the cortex plays a major role in the epileptogenicity of IS. In contrast, the scarcity of subcortical and particularly brainstem lesions is striking, since the disorder has long been believed to originate at subcortical levels of the brain.

Although a genetic contribution to IS seems to be absent in most patients, there is growing evidence that in selective and recognizable cases, a specific genetic background plays a major role via several mechanisms. A few genetically determined congenital encephalopathies are usually associated with IS; a Finnish disorder of this type has been reported. Several types of brain dysplasia producing IS are genetically determined, following a Mendelian transmission or due to chromosomal aberration. In idiopathic WS, a genetic contribution linked to other types of idiopathic epilepsy syndromes still awaits investigation.

Differential diagnosis includes nonepileptic paroxysmal events, the most peculiar of which is "benign nonepileptic infantile spasms" (otherwise known as "benign myoclonus of early infancy"), and various epilepsy syndromes occurring in infancy. The limits between early infantile epileptic encephalopathy and IS remain unclear, and the concept of periodic spasms is increasingly accepted.

New concepts in the treatment of IS have emerged. Depending on the etiology, different regimens for steroid therapy have been proposed (i.e. high versus low doses), thus reducing the risk of side-effects in the majority of patients without reducing overall efficacy. The idea that steroids should not be administered to patients with symptomatic IS would appear to be inadequate, since some etiologies, such as periventricular leukomalacia and various postnatal disorders, seem to respond well to steroids.

New drugs have been used, not only when steroids have proved not to be effective, but as the drug of choice in some etiologies. Idiopathic cases may be good candidates for the use of pyridoxal phosphate or valproate, and tuberous sclerosis may be the best indication for vigabatrin as initial treatment. Various types of surgical treatment have been developed and one of the major issues is the timing of such procedures, that is, whether patients should undergo surgery soon after the onset of IS, after a few months, or only after various drug combinations have failed.

Before the development of specific treatment schedules, the incidence of spontaneous recovery increased over a period of several years. In individual cases, and according to etiology, the outcome in IS varies greatly: a small proportion of patients recover spontaneously or with a short treatment schedule; others stop having seizures but are left with a mental, sensory or motor handicap, and in a significant proportion intractable focal or generalized epilepsy persists. The factors that determine the type of outcome are of crucial importance for prognosis and therapeutic decisions.

Cognitive disorders associated with IS are heterogeneous. They consist of a variable combination of mental retardation, speech delay, visuomotor dyspraxia and autistic features. Several mechanisms are involved which have been clarified by neuropsychological evaluation and functional imaging. For example, brain lesions can produce selective neuropsychological disorders depending upon their topography. The major involvement of posterior areas contributes to the understanding of predominant communication, including visual disorders. In addition, neuropsychological follow-up helps to determine the role played by brain lesions, persisting seizures, the persistence of major interictal EEG spiking including hypsarrhythmia that should be considered a nonconvulsive status epilepticus, and aggressive schedules of drug treatment. One major issue is to what extent the transient hypsarrhythmic phenomenon may contribute to the worsening of the long-term cognitive disorders produced by focal brain lesions.

Given the clear variability in clinical and EEG expression, and in the response to treatment according to etiology, one may be justified in splitting the syndrome. However, the various causes share a common age of occurrence, a common type of seizures and diffuse EEG abnormalities, thus suggesting that common pathophysiological mechanisms are involved whatever the etiology.

Major progress has been achieved in the understanding of seizure disorders in the developing brain. Animal models have shown that there is an excess of N-methyl-D-aspartate (NMDA) receptors postnatally, which not only play an important role in the development of sensorial pathways but also in the excitability of the brain. There is also an excess of corticocortical axons that contribute to generalization of epileptic phenomena, although the latter are asynchronous due to delayed myelination. Kindling studies in pups show that generalization occurs after fewer stimulations than in adult rats, but that jerks are asynchronous, thus expressing the paradox of increased number of fibers but also increased conduction velocity due to delayed myelination. Alternate stimulation in both hemispheres also enhances kindling. In addition, there is an excess of $GABA_B$ receptors in the substantia nigra.

In IS, the age-relationship points to the structures that undergo the most rapid maturation during infancy – the cortex and in particular the posterior portion of the cerebral hemispheres – and indeed these are the most frequent locations of focal brain lesions in symptomatic IS. Both new drugs and the surgical approach have contributed to the understanding of pathophysiology in patients with focal cortical lesions by demonstrating that IS may be no more than a particular type of generalization of epileptogenesis from a focal cortical disorder at a certain stage of brain development.

However, the structures involved in producing the IS remain undetermined, and the relationship between cortical abnormalities, hypsarrhythmia, focal discharges and the spasms are still not clearly understood. One possibility is that a focal cortical epileptogenic area triggers subcortical areas that produce both spasms and hypsarrhythmia. Another possibility is that redundant but nonmyelinized corticocortical pathways produce generalization from one or several cortical areas resulting in the hypsarrhythmic pattern, a nonconvulsive status causing continuous inhibition of cortical activity. Disinhibition of subcortical areas would then cause them to produce spasms. Later, maturation of the cortex and the disappearance of redundant corticocortical fibers would prevent generalization into hypsarrhythmia, explaining the age-relationship.

The causes of the eventual persistence of a severe generalized epilepsy remain unclear and IS is a valuable model for the study of seizure intractability. Mechanisms such as the kindling of cortical structures may be involved, although the conditions under which they occur are different in infancy and in adulthood. In addition, other neurobiological phenomena may play a role: the relative contribution of the topography of brain lesions, the ontogeny of various neurotransmitter receptors, the transient presence of redundant fibers and synapses at the age of onset of IS, the lack of maturation of wide dysplastic cortical areas, all remain to be determined for given etiologies.

This book comprises five parts. (1) The general characteristics of the syndrome are studied – its history, nosology and epidemiology – and the basic mechanisms are discussed according to experimental data. (2) We then consider the variable aspects of each component of the syndrome (i.e. types of seizures, interictal EEG and cognitive disorders) and discuss the differential diagnoses. (3) The next part of the book is devoted to morphology and imaging, both of which have been central to our understanding and management of the syndrome. (4) Next, according to each major etiology, we review the special characteristics of each component of the syndrome. (5) Finally, we consider both medical and surgical treatments.

1

West Syndrome: History and Nosology

J. ROGER, O. DULAC

HISTORY

As shown in great detail by Gastaut and Poirier (1964), the identification of clusters of spasms as a subacute epileptic condition comprise two periods. The clinical period was initiated by West (1841), an English pediatrician who witnessed the condition for the first time in his own child. He gave a most complete and precise description, mentioning that the movements were brief, flexor and axial, mainly involving the neck, and that they occurred in clusters. He described the mental deterioration and emphasized intractability, noting that all his therapeutic trials had been "without any benefit". In addition, he recognized the convulsive nature of the disorder, although at onset he had "thought the child had learned a new tick".

Following West, a number of reports appeared over the following 80 years. The condition was discovered in Germany 10 years after West's report (Willshire, 1851) and in France 30 years later (Féré, 1883), although Herpin from Geneva mentioned it in his 1867 textbook, recognizing that "minor" forms of epilepsy could produce cognitive deterioration. It had been considered a rare condition, because by 1941 only 68 cases had been reported in the literature (Wöhler, 1941). Zellweger (1948) was the first to suspect a higher incidence, as he was able to report on 32 cases personally witnessed over a period of 20 years.

There was no major improvement in clinical knowledge during this period. The most striking feature is the spectrum of names given to the condition, and therefore its nosological understanding (Table 1.1). The terms placed emphasis on the *flexion* that predominates at the head, and to some these movements suggested a *greeting* (e.g. "Salaam convulsions", "Komplimentierkrämpfe", "spasmes salutatoires"); other terms stressed the *brevity* of the movements (e.g. "lightning major seizures", "startle seizures"). Most unfortunate among this profusion of terms was the use of the term "tic", which suggests a nonconvulsive phenomenon: it may be one reason why the condition was for a long time confused with stereotyped movements of mentally retarded children. Zellweger, who had the most precise perception of the condition as a nosological

Table 1.1 Early names for West syndrome

Name	Reference
Eclampsia nutans	Newnham (1849)
Nodding convulsions of infancy	Barnes (1873)
Nickkrämpfe	Lederer (1926)
Tics d'inclination de la tête	Marchand and De Ajuriaguerra (1948)
Salaam convulsions	Clarke (cited in West, 1841)
Komplimentierkrämpfe	Willshire (1851)
Salaamkrämpfe	Knauer (1925)
Tic de salaam	Féré (1883)
Spasmes salutoires	Jacquet (1903)
Blitzkrämpfe	Asal and Moro (1925)
Lightning major seizures	Buchanan (1946)
Startle seizures	Bridge (1949)
Blitz- Nick- und Salaamkrämpfe	Zellweger (1948)

entity at the end of the clinical period, created the term "Blitz- Nick- und Salaamkrämpfe" (1948), thus synthesizing all previous concepts. Therefore, at the end of the clinical period, clusters of epileptic spasms often remained confused with other epileptic (Barnes, 1873; Descroizilles, 1886) or nonepileptic (Schachter, 1954) conditions.

In the early 1950s, electroencephalography (EEG) changed the way in which paroxysmal motor phenomena were studied. Neurophysiologists believed they had discovered a previously unknown condition. They reported slow dysrhythmia with diffuse spike waves in infants with "epilepsia en flexion generalizada" (Vasquez and Turner, 1951), or "myoclonic phenomena in infants" (Kellaway, 1952). In addition, the "petit mal variant" tracing was first reported by Lennox and Davis (1950) in young children who exhibited "massive myoclonic jerks, jacknife movements", often in clusters during sleep. Evidently, there was some confusion between what were to become the "West" and "Lennox-Gastaut" syndromes.

There were two major contributions to the identification of West syndrome. Gastaut and Rémond (1952) distinguished two types of epileptic jerks: the "myoclonies A", corresponding to the massive myoclonus of the present classification (Classification, 1981), and the "myoclonies B", which are more prolonged and often occur in clusters during the first 2 years of life, thus corresponding to clusters of epileptic spasms. The latter were associated with "diffuse dysrhythmic delta and theta activity intermingled with slow spike waves of variable topography". Gibbs and Gibbs (1952) provided the classic description of the interictal EEG tracing, and invented the term "hypsarrhythmia". They proposed to name the ictal events "spasms", noting that the concomitant EEG recording consisted of a rapid low-amplitude discharge.

Thus, the various components of the syndrome were identified by neurophysiologists long before pediatricians became interested in studying the EEG correspondence of what their predecessors had identified on a clinical basis a century earlier. One remarkable exception was Hess, who recognized the condition he had previously studied with Zellweger and reported with Neuhaus on "Bltiz- Nick- Salaam Krämpfe mit diffuse gemische Krämpfe potentiale" (Zellweger and Hess, 1950).

Although the condition had long been known to a number of clinicians, its recognition in a given infant remained problematic on clinical grounds. The role played by EEG in its diagnosis is expressed by the confusion that is still often made between the terms "infantile spasms" and "hypsarrhythmia". Indeed, the present classification (1981) of epileptic seizures does not consider clusters of spasms as a type of epileptic seizures.

Sorel and Dusaucy-Bauloye (1958) increased significantly interest in this condition with their report on the efficacy of adrenocorticotrophic hormone (ACTH). Since there seemed to be a rather specific treatment, clusters of spasms and hypsarrhythmia were considered to be either a disease or a syndrome, often called "West syndrome".

The precise nosological limits, etiology and variable expression of the condition became the subject of study. For example, although some infants had previously been retarded, West noted that his child had experienced normal development. From a meeting in Marseille (Gastaut et al., 1964a), it appeared that the interictal pattern was variable, and several variants of "atypical hypsarrhythmia" were described. They included fragmented, slow, rapid asymmetric and focal variants. The distinction emerged between cryptogenic and symptomatic cases, the latter comprising pre-, peri- and post-natal causes. Tuberous sclerosis had been recognized in 1955 (Janz and Matthes, 1955), but its frequency was underestimated until Pampiglione and Pugh (1975) reported the achromic nevus as the earliest cutaneous stigma of the disease. Neuroradiology contributed to the identification of specific malformations, such as the Aicardi syndrome of callosal agenesis and ocular lacunae in girls (Aicardi et al., 1969) and agyria-lissencephaly (Goutieres and Aicardi, 1971) as causes of spasms in clusters. In addition, it appeared paradoxically that focal brain lesions could be involved in this generalized epilepsy. The best prognosis involved the primary cases, labelled "idiopathic" (Jeavons and Bower, 1964) or "cryptogenic" (Gastaut et al., 1964b). The distinction between the two terms only appeared later (Commission 1989). Whatever the cause, the disorder was thought to result from brainstem dysfunction because of the diffuse involvement of the brain.

From the late 1970s, other conditions of severe generalized epilepsy of early infancy, resembling West syndrome from a clinical or EEG point of view, have been recognized. Two of these comprised a suppression burst pattern for which Maheshwari and Jeavons (1975) had previously stressed poor prognostic significance. A non-progressive condition described by Ohtahara (1978) combining spasms and focal seizures without myoclonus, was mainly due to malformations. Ohtahara believed it often evolved to West syndrome. Another progressive condition combining myoclonus and focal seizures, with (Aicardi, 1985) or without (Schlumberger et al., 1992) spasms, was supposed to result from an inborn error in metabolism. Dalla Bernardina *et al.* (1985) described myoclonic epilepsy in nonprogressive encephalopathy of infancy. A non-epileptic condition, "benign myoclonus of infancy", was also identified (Lombroso and Fejerman, 1977).

Four new methods of investigation helped to improve our understanding of the disorder. First, with the advent of *computerized neuroradiology*, it was possible to recognize differences in the clinical and EEG characteristics of different etiologies, particularly Aicardi syndrome (Fariello *et al.*, 1977), agyria (Dulac *et al.*, 1983a) and tuberous sclerosis (Dulac *et al.*, 1984). It was shown that patients with tuberous sclerosis rarely exhibited hypsarrhythmia, but did exhibit focal spikes, the "focal" variant of hypsarrhythmia (Gastaut *et al.*, 1964a), and that they suffered from secondary generalized epilepsy produced by the major cortical tubers. The interictal tracing of agyria corresponded to the "rapid" variant of hypsarrhythmia reported by Gastaut *et al.* (1964a).

Second, the systematic use of *polygraphy* and *video monitoring* showed that in patients with malformations, clusters of spasms could be combined with a focal cortical discharge, and that the whole cluster of spasms consisted of a single seizure, thus demonstrating the contribution of the cortex to epilepsy (Bour *et al.*, 1986). Video-recordings showed that in symptomatic cases, patients often had asymmetric spasms with eye of head lateral deviation. Ambulatory 24 hour recordings revealed frequent focal discharges (Plouin *et al.*, 1993). In contrast with symptomatic cases, it appeared that 5–10% of cases had no evidence of brain lesion, even on long-term follow-up, and that these "idiopathic" cases had specific clinical and EEG characteristics (Dulac *et al.*, 1986a; Vigevano *et al.*, 1993). On the other hand, Gobbi *et al.* (1987) showed that clusters of spasms could appear in childhood, without hypsarrhythmia. They called these later occurring spasms "periodic spasms".

Third, *neuropsychological* evaluation showed that cognitive problems are varied but quite specific, and that they correlate with the topography of cortical involvement (Jambaqué *et al.*, 1989). Fourth, *functional imaging* helped to demonstrate local abnormalities in cryptogenic cases, using single photon emission tomography (Dulac *et al.*, 1987a) and positron emission tomography (PET: Chugani *et al.*, 1990). PET showed local abnormalities in cryptogenic cases that consist of focal dysplasia and that such patients can be considerably improved by surgical resection. Functional imaging also contributed to the understanding of pathophysiology of seizures (Chugani *et al.*, 1992).

From the therapeutic point of view, it is striking that no controlled study has demonstrated the efficacy of steroids on seizures, compared with a placebo or a reference drug. The need for controlled studies has been stressed by retro-spective studies of spontaneous remission and long-term outcome in patients with infantile spasms, which have shown that in older series prior to steroid treatment, the cumulative spontaneous remission rate was 25% during the first 12 months after onset (Hrachovy *et al.*, 1991). Paradoxically, many open studies have attempted to determine the optimal doses of steroids, based on their effect on seizures, but efficacy still remains a matter for debate, particularly in terms of cognitive function (Jeavons *et al.*, 1973). Progress in therapy has also included the administration of conventional drugs such as benzodiazepines, valproate or vigabatrin, and also surgery. It would appear at present that therapeutic decisions should be based on etiology.

NOSOLOGICAL CONSIDERATIONS

The present understanding of nosology can be synthesized as follows. *Epileptic spasms* usually occur in clusters. A given cluster may consist of a series of independent seizures or of a single seizure. In the latter case, the cluster may be initiated, combined or followed by a focal discharge. Therefore, epileptic spasms are particular seizure types, but not a single and homogeneous type of epileptic seizure. This should be taken into account when classifying epileptic seizures.

Epileptic spasms most often occur in the first year of life, thus justifying the term *infantile spasms*; and in combination with interictal diffuse asynchronous paroxysmal activity. However, epileptic spasms are occasionally observed later in the first decade of life. Thus, the term infantile spasms involves a syndromic condition comprising three components: particular seizure types, interictal EEG and age of occurrence.

The *hypsarrhythmic* pattern defined by Gibbs and Gibbs (1952) is age-related. It is fragmented by sleep and may be modified by underlying pathology. However, it is different from the specific pattern produced by brain malformations such as Aicardi's callosal agenesis or agyria. In tuberous sclerosis and various focal brain lesions, it is usual to see focal spikes with secondary generalization, a tracing different from hypsarrhythmia. However, the spike activity is age-related (see Chapter 3), and correlates with the peak incidence of epileptic spasms in infancy.

According to the type of interictal activity, epileptic spasms may therefore consist of a focal epilepsy with secondary generalization, of a symptomatic generalized epilepsy, or of a primary condition. The latter does not, however, meet the other characteristics of primary generalized epilepsy – generalized synchronous 3 Hz spike wave activity, generalized tonic clonic, absence of myoclonic seizures, and genetic predisposition. Only the patients with epileptic spasms and either typical hypsarrhythmia or hypsarrhythmia modified by the underlying pathology should be included under the term "West syndrome" and considered as suffering from primary ("idiopathic West syndrome"), cryptogenic or symptomatic generalized epilepsy. Mental retardation is not a consistent feature of West syndrome, even at follow-up. There is growing evidence that the distinction between various types of infantile spasms – focal or generalized epilepsy – has practical therapeutic implications.

Whether West syndrome should be considered a type of nonconvulsive status epilepticus or a chronic disorder consisting of recurring epileptic seizures remains unclear. It shares with epilepsy the recurrence of seizures, but with status epilepticus the deterioration of cognitive and neurological function. This type of condition, usually called *epileptic encephalopathy*, also comprises Lennox-Gastaut syndrome and continuous spike waves in slow sleep. All these conditions may lead to a worsening of the patient's condition as a consequence of frequent seizures and major interictal spike activity.

The relationship between the Ohtahara and West syndromes remains confused. Follow-up of patients with Ohtahara syndrome shows that the suppression of activity between bursts decreases progressively to a point where the tracing resembles fragmentation of interictal activity in sleep that is so usual in West syndrome (Lombroso, 1990). The confusion between the syndromes is increased by the heterogeneous etiology of West syndrome. Most patients with suppression bursts, spasms and focal seizures due to Aicardi syndrome never exhibit hypsarrhythmia, whereas patients with tuberous sclerosis never exhibit suppression bursts. Therefore, the time has come to base diagnosis as much as possible on etiology. On the other hand, there is growing evidence that neonatal myoclonic encephalopathy is an autonomous condition (Lombroso, 1990).

DEFINITIONS

In this volume, the term *epileptic spasms* will address a seizure type of brief axial muscular contraction often occurring in clusters. It will be used in a broad sense, whatever the age of occurrence, and including the so-called periodic spasms (Gobbi *et al.*, 1987). The term *infantile spasms* will address an epilepsy syndrome of epileptic spasms beginning in infancy and combined with interictal activity, be it focal or diffuse. *Hypsarrhythmia*, a particular type of interictal EEG, will be used according to its classical definition of generalized interictal paroxysmal activity, eventually modified, but not as a secondary generalized phenomenon, and it will not include the tracings that are specific to particular cortical malformations. *West syndrome* will relate to the combination of infantile spasms and hypsarrhythmia, with or without cognitive impairment.

2

Epidemiology

D.L. HURST

OVERVIEW

Previous epidemiological reviews of West syndrome have unfortunately pre-dated the 1985 definition of infantile spasms as determined by the Commission on Classification and Terminology of the International League Against Epilepsy (Commission, 1985). However, the following three large studies do allow for a calculation of incidence rates in infantile spasms: the National Institute of Neurologic and Communicative Disorders Perinatal Collaborative Study (NCPP) performed in the USA between 1959 and 1966; a review of infantile spasms from Denmark covering the years 1957–75; and a study from Finland covering the years 1960–76 (Nelson, 1972; Ellenberg *et al.*, 1984; Shields *et al.*, 1988; Riikonen and Donner, 1979). Four smaller studies from France, Denmark and Sweden have calculated incidences for infantile spasms (Luna *et al.*, 1988; Howitz and Platz, 1978; Loiseau *et al.*, 1990; Eeg-Olofsson and Sidenvall, 1992). Although the National Childhood Encephalopathy Study from Great Britain yields some epidemiologic data, an incidence cannot be calculated from its data (Bellman *et al.*, 1983; Miller *et al.*, 1981; Committee, 1981). A number of other studies from Italy, Japan, the USA, Sweden and Saudi Arabia also allow for the calculation of some epidemiological data but are too small in size to allow for reliable incidence rates to be calculated (Maremmani *et al.*, 1991; Tsuboi, 1988; Van den Berg and Yarushalmy, 1969; Heijbel *et al.*, 1975; Al-Rajeh *et al.*, 1990; Ohtahara *et al.*, 1981; Cowan *et al.*, 1989). Besides calculating an incidence, at least two notable observations can be made from a review of these prior studies. First, multiple studies have identified a higher male-to-female ratio in infantile spasms (Jeavons, 1985). Second, the epidemiological data available at this time do not support a causative association between immunizations and infantile spasms (AAP, 1991). A recent review of infantile spasms discussed other aspects, such as the epidemiology of etiologies and differences related to genetic background and environmental factors (Cowan and Hudson, 1991).

12

INTRODUCTION

Although West syndrome is a well-recognized entity which has been identified and discussed for some time (Jeavons and Bower, 1964; Dreifuss, 1983a), its age of onset has recently been redefined to a more narrow period and its characteristics have been more closely delineated (Commission, 1989). As stated by the Commission on Classification and Terminology of the International League Against Epilepsy, "Onset peaks between the ages of four and seven months and always occurs before the age of one year," (Commission, 1989). Previous to 1985, a broader definition of infantile spasms was used and cases of infantile spasms were accepted with onset after 1 year of age (Commission, 1985; Jeavons *et al.*, 1973). Furthermore, the spasms of seizures of West syndrome are now recognized to be of several types and to be associated with hypsarrhythmia (Commission, 1989; Bobele and Bodensteiner, 1990). Until now, there has been no epidemiological review of infantile spasms within a general population base using the 1985 definition or understanding of West syndrome (Commission, 1985). Some pre-1985 studies of infantile spasms are, however, available for review and contain enough information for a discriminating and current epidemiological analysis. It must be accepted for purposes of this discussion that the authors of these earlier studies appropriately identified their patients with infantile spasms (Cowan *et al.*, 1989; Melchior, 1977). It is acknowledged that the definitions earlier studies used may be somewhat more flexible than the current definition. For some it may seem more reasonable to use the previous broader definitions, since only the International League used such a strict definition.

Since "incidence is the rate at which new cases of a condition occur in a population" and "prevalence of epilepsy is a measure of the proportion of patients currently suffering from an active epilepsy", then only studies which have a general population base can give rise to incidence and prevalence figures (Melchior, 1977). It is unfortunate that so many studies have given only the number of children with West syndrome in a given selected epilepsy population, since these studies do not leave themselves open for the calculation of an incidence or prevalence rate of infantile spasms (Dreifuss, 1983a; Commission, 1989; Jeavons *et al.*, 1973; Bobele and Bodensteiner, 1990). Those studies which were population-based did not necessarily use uniform definitions or large general population bases, but at least nine studies from various countries do lend themselves to the generation of epidemiological data such as prevalence and incidence rates for infantile spasms (Howitz and Platz, 1978; Loiseau *et al.*, 1990; Eeg-Olofsson and Sidenvall, 1992; Bellman *et al.*, 1983; Miller *et al.*, 1981; Committee, 1981; Maremmani *et al.*, 1991; Tsuboi, 1958; Van den Berg and Yerushalmy, 1969; Heijbel *et al.*, 1975; Al-Rajeh *et al.*, 1990; Ohtahara *et al.*, 1981; Cowan *et al.*, 1989).

Past reviews of infantile spasms have stated the frequency to range between 1 in 1700–4000 or 1 in 4000–6000 live births (Melchior, 1977; Hrachovy *et al.*, 1981; Holmes, 1987). Although many excellent reviews about infantile spasms have been published, no-one has analyzed all available epidemiological data for which a prevalence or incidence rate in infantile spasms can be calculated (Jeavons, 1985; Melchior, 1977; Hrachovy *et al.*, 1981; Holmes, 1987; Aicardi, 1986a). Multiple studies from pediatric and adult epilepsy groups have identified children with West syndrome, and the prevalence of infantile spasms among patients with epilepsy at some particular clinics can be calculated (Loiseau *et al.*, 1991; Todt, 1984; Viani *et al.*, 1988; Sofijanov, 1982). However, since these studies are not population-based, they unfortunately do not give rise to data which produce an incidence rate for infantile spasms. In other words, they contain a numerator (i.e. the number of children identified with infantile spasms), but lack a denominator (i.e. the total number of children at risk for infantile spasms in a general population).

General prevalence rates for epilepsy in children are known but do vary widely (from 2 in 1000 to 37 in 1000) among populations (Hauser and Nelson, 1988). Since "incidence is the rate at which new cases of a condition occur in a population" during a given period of time, and prevalence is the number of existing cases in the total study population, then only studies which have a general population base can give rise to incidence and prevalence rates which are meaningful for infantile spasms (Hauser and Nelson, 1988). It is unfortunate that so many studies have given only the number of children with infantile spasms in a given selected epilepsy population rather than in a general pediatric population. Prevalence rates of infantile spasms in specialized epilepsy referral clinics are not very useful unless they can be tied to the known general incidence or prevalence rates of epilepsy, or other epileptic syndromes.

REVIEWS

Those studies which are population based have not necessarily used uniform definitions or large general population bases, but at least 14 studies from various countries do lend themselves to the generation of epidemiological data, such as prevalence and incidence rates for infantile spasms (Jeavons, 1985; Melchior *et al.*, 1977). The collaborative perinatal project of the National Institute of Neurological and Communicative Disorders (NCPP) was a study which enrolled pregnant women from 12 American urban teaching hospitals between the years 1959 and 1966 (Ellenberg *et al.*, 1984). The study registered 52,360 live births. Approximately 90% of these children were followed to 1 year of age, and 75% were followed to 7 years of age. The collaborative perinatal project (NCPP) has been intensely studied for a number of disorders including infantile spasms (Nelson, 1972; Ellenberg *et al.*, 1984). The NCPP has an abundance of medical information on those children in the study suffering from seizures. In addition, extensive developmental and neurological status data are known on all the children followed to the age of 7 years, and access to EEG reports is available. This allows for the identification of seizure events which meet the current clinical criteria for infantile spasms. Thus, due to its design, the NCPP ought to allow for excellent incidence and prevalence statistics, since extensive data are available for individual cases, and since the total study population (denominator) is well-defined.

In their article concerning the NCPP data, Ellenberg, Hirtz and Nelson identified 29 individuals with "minor motor seizures, including infantile spasms" (Ellenberg *et al.*, 1984). Minor motor seizures were further defined in their article as "tonic, hemitonic, myoclonic, or akinetic seizures, or mixtures of these". Since the children with infantile spasms are mixed with a large seizure category in this major review of the NCPP data, the numerator for this group could not be accurately determined. Furthermore, another study examining the epidemiology of severe myoclonic epilepsy reviewed data on NCPP infants with minor motor seizures and found that the majority of the cases did not have infantile spasms (Hurst, 1990). Thus, an incidence figure for infantile spasms in the NCPP population cannot be calculated based on the analysis by Ellenberg and colleagues (1984).

In a brief report by Nelson, 12 infantile spasm cases are identified in the NCPP data, though no details about the patients are given (Nelson, 1972). Again, of the 52 360 live births in the NCPP, 90% were followed to 1 year of age. So, using the 12 infantile spasm cases identified by Nelson from the first year NCPP data with a total study population of approximately 47 000, the incidence of infantile spasms during the first year of life would be 12 in 47 000 or approximately 1 in 3900 children (Nelson, 1972). The possibility exists that some children in the study had infantile spasms at an earlier date but died or were lost to follow-up before the end of the first year, since a total of 52 360 live births were registered but only 47 000 1-year-olds were examined in the NCPP. Yet even given the concerns about the total number of cases, the NCPP data would seem to allow the calculation of an estimated incidence of infantile spasms during the first year of life.

In Melchior's study in Denmark from 1970 to 1975, a large number of cases of infantile spasms were identified, though 3–4% of the cases had onset of spasms after 1 year of age (Melchior, 1977). This is a well-known article on infantile spasms because it explores the relationship of infantile spasms to early immunization against whooping cough. Since it was not Melchior's intent to look at the incidence or prevalence of infantile spasms in Denmark during the study period, he did not report the total population at risk for infantile spasms (the denominator).

Nevertheless, a further study of the Danish data allows a calculation of the incidence of infantile spasms within its population. Shields and colleagues, reviewing the same data as Melchior, focused on the relationship of the pertussis immunization to the onset of neurological disorders (Shields *et al.*, 1988). Shields *et al.* compared two 1-year periods, 1967–68 and 1972–73. A total number of 80 cases of infantile spasms were identified during the study years. The stated population for the study was about 150 000 children. Thus, the prevalence of infantile spasms in the Danish population as studied by Shields *et al.* is 80 in 150 000 or approximately 1 in 1875 children. Since this study followed its subjects from birth through the first 2 years of life, the incidence figures on infantile spasms should be approximately the same as the prevalence. Because, as Melchior noted, 3%–4% of the children with infantile spasms were over 1 year of age, the numerator generated from the data of Shields *et al.* would need to be reduced by 3–4% to fit the 1985 guidelines (Melchior, 1977). Such a reduction would result in only a slightly different prevalence in incidence calculation for the Danish study (1 in 1948). In sum, the incidence from the Danish study can be assumed to be approximately 1 in 1900 cases.

In a smaller study, Howitz and Platz (1978) prospectively identified all children with infantile spasms reported by each pediatric department in Denmark during 1976. The authors conclude that the cases identified give an incidence of about 1 in 3000–4000 live births. They do not report their denominator, the number of live births in Denmark during 1976, but do state that their results agree with the "reported incidence" of infantile spasms.

Riikonen and Donner (1979) undertook a major epidemiological study of infantile spasms in Finland between 1960 and 1976. They collected cases from Uusimaa County, Finland, identifying 107 children with infantile spasms admitted to three hospitals during that time period. The authors calculated incidence rates for three separate periods (1960–66, 1966–71 and 1972–76) to look at changes in incidence over time. They conclude that "the incidence of infantile spasms remained almost unchanged over the 17 years covered by this study" (Riikonen and Donner, 1979). From 1960 to 1966, 46 cases were reported in a total number of 109 478 live births. This gives an approximate incidence of 1 in 2300. From 1966 to 1971, 29 cases were identified in 76 082 live births for an approximate incidence of 1 in 2900. From 1972 to 1976, 33 cases of infantile spasms were noted in 75 217 live births for an approximate incidence of 1 in 2300. Riikonen and Donner discuss a wide range of etiological categories for infantile spasms in their article. They conclude that for the time period of study in Uusimaa County, the approximate incidence of infantile spasms was 1 in 2500 live births (Riikonen and Donner, 1979). Of the available literature, this Finnish study is the only one to look specifically at epidemiological data for a single population over time.

The National Childhood Encephalopathy Study (NCES) is a well-known British study undertaken to assess the potential relationship of neurological disorders to immunizations (Bellman *et al.*, 1983; Miller *et al.*, 1981; Committee, 1981). One of the disorders identified during the study period, 1976–79, was infantile spasms (Bellman *et al.*, 1983). Since the primary purpose of this study was to generate epidemiological information about immunizations, the total childhood population of immunization age in Great Britain (between 2 months and 3 years) was included in the study. No population numbers are given for 1976, but for 1977 the study population was 1 844 387, and for 1978 it was 1 792 546, as determined by mid-year estimates for the NCES. During the study, 269 infants were diagnosed with infantile spasms. In their review of NCES data, Bellman *et al.* (1983) use a definition of infantile spasms which includes myoclonic seizures, hypsarrythmia and developmental retardation. A graph provided in the article by Bellman *et al.* indicates that 10 of the 269 infantile spasm cases had their onset after 1 year of age. Thus, 259 cases of epileptic spasms from the NCES study can be considered to meet the criteria for the diagnosis of infantile spasms (Commission, 1989).

It is difficult to calculate the denominator (prevalence or incidence) for the NCES. Since the childhood population in Great Britain aged 2 months to 3 years by "mid-year estimates" was 1 844 387 in 1977 and 1 792 546 in 1978, the average number of children followed during the 2 years of the NCES is 1 818 466 (1 844 387 + 1 792 546 = 3 636 933 ÷ 2 = 1 818 466). In order to calculate a prevalence, this number must be assumed to be representative of 1976 also.

To calculate NCES incidence and prevalence rates under current definitions of West syndrome, it is necessary to include the children presenting with infantile spasms before the age of 2 months. Since the general population figures are not given for infants under 2 months, that population could be estimated to be 2/34 months, or 2/36 months − 2 months, or 1/17th of the NCES average total (1 818 466 = population 2 months to 3 years) as so far calculated. The additional estimated number of children under 2 months is 106 956. The "average" prevalence of infantile spasms in the NCES would then be roughly 259 in 1 925 422 (1 818 466 + 106 956) or approximately 1 in 7434. This has been a tedious calculation with many assumptions, and the prevalence figure includes not the actual study population but only the estimated average study population. Hence an accurate incidence rate cannot be calculated from the NCES data as it now exists, since the total population of children aged 1 year or less during the study is unknown.

Two studies from France produced data which allow for approximate incidence figures to be calculated (Luna *et al.*, 1988; Loiseau *et al.*, 1990). In a study from Bordeaux, all neurologists and electroencephalographers of the department of Gironde were asked to obtain information by questionnaire from all persons with new epileptic seizures commencing March 1, 1984 until February 28, 1985 (Loiseau *et al.*, 1990). The total study population for this area was 1 128 164. Eight cases of infantile spasms were identified for an incidence of 0.7 per 100 000 (all ages). If this number is divided by 70, the estimated incidence for infantile spasms during the first year is approximately 1 in 2000.

In a study from Oise between 1980 and 1984, Luna also registered all cases of epilepsy aged 10 years and under identified by the region's neurologists and EEG laboratories (Luna *et al.*, 1988). The total general population during the study was 107 562. This group identified cases of infantile spasms during the first 2 years of life. Statistics are given which suggest six cases of infantile spasms were identified. The study noted 10 726 children aged 0–1 year of age and 21 526 children aged 0–2 years of age. This gives an incidence figure of 1 in 1800–3600 or a mean of 1 in 2700.

A recently published epidemiological study of epileptic syndromes for the District of Northwest Tuscany (Vecchiano) did not report any cases of infantile spasms among 9952 inhabitants (Maremmani *et al.*, 1991). Since no children with infantile spasms could be identified, then the incidence was 0. The authors felt that with a relatively small population of approximately 10 000 the study would allow for intensive evaluation of those patients with epilepsy, resulting in a highly accurate classification of epileptic syndromes (Maremmani *et al.*, 1991). For small areas, the incidence may be low as in Vecchiano, but other cities in Italy such as Milan have identified cases of infantile spasms. Thus, the incidence of infantile spasms in Italy is not 0. This study illustrates the problem of looking for relatively uncommon epileptic syndromes in small general populations. With this in mind, another four relatively small study populations will be reviewed.

Tsuboi (1988) has reviewed the prevalence and incidence of epilepsy in Tokyo. He aimed to identify all 3-year-old children in Fuchu City, Tokyo who were seen at the Fuchu Health Center for regular health examinations during a 5-year period from 1974 to 1980. The total number of children examined was 17 044, and the examinations were usually conducted at 37 months of age. The author felt that the investigation covered 95% of the total population aged 3 years in the Fuchu area. The prevalence of seizures of any type in the 3-year-old population in Fuchu was 1649 in 17 044. Three children were identified as having infantile spasms. Three cases of Lennox-Gastaut syndrome were identified without comment about previous seizures being infantile spasms. Since infantile spasms are identified separately from Lennox-Gastaut syndrome, the assumption is that only three children were identified as having infantile spasms and that none of the Lennox-Gastaut syndrome patients started out with West syndrome. This results in a prevalence rate of 3 in 17 044, or 1 in 5681 for the 5-year period. Since examinations were not conducted in these children earlier than 3 years of age, an incidence figure for the onset of infantile spasms in the first year of life cannot be accurately calculated from this data.

Eeg-Olofsson and Sidenvall (1992) report the incidence of infantile spasms in the Uppsala region of Sweden between 1986 and 1991. The authors report an incidence of 1.4 in 1000 newborns per year in one of the north-eastern counties of this district. They suggest a possible relationship with the 1987 Russian Chernobyl nuclear plant catastrophe. A prospective study in this area is now in progress.

Matsumoto and colleagues (1981a) have published an account of a large series of cases with infantile spasms. Unfortunately, these are specialized referrals for in-hospital epilepsy treatment, and the general population database, or denominator, is unknown for the Matsumoto series. Ohtahara has reviewed the prevalence of epilepsy and febrile convulsions in Okayama Prefecture (Ohtahara *et al.*, 1981). This study was for the first 10 years of life and noted an annual prevalence rate of 0.14 per 1000 children.

In a study from the USA on convulsive disorders in young children, a cohort of 18 500 newborn infants were systematically followed through the Kaiser Foundation Hospital in Oakland, California between the years 1960 and 1967 for the development of febrile and nonfebrile convulsions. In total, 113 children were identified with nonfebrile convulsions. Van den Berg and Yerushalmy (1969) state that 3%, or 3 individuals, were identified as having infantile spasms. The prevalence of infantile spasms in this population is thus 1 in approximately 6200. A second US study from Oklahoma reported a 0.19 per 1000 (1 in 5273) prevalence of infantile spasms during the first 10 years of life (Cowan *et al.*, 1989).

A study by Heijbel *et al.* (1975) looked at epilepsy in northern Sweden for the year 1974. The number of children aged 0–4 years was 18 578. For the classification of epileptic seizures, one infant was noted to have infantile spasms. This gives a prevalence rate of 1 in 18,578, with an estimated incidence of 1 in 4644 (18 578 ÷ 4) for the children under 1 year of age. Unfortunately, the age of the child with infantile spasms was not identified and with such small numbers much caution in interpreting these data is required (Heijbel *et al.*, 1975).

Al-Rajeh and colleagues (1990) reviewed the prevalence of seizure disorders in a hospital-based population at the King Fahd Hospital, Al-Khobar in Saudi Arabia. The estimated Saudi referral population for this hospital is 1.2 million inhabitants, though this population is not broken down by age. Including only Saudi nationals in their review, the authors identified 1000 consecutive epilepsy admissions from 1984 to 1987. During that time, 8 of every 1000 patients admitted to the hospital were admitted for epilepsy. Infantile spasms were found to represent 3% of the 1000 epilepsy admissions, or 30 cases. This represents a prevalence of approximately 1 in 4200 of the hospital-based general population. The number of admissions for this period does seem to be quite large and works out to be 125 000, which represents 10% of the population. Unfortunately, a breakdown of the demographics by age is not available (Al-Rajeh *et al.*, 1990). So, the incidence of infantile spasms in the first year of life cannot be calculated from these data.

The four small epidemiologic studies from Tokyo, California, Sweden and Saudi Arabia all yielded 2–3% prevalence rates of infantile spasms in those cases identified with nonfebrile seizures or epilepsy (Tsuboi, 1988; Van den Berg and Yerushalmy, 1969; Heijbel *et al.*, 1975; Al-Rajeh *et al.*, 1990). According to Hauser and Nelson (1988), the overall incidence of epilepsy for all age groups is about 40 per 100 000 person years with 50% of all epilepsies starting in childhood. This suggests that the prevalence of infantile spasms in the general population is approximately 1 in 100 000. These small studies do yield some epidemiological information. The Ohtahara and Cowan studies yield "annual prevalence rates" of 0.14–0.19 per 1000 children during the first 10 years of life (Ohtahara *et al.*, 1981; Cowan *et al.*, 1989; Cowan and Hudson, 1991).

Two additional articles contained data for regional epilepsy clinics based on diagnosis by the international classification of epileptic syndromes (Loiseau *et al.*, 1991; Viani *et al.*, 1988). In these articles, patients with infantile spasms and severe myoclonic epilepsy of infancy (SMEI) were identified. Infantile spasms were identified 2–3 times more frequently than severe myoclonic epilepsy. One estimate of the incidence of SMEI is 1 in 20 000 (Hurst, 1990). Comparing relative frequencies of infantile spasms and severe myoclonic epilepsies suggests a possible incidence of infantile spasms in the 1 in 6000 range. It could be argued, however, that epilepsy clinics have a referral bias and therefore may not lead to consistent ratios between different identified epileptic syndromes.

Most studies have found infantile spasms to occur more frequently in males than in females (Riikonen and Donner, 1979; Jeavons, 1985; Bobele and Bodensteiner, 1990; Bellman *et al.*, 1983; Matsumoto *et al.*, 1981b; Lombroso, 1983a). Jeavons (1985), in his review of 1245 patients, found a male-to-female ratio of 1.5 to 1. This calculated figure is close to the epidemiological study results obtained by Riikonen and Donner (1979) in their Finnish study in which 62 boys and 45 girls were identified with infantile spasms. The ratio was somewhat less in the NCES study, in which 148 boys and 121 girls were identified as having infantile spasms (Bellman *et al.*, 1983). However, other studies have not found such a large difference (Jeavons and Bower, 1964; Melchior, 1977). Melchior, for example, in his Danish study, identified 56 boys and 53 girls with infantile spasms between 1970 and 1975 (Melchior, 1977). Also, Bernard *et al.* found no sex difference in their patient populations (Jeavons and Bower, 1964).

Many different aspects of infantile spasms have been investigated, but, despite their interesting features, a lengthy review of every prior study is unwarranted. However, the connection between infantile spasms and immunizations has been the subject of two major studies of West syndrome cited in this review and merits further comment (Shields *et al.*, 1988; Bellman *et al.*, 1983). Immunizations and infantile spasms have been a matter for discussion for some time (Miller *et al.*, 1981; AAP, 1991; Bobele and Bodensteiner, 1990; Hrachovy *et al.*, 1981). The current consensus appears to be that immunizations and infantile spasms are not causally related (AAP, 1991; Bobele and Bodensteiner, 1990; Melchior, 1977; Hrachovy *et al.*, 1981). Using the NCES data, Bellman *et al.* (1983) suggested a possible association between infantile spasms and immunizations in the first 7 days after diphtheria-pertussis-tetanus (DPT) immunization. Bellman *et al.* plotted the onset of infantile spasms in their population and their Table 2 offers a breakdown of the onset of infantile spasms by week after DTP and diphtheria-tetanus (DT) immunizations. In their analysis of their data they state that, in the first week after immunization, more cases of infantile spasms occurred than were expected, whereas in the next 3 weeks, fewer cases than expected were noted. By their own assessment, then, the association between infantile spasms and immunizations is, at best, unclear.

When reading Bellman and colleagues' (1983) review, one is struck by the fact that the large majority of cases of infantile spasms were not associated with immunizations. The probability of the random onset of infantile spasms in the NCES within 1 week following an immunization can be determined from Bellman and colleagues' data by two statistical models: a discrete random variable distribution and by a Poisson variable distribution (Larson, 1969, pp. 68–80, 120–129). Using both distributions, one can calculate the mean value or the expected number of cases of infantile spasms with onset within 1 week of a given date, like an immunization, due to random chance alone (Larson, 1969, pp. 68–80, 120–129). These numbers can then be compared with the number of cases of infantile spasms so identified in the NCES.

Bellman *et al.* (1983) identified the onset of infantile spasms in 152 previously normal cases. Of these, 131 occurred between the ages of 2 and 8 months. If an equal number of new onset infantile spasm cases occurred each week over the course of 6 months or 26 weeks, then approximately five new cases would occur each week (Larson, 1969, pp. 68–80). With three immunizations given, then 3 weeks, or 15 cases, would follow the time of immunization. If a Poisson distribution – the observation of discrete events over a continuous interval – is considered, then the numbers of cases occurring within 1 week of immunizations given at 2, 4 and 6 months can be calculated (Larson, 1969, pp. 120–129). Using Bellman's graph with DPT 1, 3.5 cases would be expected; 5.75 cases would be expected with DPT 2 and 6.75 cases would be expected with DPT 3 (Bellman *et al.*, 1983; Larson, 1969, pp. 120–129). As just calculated, between 15 and 16 new cases of infantile spasms would be expected to occur within 7 days after three immunizations given between 2 and 8 months in 131 children with infantile spasms (Bellman *et al.*, 1983; Larson, 1969, pp. 68–80, 120–129). Bellman *et al.* (1983, table 2), however, identified seven cases only.

In their discussion of infantile spasms, Bellman *et al.* (1983) noted no significant association between infantile spasms and immunization within 28 days before onset. They concluded that a deficit of cases was noted between 7 and 28 days, which they thought was compensated for by a slight excess noted in the first 7 days. The calculations just performed would suggest that approximately 15 cases in the NCES should have been identified by Bellman as vaccine-associated based on random chance occurrence alone. Since only seven cases were noted by Bellman *et al.*, this does not support an association between immunization and infantile spasms other than random chance.

A number of problems exist when evaluating the available epidemiological data concerning infantile spasms. Uppermost is the fact that the current definition of infantile spasms does not include the onset of infantile spasms after 1 year of age. All three major studies cited in this review were performed prior to the new definition and therefore may have included some cases which had their onset after 1 year of age (Nelson, 1972; Ellenberg *et al.*, 1984; Shields *et al.*, 1988; Riikonen and Donner, 1979). The data obtained from the NCPP study lack detailed information about the 12 infantile spasm cases identified, so although the study has an excellent denominator, the numerator is therefore at least somewhat suspect (Nelson, 1972). The calculations from the Danish study in this review used Shield and co-workers' (1988) data. Unfortunately, Melchior's (1977) study, which was obviously much larger, did not note the size of the study population. The numbers obtained from Melchior's study should have been larger and more reliable, but they are not available. The smaller studies from France and Denmark lack large numbers but give relatively consistent results (Luna *et al.*, 1988; Howitz and Platz, 1978; Loiseau *et al.*, 1988). The study from Sweden which noted an incidence of 1.4 in 1000 focused on a small isolated region and may have recorded a special environmental effect (Eeg-Olofsson and Sidenvall, 1992). The studies from Japan, California,

Sweden and Saudi Arabia are such that they preclude calculation of an incidence (Tsuboi, 1988; Van den Berg and Yerushalmy, 1969; Heijbel *et al.*, 1975; Al-Rajeh *et al.*, 1990). In the National Childhood Encephalopathy Study, data are available to calculate the denominator for prevalence, but the basic data are not presented in such a way as to permit calculation of the incidence (Committee, 1981). Despite all these drawbacks, useful epidemiological information can be gleaned from these studies if one is aware of the problematic status of the data.

In summary, the Finnish, NCPP and Danish studies were the largest and allow for the most accurate calculations of incidence ratios for infantile spasms using the 1985 criteria (Commission, 1985; Nelson, 1972; Ellenberg *et al.*, 1984; Shields *et al.*, 1988; Riikonen and Donner, 1979): approximately 1 in 1900 to 1 in 3900. The French and 1976 Danish studies noted an incidence of 1 in 1800 to 1 in 4000 (Luna *et al.*, 1988; Howitz and Platz, 1978; Loiseau *et al.*, 1990). The calculation of incidence from the Danish data (1 in 1900) yields a substantially different number than from the NCPP data (1 in 3900) (Nelson, 1972; Shields *et al.*, 1988). One possibility is that major differences in incidence occur among different ethnic and national groups. Larger studies from other countries will be needed to confirm this hypothesis. These epidemiological studies show the possibility of varying incidences between national groups, but they also suggest that within a given stable population nonvarying incidence ratios can be obtained for infantile spasms (Riikonen and Donner, 1979). Until better studies of infantile spasms are conducted, those cited here provide the best incidence rates. The sex ratio in infantile spasms appears to support an excess of males but the ratio has varied between 1.5:1 and 1:1 in different series. A close statistical look at the NCES data argues against an association between the DPT immunization and infantile spasms.

3

Basic Mechanisms

S.L. MOSHÉ, D.S. GARANT, E.F. SPERBER, S.G. XU, L.L. BROWN

INTRODUCTION

Epidemiological studies indicate that human seizure disorders frequently have their onset early in life (Hauser and Kurland, 1975; Woodbury, 1977). The West syndrome occurs exclusively in infancy (Kellaway *et al.*, 1983) and may represent an age-specific expression of multifocal seizures (Haas *et al.*, 1990). The multifocal nature of this disorder can be best seen in its EEG pattern, hypsarrhythmia. Hypsarrhythmia is characterized by the presence of mountainous randomly distributed spikes and slow waves, recorded from all sampled brain regions (Hrachovy and Frost, 1989b). The clinical spasms can be either symmetrical or, less often, asynchronous. The reasons why infantile spasms occur during a certain period of development are not clear. Recent experimental evidence suggests that the immature central nervous system (CNS) is more susceptible to seizures than its mature counterpart (Albala *et al.*, 1984; Cavalheiro *et al.*, 1987; Moshé, 1987; Schwartzkroin, 1984; Sperber and Moshé, 1988; Swann and Brady, 1984). Ontogenetic seizure studies have demonstrated that 15 to 16-day-old rat pups are more prone to the development of bilateral, initially asynchronous convulsions and status epilepticus than adult rats regardless of the seizure model used to induce the seizures. These behavioral observations parallel the human epidemiological and behavioral data concerning the expression of seizures as a function of age (Moshé, 1989). The similarities between human and animal data permit the use of developmental studies in rats in an attempt to understand the human condition, although a distinct model of infantile spasms is not yet available.

DEVELOPMENTAL ANIMAL MODELS OF EPILEPSY

Kindling is probably the best model of epilepsy to study how seizures propagate from the focus and progressively recruit many additional brain structures, culminating in the emergence of a generalized seizure (Goddard *et* al., 1969). In kindling, repetitive, discrete, low-intensity electrical stimuli induce initially focal electrographic seizures (afterdischarges, ADs). The occurrence of focal ADs is necessary for kindling to develop. If ADs are not triggered, kindling does not occur. With time, focal motor seizures and finally generalized, mostly clonic, seizures occur (Goddard et al., 1969; Racine, 1972a,b). Kindling, once induced, permanently changes the brain in that generalized seizures will be triggered anytime the initially subthreshold for seizures stimulus is delivered (Goddard et al., 1969). Occasionally, spontaneous seizures occur (Pinel and Rovner, 1978; Wada and Osawa, 1976; Wada et al., 1974).

The behavioral manifestations of kindled seizures induced by stimulating limbic structures have been described in adult and immature rats (Table 3.1). The behavioral manifestations of the kindled seizures are the same in prepubescent and adult rats but have age-specific characteristics in rat pups. In adult

Table 3.1 Behavioral manifestations of amygdala kindled seizures as a function of age

Kindling stages	Pups (2 weeks old)	Pubescents (4–5 weeks old)	Adults (older than 9 weeks)
0	Arrest	Arrest	Arrest
1	Facial movements	Chewing	Chewing
2	Rhythmic head movements or turning of body to stimulated site	Head nodding	Head nodding
3	Unilateral forelimb clonus ± hindlimb clonus; "wet dog shakes"	Contralateral forelimb clonus	Contralateral forelimb clonus
3.5	Alternating forelimb clonus		
4	Bilateral forelimb clonus or rotatory movements of tonically extended forelimbs; rearing not consistent	Bilateral symmetrical forelimb clonus with rearing	Bilateral symmetrical forelimb clonus with rearing
5	Bilateral forelimb clonus with rearing and falling[a]	Bilateral forelimb clonus with rearing and falling	Bilateral forelimb clonus with rearing and falling
6	Wild running and jumping with or without vocalizations (popcorn seizures)	No available studies	Wild running and jumping with vocalizations
7	Tonus	No available studies	Tonus
8	Spontaneous seizures	No available studies	Spontaneous seizures

[a] This stage may be absent in rat pups (see text).

rats, stages 0–2 represent local events, stage 3 the involvement of the ipsilateral to the stimulation site hemisphere, stages 4–5 bilateral (generalized) seizures, while stages 6 and 7 (Haas *et al.*, 1990; Sperber *et al.*, 1990) resemble seizures elicited by direct stimulation of the brainstem (Browning, 1985; Burnham, 1985; Gale, 1989).

The administration of a repetitive suprathreshold for ADs stimuli leads to the progressive intensification of kindled seizures in rat pups (Moshé and Albala, 1982). There are several differences from the seizures observed in adult animals. Pups have either alternating forelimb clonus or bilateral and asymmetric clonus. Haas *et al.* (1990) called this stage 3.5, since it falls between unilateral forelimb clonus of stage 3 and bilateral symmetrical forelimb clonus of stage 4, in an attempt to maintain the continuity of the pup and adult scales. Seizures similar to the pub stage 3.5, called "see-saw seizures", are seen in human infants (Gastaut *et al.*, 1974). The ability of immature, but not adult rats, to exhibit bilateral asymmetrical seizures may reflect a lack of complete myelination of the corpus callosum (Agrawal and Davison, 1973; Carey, 1982; Davison, 1970; DeMeyer, 1967). Compared with older rats, pups spend proportionally less time in the early stages of kindling (stages 0–2), which are associated with focal seizures. Furthermore, in rat pups, the early appearance of bilateral although often asynchronous manifestations indicates a tendency for seizure generalization.

In the older age groups, hindlimb clonus is a late manifestation of generalized kindled seizures and occurs after repeated stage 5 seizures. This is not the case with rat pups, in which hindlimb clonus may be a part of the "migratory" clonic seizures that can affect any limb during stage 3.5. Additionally, in rat pups, from stage 3 on there are frequent "wet dog shakes" during the seizure. "Wet dog shakes" rarely occur during amygdala-kindled seizures in adult rats, and when they do, they are usually observed towards the end of the ADs. In stage 4, rat pups exhibit rotatory movements of rigidly held forelimbs and/or bilateral clonus; rearing is infrequent in pups younger than 16 days. Pups do not often experience stage 5 seizures, which are characterized by falling. Instead, they experience many stage 3–4 seizures intermixed with isolated stage 5 seizures followed by the explosive onset of stage 6 and stage 7 seizures (Haas *et al.*, 1990; Sperber *et al.*, 1990). Stage 6 is characterized by wild running and jumping with or without vocalization. Stage 7 is characterized by tonus and appears at the end of stage 6 seizures. Stages 6 and 7 are dramatically more severe than the usual kindled motor behaviors. Because of the explosive nature of stage 6 seizures, Haas *et al.* (1990) proposed the name "popcorn" seizures. They resemble descriptions of "brainstem" seizures produced by direct brainstem stimulation (Browning, 1985; Burnham, 1985; Gale, 1989). Although preliminary deoxyglucose studies of stage 6 and 7, however, do not reveal any significant increases in deoxyglucose uptake in brainstem regions (Ackermann *et al.*, 1990), brainstem involvement cannot be ruled out. In contrast to pups, in which severe seizures can be elicited with an average of 26 stimulations, in adults, seizures similar to stage 6 and 7 have been observed only after prolonged kindling with more than 80 stimulations (Pinel and Rovner, 1978). We have failed to elicit severe seizures in adult Sprague-Dawley rats after more than 90 stimulations (unpublished).

During kindling, the ADs grow in duration and complexity in all age groups but the morphology of the ADs is somewhat different. At comparable stages, the ADs, in 15-day-old pups, are slower, less rhythmic and of lower amplitude than the ADs in older rats (Moshé, 1981). The amygdala ADs quickly spread into the contralateral amygdala or hippocampus as well as "downstream" to involve the striatum and the substantia nigra (SN) (Moshé et al., 1988). Few postictal spikes occur in pups (Ackermann and Moshé, unpublished).

Amygdala or hippocampal kindling can be produced in 15-day-old pups using frequent stimulations, for example every 15 min (Lee et al., 1989; Moshé and Albala, 1983; Moshé et al., 1983). In adults, stimulations delivered every 15 min either significantly retard or fail to induce kindling (Goddard et al., 1969; Moshé et al., 1983; Peterson et al., 1981; Racine, 1972b). Hippocampal-stimulated rat pups have the same kindling stages as amygdala-stimulated pups with the exception of "wet dog shakes" (Haas et al., 1990). In hippocampal-stimulated pups, "wet dog shakes" are the first behavior; as the other ictal events emerge, the incidence of "wet dog shakes" is reduced. In amygdala-kindled rats, "wet dog shakes" appear after the pups experience stage 3 or higher. However, hippocampal kindling progresses at the same rate as amygdala kindling. This is different from adult kindling of these two sites; in adults, the amygdala kindles faster than the dorsal hippocampus (Goddard et al., 1969). Thus, the immature hippocampus appears to be more susceptible to the development of kindled seizures than the adult (see also Haas et al., 1990; Lee et al., 1989).

There is another difference between adults and rat pups, concerning the phenomenon of "kindling antagonism" (Applegate and Burchfiel, 1990; Burchfiel and Applegate, 1989). In adults, concurrent kindling of two limbic foci, obtained by delivering alternating stimulations between the two sites, results in the suppression of generalized seizures from one or both sites. One limbic site may become dominant, while the other site may be suppressed, with the stimulations producing only focal seizures. Pups do not show kindling antagonism to the development of generalized seizures between the amygdala and hippocampus, or between the amygdala (Haas et al., 1990; Sperber et al., 1990). Alternating stimulations enhance the kindling development of both sites and each site develops generalized seizures twice as fast as a site receiving single stimulations. These data indicate that, in rat pups, the mechanisms underlying positive transfer are more powerful than the mechanisms underlying the suppression of the kindling process. This augmented positive transfer may be unique for the developing brain, since it has not been reported in adult rats.

These data indicate that during the critical period, the immature CNS is more prone to the development of secondarily generalized seizures that may have their onset from multiple seizure limbic foci. This increase in seizures susceptibility extends beyond the local generation of epileptic discharges and involves the mechanisms that participate in the propagation of seizures from the focus to recruit additional structures that may increase seizure severity. In rats, the increase in overall seizure susceptibility is predominantly seen during the second and third postnatal week (Moshé *et al.*, 1990, 1991); but, in kittens, the period of increased seizure susceptibility lasts till the sixth postnatal month (Shouse *et al.*, 1990). Although the exact human age equivalent is unknown, correlative ontogenetic studies suggest that the period during which infantile spasms are expressed (the first year of life) may be related to the second and third postnatal weeks in the rat (Gottlieb *et al.*, 1977; Moshé, 1987; Moshé *et al.*, 1992).

Shouse *et al.* (1990, 1992) have described the kindling of spontaneous, multifocal epilepsy in immature cats. Their data suggest several similarities to the electroclinical, sleep and pathologic characteristics of West syndrome. These authors studied 26 amygdala-kindled preadolescent or adult cats. The kittens ranged in age from 2.5 to 6.5 months, and the adults were 1–3 years old at the beginning of kindling, as identified by initial focal ADs. Spontaneous seizures occurred more frequently in kittens (62%) than in adult cats (8%). Half the kittens exhibited more than one seizure type; their EEGs contained multifocal paroxysms, including posterior cortical involvement. Jack-knife seizures were detected in one kitten. In this kitten, the following behaviors were noted. Initially, there was absence-like staring and purring which persisted for up to 1.5 h at a time ("catnip" seizures). Afterwards, there was head nodding, sometimes followed by jack-knife seizures, accompanied by multi-spike or multiple sharp-and-wave transients in the EEG. These seizures were noted during quiet waking, and slow-wave sleep, including the transition to rapid eye movement (REM) sleep. They stopped only during rare periods of active waking and stable REM sleep.

There are few interesting similarities between the kindling data and the expression of infantile spasms. As with developmental kindling, infantile spasms are often asymmetric and the EEG (at least during wakefulness) multifocal. The ongoing myelination may account for these phenomena; as myelination progresses, the seizure patterns become more symmetric. In addition, the propensity of the immature CNS to express multifocal seizures may be an important variable accounting for the appearance of infantile spasms in patients with presumed focal lesions (Dulac and Schlumberger, 1993).

FACTORS INFLUENCING SEIZURE SUSCEPTIBILITY WITH AGE

There are several factors which may be responsible for the enhanced seizure susceptibility of the immature CNS. These include developmental features of neurons, myelination, neurotransmission, and neuronal circuits involved in the suppression of seizures.

Local Features

Immature neurons may have different intrinsic cell properties than mature neurons (Kriegstein *et al.*, 1987). Differences in the rate of maturation of synapses may also be important. Early in life, in some structures such as the CA1 region of the hippocampus, asymmetric (presumably excitatory) synapses are more abundant, while symmetric (presumably inhibitory) synapses increase in number with development (Schwartzkroin *et al.*, 1982; Swann *et al.*, 1990). In addition, the biological markers of GABA activity, although present at birth, increase significantly with maturation (Seress and Ribak, 1988; Swann *et al.*, 1990). GABA is considered to be the predominant inhibitory neurotransmitter. In other areas, such as the CA3 region of the hippocampus, critical factors may be the abundance of recurrent excitatory synapses (Swann *et al.*, 1990, 1991) and the calcium-mediated voltage-dependency of the NMDA receptors (Brady *et al.*, 1991).

Myelination

Incomplete myelination may explain the age-specific differences in the expression of the motor seizures and electrographic seizure patterns, as well as the poor inter-hemispheric synchrony of the ADs. Myelin assembles slowly during the last part of gestation and more rapidly afterwards. Myelination occurs first in the phylogenetically older parts of the brain such as the brainstem and later in the corpus callosum and frontopontine tracts (Agrawal and Davison, 1973; Davison, 1970; Eayrs and Goodhead, 1959). Characteristic features of generalized kindled seizures in 15-day-old pups include the asymmetric involvement of the limbs, inconsistent rearing and falling (see Table 3.1), and the observation that stage 5 seizures are rare. Rat pups experience many stage 3–4 seizures intermixed with isolated stage 5 seizures followed by the explosive onset of stage 6 and stage 7 seizures. One possible explanation for the relatively infrequent stage 5 seizures may be the inability of some pups to rear and thus they do not fall. However, while other pups rear they do not fall. From this aspect, 15-day-old pups resemble adult rats with prefrontal lesions (Corcoran *et al.*, 1976), which tend to remain in stage 4 despite numerous stimulations. This observation may suggest that prefrontal inputs are necessary for the expression of adult-like seizure stage 5 patterns. In humans, a similar immaturity of prefrontal inputs along with the incomplete myelination may account for the characteristic clinical phenomenology of infantile spasms.

Neurotransmission

Changes in the levels of neurotransmitters may be relevant. Catecholamines and especially norepinephrine have an important role in containing kindled seizures within the focus. Norepinephrine depletions accelerate the development of kindling in adults (Corcoran and Weiss, 1990; McIntyre, 1981; McIntyre *et al.*, 1987) and pubescent rats (Michelson and Butterbaugh, 1985). Norepinephrine-depleted adults develop generalized kindled seizures faster than controls even when stimulated with short interstimulus intervals (McIntyre *et al.*, 1987) that, otherwise, do not include kindling (Goddard *et al.*, 1969; Moshé *et al.*, 1983; Peterson *et al.*, 1981; Racine, 1927b). The acceleration mainly affects the early kindling stages and, in this respect, these rats resemble 15 to 18-day-old rat pups. In pups, the levels of norepinephrine are lower than in older rats (Moshé *et al.*, 1981), and this may in part be responsible for the facilitation of kindled seizures. On the other hand, pubescent (35-day-old) rats have lower norepinephrine levels than adults but kindle slower than adults (additional factors that may play a role include hormonal influences, since gonadal steroid hormones can suppress kindling in the young but not in adults: (Holmes and Weber, 1986). Norepinephrine has been implicated as the neurotransmitter responsible for determining whether focal seizures can spread to other brain areas and, in adults, total brain norepinephrine depletion results in the loss of kindling antagonism (Applegate and Burchfiel, 1990; Burchfiel and Applegate, 1989; Corcoran and Weiss, 1990; Moshé *et al.*, 1991). Thus, the lack of kindling antagonism in pups can be partly attributed to the low norepinephrine levels in this age group (Konkol *et al.*, 1990; Moshé *et al.*, 1981).

It has been proposed that the West syndrome may be associated with a dysfunction of central monoaminergic systems. Hrachovy and Frost, 1989b) have reviewed the evidence suggesting a role for either serotonin or norepinephrine. In most quoted studies, the cerebrospinal fluid (CSF) levels of either serotonin or norepinephrine or their metabolites were increased, although Hrachovy and Frost (1989b) were not able to reproduce these findings. If the clinical laboratory findings prove to be correct, they would seem to contradict the basic observation that depletion of norepinephrine is proconvulsive. However, it is unclear whether the CSF monoamine level changes precede or are a sequel to the spasms.

Neuronal Circuits

There is evidence to suggest the existence of seizure-modifying circuits which include several subcortical nuclei. One such system may include a GABA-sensitive substantia nigra (SN) based circuit. The SN, and the pars reticulata (SNR) in particular, may be critically involved in the expression and control of generalized seizures in rats (for a review, see Moshé and Sperber, 1990). The potentially crucial role of the SN was first suspected from the results of deoxyglucose autoradiographic studies performed in 16-day-old rats to determine the patterns of seizure propagation. Rat pups, kindled from the amygdala, show age-characteristic patterns of glucose utilization (Ackermann *et al.*, 1989). The basolateral amygdala may be the initial pacemaker. As seizure activity spreads, deoxyglucose utilization increases in the adjacent piriform cortex and then longitudinally through the paleocortex, first caudally to the entorhinal cortex and then rostrally to the olfactory bulb. As kindling becomes progressively more severe, deoxyglucose utilization disseminates into rhinencephalic projection areas including the subiculum and hippocampus, nucleus accumbens and diagonal band. One remarkable feature of the deoxyglucose utilization studies in rat pups is the lack of increased deoxyglucose accumulation in the SN. This nucleus consistently demonstrates increased deoxyglucose utilization in kindling of adult rats (Ackermann *et al.*, 1989, 1990; Moshé *et al.*, 1988).

Are the SN changes specific for the kindling model? To answer this question, we performed deoxyglucose studies in animals exposed to other models of epilepsy. These included kainic acid induced seizures and flurothyl seizures. Kainic acid seizures are actually a model of limbic seizures culminating in status epilepticus (Albala *et al.*, 1984). Flurothyl seizures are seizures generalized from the onset, which consist of forelimb clonic movements followed by generalized tonic contractions and loss of posture (Prichard *et al.*, 1969; Sperber and Moshé, 1988). Immature animals are more susceptible than adults to the development of either kainic acid or flurothyl seizures (Albala *et al.*, 1984; Sperber and Moshé, 1988). Both agents are administered systemically, thus age-related differences in seizure suceptibility may be confounded by several factors such as drug absorption, distribution, metabolism and permeability of the blood–brain barrier. Kainic acid, flurothyl and kindling probably have different substrates of seizure initiation, yet all three models have one thing in common: decreased glucose utilization of the SN during these seizures even when the rat pup is experiencing severe seizures (Ackermann *et al.*, 1989; Albala *et al.*, 1984; Sperber *et al.*, 1992). This is not the case with adult rats under similar experimental conditions.

SUPPORTIVE DATA RECORDING THE ROLE OF THE SN IN SEIZURES

The nigral effects on seizures are age-specific. Our working hypothesis is that some of the age-related differences in seizure susceptibility may be due, in part, to functional differences of the SN GABA receptors and its GABA-sensitive output pathways. In the CNS, there are several types of GABA receptors: $GABA_A$, which are bicuculline-sensitive, and $GABA_B$, which are bicuculline-insensitive but sensitive to baclofen (Bowery *et al.*, 1983, 1984). A putative $GABA_C$ receptor insensitive to both bicuculline and baclofen has also been proposed but not widely accepted (Bartholini *et al.*, 1985; Bowery *et al.*, 1984, 1987; Hill and Bowery, 1981; Wamsley *et al.*, 1988). Muscimol is mainly a $GABA_A$ receptor agonist binding to both the high- and low-affinity site (Enna, 1988). Bicuculline is the classic $GABA_A$ receptor antagonist and exerts its effects by blocking the receptor to endogenous GABA (Olsen *et al.*, 1976, 1978, 1983, 1990). Recent studies indicate that bicuculline binds to low-affinity $GABA_A$ receptor subtype (Bowery *et al.*, 1984; Enna, 1988; Olsen *et al.*, 1983, 1990; Unerstall *et al.*, 1981). Baclofen is the prototypic $GABA_B$ agonist and has no

Table 3.2 Adult rats: Effects of intranigral infusions of specific GABAergic agents on seizures

Drug	GABA receptor action	Effect on seizures
Single drug infusions		
Muscimol	GABA$_A$ agonist	Suppression
Bicuculline	GABA$_A$ low-affinity antagonist	Facilitation
Baclofen	GABA$_B$ agonist	No effect
GVG	GABA$_A$ and GABA$_B$ agonist	Suppression
Two-drug infusions		
GVG/bicuculline		Blockade of GVG anticonvulsant effect
GVG/muscimol		Suppression but GVG effect attenuated

effects on the GABA$_A$ receptor (Bowery *et al.*, 1983, 1984, 1987). The irreversible inhibitor of the GABA-degradating enzyme GABA transaminase, γ-vinyl GABA (GVG), increases the concentration of endogenous GABA, which in turn can bind to both GABA receptors (Gale, 1989; Iadarola and Gale, 1982).

Adult Pharmacological Studies

Table 3.2 summarizes the effects of site-specific SNR bilateral GABAergic drug infusions on flurothyl-induced seizures. The data suggest that in adults, the nigral effects on seizures are mediated by the GABA$_A$ receptor, since an agonist (muscimol) and an antagonist (bicuculline) produce opposing effects on seizures (Sperber *et al.*, 1989c). Both subtypes of GABA$_A$ receptor may be involved because bicuculline is an antagonist of the low-affinity site, while muscimol acts on both the high- and low affinity sites. The importance of the low-affinity site is also reflected from GVG/bicuculline infusion data, in which bicuculline abolishes the anticonvulsant effect of GVG (Xu *et al.*, 1991a,b). In adult rats, the GABA$_B$ receptor does not appear to participate because baclofen infusions have no effect on seizures (Sperber *et al.*, 1989a). The indirect effect of GVG must then be the result of GABA$_A$ receptor activation (Xu *et al.*, 1991a,b).

Pup Pharmacological Studies

Table 3.3 summarizes the effects of site-specific SNR bilateral GABAergic drug infusions on flurothyl-induced seizures in 16-day-old pups. The pup data show some similarities with the adult effects, as well as marked differences (Sperber *et al.*, 1987, 1989a; Xu *et al.*, 1991b). For example, bicuculline has a proconvulsant effect in the two age groups, suggesting that the GABA$_A$ low-affinity receptor

Table 3.3   Rat pups: Effects of intranigral infusions of specific GABAergic agents on seizures

Drug	GABA receptor action	Effect on seizures[a]
Single drug infusions		
Muscimol	$GABA_A$ agonist	**Facilitation**
THIP	$GABA_A$ high-affinity agonist	Facilitation
Bicuculline	$GABA_A$ low-affinity antagonist	*Facilitation*
Baclofen	$GABA_B$ agonist	**Suppression**
GVG	$GABA_A$ and $GABA_B$ agonist	*Suppression*
Two-drug infusions		
GVG/Bicuculline		*Blockade of anticonvulsant GVG effect*
GVG/muscimol		**Blockade of anticonvulsant GVG effect**

[a] **Bold** font depicts age-specific differences, whereas *italic* font depicts similarities between adult and rat pups.

acts in the same fashion regardless of the age of the rats. This observation is verified by GVG/bicuculline infusions experiments in which bicuculline, by blocking the $GABA_A$ low-affinity receptor, prevented the anticonvulsant action of GVG. Interestingly, in pups, baclofen has also been shown to be capable of suppressing seizures. This appears to be unique for the developing SN since, in adults, baclofen infusions are ineffective (Sperber *et al.*, 1989a). Finally, the effects of GVG infusions may require both $GABA_A$ low-affinity receptor and $GABA_B$ receptors.

To explain the opposing actions of muscimol in the two age groups – anticonvulsant in adults and proconvulsant in rat pups – the following possibilities were considered:

1. Muscimol has been reported to have a weak $GABA_B$ action (Hill and Bowery, 1981), and therefore it is conceivable that its proconvulsant effect in pups could be mediated via the $GABA_B$ receptor. This is improbable because the effects of baclofen, the classic $GABA_B$ agonist, do not agree with the muscimol effects in either age group (Sperber *et al.*, 1989a,b).
2. Muscimol's effect is not mediated by the GABA system (Brown, 1979; Heyer *et al.*, 1981). This is unlikely because preliminary results suggest that THIP, a $GABA_A$ high-affinity receptor agonist, has a similar proconvulsant effect to muscimol (Xu *et al.*, 1992).
3. Muscimol's effects may be predominantly mediated by the $GABA_A$ high-affinity receptor, which may be functionally different in adults and pups. This may also partially explain the results obtained with the two drug infusions studies (see Tables 2 and 3) using GVG and muscimol in both age groups (Xu *et al.*, 1991a,b).

Table 3.4 Age-related differences in nigral GABA receptors

GABA$_A$ high-affinity receptors	GABA$_A$ low-affinity receptors	GABA$_B$ receptors
Adults 100%	100%	100%
Pups 13%[a]	130%	311%[a]

[a] Statistically significant differences are based on raw data and not on percentages.

GABA Receptor Studies

In a previous study (Wurpel *et al.*, 1988), we performed *in vitro* muscimol receptor binding studies of the SN region and found that there were no differences in the receptor density of the GABA$_A$ low-affinity site as a function of age. However, there were differences in the density of high-affinity receptors. The SN of immature rats had only 13% of the adult level of high-affinity receptors.

To determine the developmental changes in GABA$_B$ receptors in the SN, we performed *in vitro* binding studies (Garant *et al.*, 1992). Tissue from the SN, hippocampus and cerebellum was obtained from adults and pups. While there were no differences in receptor affinity between the two ages in each site, there were site-specific, age-specific differences in GABA$_B$ receptor density. The receptor density (B_{max}) in pup SN was significantly different from that in adult SN (Table 3.4). In contrast, the B_{max} values for hippocampal and cerebellar tissue from rat pups were significantly lower, both about two-thirds of the corresponding adult values. The data indicate that there is a significant developmental difference in GABA$_B$ binding density for all three brain structures assayed. The results from the SN stand out for two reasons. First, because there is an order of magnitude greater difference in B_{max} between pup and adult, and second, because the GABA$_B$ density is *higher* in the pup SN than in the adult.

SUMMARY AND HYPOTHESES

Our GABA receptor data suggest that there are differences between pups and adults at the receptor level in the SN (Table 3.4). The 16-day-old pup values are depicted as a percentage of adult values. The GABA$_B$ receptor data may explain the age-specific effects of baclofen – anticonvulsant in pups and no effect in adults. Is the lower density of nigral high-affinity receptors sufficient explanation for the proconvulsant effects of muscimol and THIP in pups? It would appear not, as the binding data support only a decreased anticonvulsant action of muscimol in pups, not a proconvulsant action. Furthermore, the developmental changes in nigral high-affinity receptors cannot explain why in adults muscimol attenuates the anticonvulsant effect of GVG. Therefore, we suggest that, in addition, the nigral GABA$_A$ high-affinity receptor may be developmentally heterogeneous in terms of subunit isoforms.

Molecular cloning techniques have identified the cDNAs that encode the various α, β, γ and δ polypeptides of GABA$_A$ receptors and confirmed the suggestion that central GABA$_A$ receptors are a heterogeneous family of related proteins (Bovolin et al., 1990; Levitan et al., 1988b; Möhler et al., 1990; Schofield et al., 1987; Siegel, 1988). This molecular divergence may be partly responsible for the diverse pharmacological effects. Three factors support this notion. First, different isoforms form functionally distinct receptors when expressed in Xenopus oocytes or mammalian cells (Khrestchatisky et al., 1989; Levitan et al., 1988a; Pritchett et al., 1988). Second, the mRNAs encoding the different isoforms have characteristic regional brain distribution (Khrestchatisky et al., 1989; Siegel, 1988; Wisden et al., 1988, 1989a,b). Third, the mRNAs appear to be regulated during ontogeny in a distinct fashion (Khrestchatisky et al., 1989; Laurie et al., 1992; Poulter et al., 1992; Siegel, 1988; Wisden et al., 1988, 1989a,b). Preliminary results indicate that this may be the case for the SN, at least for the GABA$_A$ α1 isoform (Sperber et al., 1991).

To explain the ontogenetic changes in the nigra-mediated seizure suppression, we suggest that there may be specific GABA$_A$ high-affinity isoforms associated with proconvulsant or anticonvulsant effects. The putative proconvulsant isoform may be expressed in the SN early in life as the predominant isoform of the limited available high-affinity sites. With maturation, the increases in nigral GABA$_A$ high-affinity binding sites may reflect the appearance of the putative anticonvulsant isoform, which in adults constitutes the majority of the high-affinity sites. In adults, GABAergic drugs that act on the GABA$_A$ high-affinity site may activate predominantly the anticonvulsant site. With larger doses, the proconvulsant site may become involved. This hypothesis could explain why muscimol partially attenuates the GVG effect in the dual infusion studies (Table 3.2).

Our ongoing metabolic studies have shown that, in pups, proconvulsant doses of muscimol produce different metabolic maps from anticonvulsant doses of baclofen and GVG (Brown et al., 1991; Sperber et al., 1989b; Sperber et al., 1988). The latter two maps are not identical, reflecting the diversity of the activated GABA receptors. In adults, anticonvulsant doses of muscimol produce maps that partly resemble the maps produced by GVG in pups. These data may suggest that activation of distinct receptors (and isoforms) produce characteristic changes in nigral output systems independent of the animal's age.

Our hypotheses offer a unique approach to the study of seizures and seizure susceptibility in young animals. The results could lead to possible new pharmacological strategies to control systems essential to seizure propagation and modification, thus aiding the development of age-appropriate treatments of seizure disorders. West syndrome is particularly difficult to treat with conventional anti-epileptic drugs, reflecting the uniqueness of the dysfunctioning developing brain. Hrachovy and Frost (1989b) have suggested that the pathophysiological substrate of infantile spasms may be found in the brainstem and have postulated "a disruption of neuronal function within the nuclei of the pontine reticular formation and surrounding areas". The experimental developmental data described in this chapter and especially the combination of monoaminergic and SN findings also suggest that brainstem mechanisms may play a crucial role in seizure expression and control. It should be noted that the effects of the SN on seizures may be mediated via the pontine reticular formation (Okada *et al.*, 1989; Sperber *et al.*, 1989b). Therefore, possible new directions in the treatment of infantile spasms may include the use of drugs that act on the SN–pontine reticular formation circuit. Dulac and Schlumberger (1993) have found that GVG can control infantile spasms in a subgroup of patients and our experimental data indicate that nigral GVG infusions alter the SN–pontine reticular formation interactions. Another drug that may be effective is the GABA$_B$ agonist, baclofen. We have reported that baclofen can suppress kindled seizures only in developing animals (Wurpel *et al.*, 1990) and that intranigral infusions of baclofen profoundly affect the metabolism of the pontine reticular formation (Sperber *et al.*, 1989b). The effectiveness of baclofen against infantile spasms should now be determined in a clinical trial.

4

Ictal Aspects with Emphasis on Unusual Variants

D.A. SHEWMON

BEHAVIORAL DOMAIN

The classical ictal features of epilectic spasms have been well documented in the literature (Fusco and Vigevano, 1993; Hrachovy and Frost, 1986; Kellaway *et al.*, 1979, 1983; King *et al.*, 1985; Lacy and Penry, 1976, pp. 9–17; Lombroso, 1983a). Behaviorally, each spasm consists of a brief flexion, extension, or mixed flexion/extension of axial and/or appendicular musculature. The most common is the mixed type, with axial flexion and arm extension and abduction (Fig. 4.1a). Axial extension occurs much less often. Smiling, grimacing and autonomic changes are frequently associated. When spasms are intense, the baby often utters a brief stereotyped cry during or immediately after each one. Whether the spasms cause some subjective discomfort or merely startle the child, or whether the crying represents a mere subconscious automatism, is an intrinsically unanswerable question.

Often the eyes transiently deviate, usually upwards, obliquely or laterally; in our experience, the direction of eye deviation often varies within the same patient and seems to imply little about the laterality of underlying brain pathology. Fusco and Vigevano (1993) observed eye deviation more frequently in symptomatic than in cryptogenic spasms. Episodes of akinesia or decreased responsiveness lasting up to 20 s may also occur (Fig. 4.1b); Donat and Wright, 1989; Kellaway *et al.*, 1983; Lombroso, 1983a).

The great majority of spasms come in clusters, especially upon awakening, although they can also be sporadic, isolated events. In the series of Kellaway *et al.* (1979), clustering occurred in 21 of 24 patients (87.5%). Spasm clusters usually last from several to 10 min, with a spasm at more or less regular intervals. The inter-spasm interval varies from patient to patient and sometimes from cluster to cluster within the same patient, ranging from 5 to 40 s, but

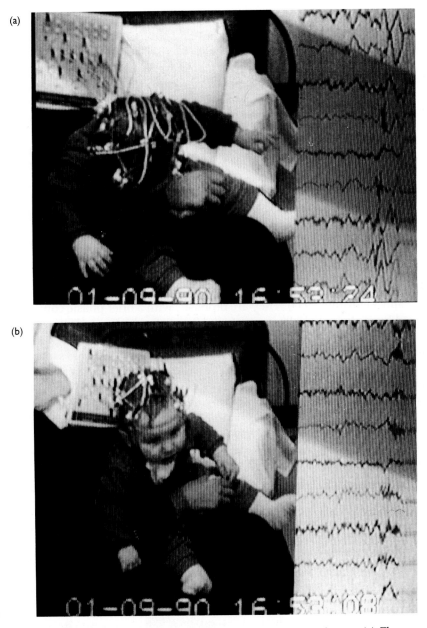

Figure 4.1 A 6-month-old child with cryptogenic West syndrome. (a) Flexor spasm with symmetrical abduction of the arms; ictal EEG pattern consists of a fast rhythm followed by a slow wave. (b) Motionless stare with ictal EEG counterpart of a fast rhythm only. Courtesy of Dr F. Vigevano.

usually around 10 s. Clusters typically evolve in a crescendo–decrescendo fashion, beginning very subtly, perhaps manifested only by periodic eye deviation, small grimaces or slight arm or hand movements. Not infrequently, a cluster will begin entirely subclinically, with a minute or so of typical repetitive ictal discharges on EEG, which only gradually become accompanied by behavioral concomitants. At the peak of a cluster the spasms can be quite violent. Then, the intensity diminishes until the spasms become very subtle again, with the whole episode perhaps terminating as purely subclinical EEG discharges, which gradually dissipate into the background activity.

The nomenclature related to the duration of spasms is still as confusing now as it was to Lacy and Penry in 1976 (p. 13). Some spasms can be extremely brief, leading to the German designation "Blitzkrämpfe" (lightning attacks), and it is difficult to formulate a consistent definitional distinction between such attacks and massive myoclonic jerks (see Chapter 1). Jeavons and Bower (1964, pp. 8–25) considered this a distinct subtype of epileptic spasms that tend not to cluster. On the other hand, the ictal EEG may serve as a distinguishing factor, as myoclonic jerks – unlike spasms – tend to be associated with spike-wave or polyspike-wave discharges (see below and Fig. 4.2).

Most spasms, however, last longer than a myoclonic jerk, typically 0.5–2 s (Fusco and Vigevano, 1993). They are biphasic, with a brief phasic contraction followed by a gradually relaxing tonic component, which may last up to 10 s (Kellaway *et al.*, 1979; King *et al.*, 1985). In a minority of cases, it can become difficult to differentiate behaviorally such spasms from brief tonic seizures on any rational basis, although the EEG correlate of tonic seizures is usually different from that of spasms (Fig. 4.2). In our experience, this kind of nosologic dilemma has been encountered mainly in older infants who are in the process of growing out of infantile spasms and into some other seizure syndrome, such as Lennox-Gastaut. The terminological confusion probably merely reflects the richness and complexity of the underlying pathophysiological reality, which refuses to be reduced to simplistic artificial categories and labels. After all, it

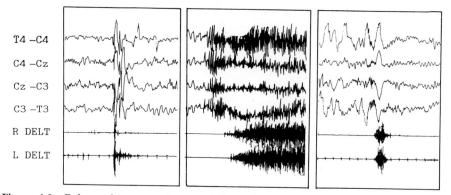

Figure 4.2 Polygraphic presentation of three different seizure types (from left to right): myoclonic jerk, tonic seizure and epilectic spasm. Courtesy of Dr F. Vigevano.

should hardly be surprising that during an age of transition from spasms to tonic seizures, there should be unclassifiable seizure types manifesting features of both (cf. Donat and Wright, 1991d; Egli *et al.*, 1985; Ikeno *et al.*, 1985; Weinmann, 1988). Rather than trying to force these into one or other category, it would seem more reasonable simply to describe them and to acknowledge their transitional character.

Spasms must also be differentiated from "benign myoclonus of early infancy" (Lombroso and Fejerman, 1977), which is a diffuse non-epileptic contraction, like a chill, without EEG abnormalities.

EEG DOMAIN

The ictal EEG patterns associated with infantile spasms have been described at length by Kellaway *et al.* (1979) and King *et al.* (1985), and include, in isolation or various combinations: a generalized high-amplitude slow wave or brief slow-wave complex, a sharp-and-slow-wave complex, diffuse attenuation, and rhythmic fast activity (sometimes called "spindle-like"). These different patterns can occur alone or together, for example rhythmic fast activity followed by a slow wave, followed by diffuse attenuation. It is often difficult in practice to distinguish the cerebral slow wave from movement-induced artifact, although at the beginning and end of clusters (when movement is typically least), the cerebral basis for the wave is usually clear. Fusco and Vigevano (1993) recently described an interesting detail of the EEG/behavioral correlation. The EEG pattern that most consistently corresponded with the clinical spasm was the slow wave; more specifically, the onset of the wave coincided with the onset of the spasm. Bursts of pure rhythmic fast activity tended to occur toward the beginning or end of a cluster, corresponding clinically to a time of decreased spontaneity or motionlessness (Fig. 4.1b). Sometimes rhythmic theta or delta activity follows the spasm-discharge for a number of seconds.

The classical electrodecrement, as a *pure* EEG event, occurred in only 12% of spasms in the series of Kellaway *et al.* (1979), the most common ictal pattern being a slow wave followed by attenuation. It is my impression that pure electrodecremental events with immediate return to the interictal pattern (typically hypsarrhythmia) are associated more often with isolated than with clustered spasms. Dulac *et al.* (1986a) referred to such spasms as "independent" and found them to be associated with a more favorable prognosis than those with attenuation of background activity throughout the inter-spasm interval (Fig. 4.3).

By contrast, the great majority of spasm clusters behave in some ways as large-scale ictal entities in themselves, rather than mere successions of brief seizures. Before the behavioral spasms or associated EEG discharges actually begin, there is typically a relative normalization of the background abnormalities, with disappearance of the otherwise abundant epileptiform discharges and replacement of the high-amplitude slowing with a low-amplitude irregular mixture of faster frequencies. Even before the spasm-associated discharges appear, this change in EEG pattern may be accompanied by clinical symptomatology if it occurs during wakefulness (spontaneous behavior may slow down and interaction with the environment diminish). Then the characteristic EEG discharges appear, sometimes entirely subclinically.

As the cluster evolves, the discharges may become more prominent, in parallel with the intensity of the behavioral manifestations. The inter-spasm EEG activity typically remains attenuated, as though the cluster itself were a kind of large-scale electrodecrement punctuated by electroclinical spasms. In cases where the cluster follows upon a partial seizure, the intra-cluster electrodecrement could even be interpreted as something closely related to the partial seizure's postictal suppression. After the peak-intensity phase has passed, the inter-spasm activity usually begins to "fill-in" with theta and delta frequencies of increasing amplitude and admixture of sharp waves, and the ictal dicharges may decrease in amplitude, eventually becoming indistinguishable from the interictal background pattern unless characterized by a distinctive overriding fast component. The discharges also tend to become subclinical again, as at the beginning of the cluster. The EEG background usually does not fully revert to the interictal baseline pattern until a minute or more after the last discernible electrographic discharge.

This large-scale electroclinical evolution, which precedes, continues through and follows the actual spasms, suggests that it might be more physiological to

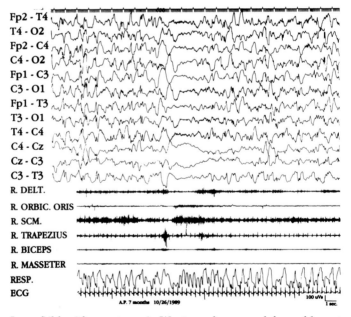

Figure 4.3 In a child with cryptogenic West syndrome and favorable outcome, the spasm is preceded and immediately followed by hypsarrhythmia. Courtesy of Dr F. Vigevano.

conceptualize "the seizure" at the level of the cluster itself rather than at that of the individual spasms. Thus, for example, the notion of "seizure count" in infantile spasms is probably more meaningful, and certainly much more reliably estimated by parents, if it is taken to mean "cluster count" rather than "spasm count".

UNUSUAL VARIATIONS

"Subclinical Electrographic Spasms"

Donat and Wright (1991b) reported 11 infants with extremely subtle behaviors associated with ictal and interictal EEG patterns characteristic of infantile spasms. Moreover, some babies with more typical spasms can have a rare cluster that is subclinical not only at the beginning and end, but remains entirely electrographic throughout. Although the notion of a "subclinical spasm" seems at face value like an oxymoron, if the ictal event is taken to be at the level of the *cluster*, there is less apparent contradiction – in fact, the phrase conveys important information.

I am not aware of any previous description of this phenomenon in the literature, but we have stumbled across it by chance on several occasions when intending to review random sleep epochs during video/EEG monitoring. At some moment the highly abnormal background EEG pattern begins to "normalize" in a fashion identical to that of the behavioral spasm clusters upon awakening in that particular child. The epileptiform discharges disappear and the background assumes a lower-amplitude, faster, nondescript pattern. Soon the characteristic ictal discharges appear – typically high-amplitude slow waves with overriding rhythmic fast activity, each lasting 1–2 s – and these repeat approximately every 10 s. But the child does not awaken, and no discernible movement accompanies any of the discharges. (Of course, it is quite possible that the discharges could have been accompanied by some eye deviation under closed lids, or by some slight tensing of musculature insufficient to produce any movement discernible on video.) After several minutes, the discharges dissipate and the EEG gradually assumes the characteristic highly abnormal sleep pattern again.

Given that we happened to observe such events only by chance, it seems likely that they occur more frequently than is generally realized. The clinical significance of a cluster of "subclinical spasms" is of course unknown, but the phenomenon should be recognized to exist and should be taken into account in formal studies of spasm phenomenology or treatment efficacy.

Asymmetry

The vast majority of spasms are symmetrical, both behaviorally and electrographically. In the series of Kellaway *et al.* (1979), only 0.6% of spasms were behaviorally asymmetrical, and the 11 ictal EEG patterns were described either as "generalized" or without mention of topographic distribution. This is consistent with other past studies which have traditionally emphasized the symmetry of spasms and the diffuseness of underlying pathology (or lack of identifiable pathology), even though asymmetries in the *interictal* EEGs of these patients have occasionally been described, even to the extreme of hemihypsarrhythmia (Altman and Shewmon, 1990; Cusmai *et al.*, 1988; Donat *et al.*, 1991; Hrachovy *et al.*, 1984; de Jong *et al.*, 1976; Lerman, 1969; Ohtahara, 1965; Parmeggiani *et al.*, 1990; Riikonen, 1982; Stafstrom *et al.*, 1989; Tjiam *et al.*, 1978).

It is now becoming common knowledge that some cases of infantile spasms are associated with focal brain pathology (Alvarez *et al.*, 1987; Ashkenasi and Snead, 1989; Cusmai *et al.*, 1988, 1990a; Dulac *et al.*, 1987b; Gabriel, 1980; Singer *et al.*, 1982; Vinters *et al.*, 1992), and that surgical resection of the lesion can result in remission of spasms and relative normalization of background EEG patterns (Branch and Dyken, 1979; Carrazana *et al.*, 1993; Chugani *et al.*, 1990, 1993; Mimaki *et al.*, 1983; Palm *et al.*, 1988; Ruggieri *et al.*, 1989; Shewmon *et al.*, 1989, 1990; Shields *et al.*, 1990, 1992; Uthman *et al.*, 1991). It should not be surprising that in such cases both the behavioral and electrographic aspect of the spasms might manifest asymmetries; in fact, at our institution, the spatial concordance of such asymmetries, when present, with other lines of evidence for localized cortical abnormality, is an important factor in the assessment of surgical candidacy (Quesney *et al.*, 1993; Shewmon *et al.*, 1990).

Over the past several years, the pattern of referral for EEG/video monitoring of infantile spasms at UCLA has shifted toward a greater proportion of medically intractable, possibly surgical cases, thereby strongly biasing our series in the direction of a higher prevalence of asymmetries. (About one-third of the cases have ended up qualifying for resective surgery.) Though not representative of the spasms population in general, this selected subpopulation has provided an exceptional opportunity to witness the richness and extent of the spectrum of spasm phenomenology.

I suspect that the true incidence of ictal asymmetries, though lower than in our series, is higher than is generally realized. We have had the chance to examine prior EEGs of referred patients, which have shown consistently lateralized or even localized areas of increased slowing, decreased beta activity, attenuation, or bursts of paroxysmal fast activity, either interictally or ictally. Such features, however, were easily overlooked in the sea of more dramatic diffuse or multifocal abnormalities, and were not mentioned in the formal reports; but they were noticeable when one looked for them.

Between the Infantile Spasms Workshop in May 1991 (Commission, 1992) and the writing of this chapter, further research in this area has been reported from our group (Gaily and Shewmon, 1992, 1993). As of December 1992, we had performed 75 EEG/video recordings on 60 patients with infantile spasms (not including 10 from an early drug study). Every behavioral spasm was reviewed, and of the more than 8000 spasms, 7327 were of sufficient recorded quality to be scored visually for symmetry and synchrony of both behavioral and EEG aspects.

One kind of ictal asymmetry, at the level of the cluster rather than of the spasms, was the concurrence of focal seizures, a phenomenon reported by others in recent years (Carrazana *et al.*, 1990, 1993; Donat *et al.*, 1991; Donat and Wright, 1991a,c; Hrachovy *et al.*, 1984; Vigevano *et al.*, 1991a; Yamamoto *et al.*, 1988) and observed in 21 of the 60 patients in our series. The focal seizures are often hemitonic but may be complex partial or even entirely subclinical. Often, the focal seizure is what initiates the entire ictal episode, as though "triggering" a cluster of spasms, which begin in the immediate postictal period. Alternatively, the spasms can begin before the focal seizure terminates, with the EEG revealing both ictal patterns simultaneously. Less commonly, the focal seizure gradually evolves into the spasms by decelerating and fragmenting. On other occasions, the focal seizure begins in the middle of a spasm cluster, which may or may not be transiently interrupted as a result.

Of equal interest are asymmetries and/or asynchronies at the level of the individual spasms (Donat *et al.*, 1991; Jeavons and Bower, 1964, p. 9; King *et al.*, 1985a; Lacy and Penry, 1976, p. 13; Lombroso, 1983a; Vigevano *et al.*, 1991a). In a recent study, Fusco and Vigevano (1993) found that cryptogenic spasms were always symmetrical, but that nearly 40% of symptomatic cases manifested asymmetry of the limb contraction (Fig. 4.4). As many as 31 of 60 patients in our series manifested some degree of asymmetry or asynchrony of behavioral spasms, including 12 in whom more than 50% of the recorded spasms were asymmetric or asynchronous. Combining patients, 35% of all behavioral spasms and 41% of ictal EEG discharges were asymmetric or asynchronous. Of

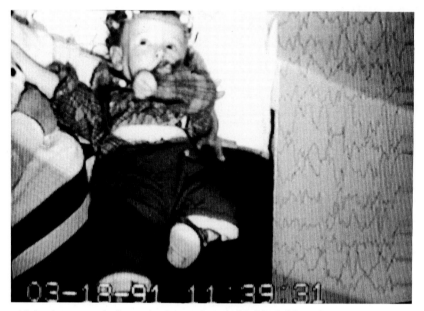

Figure 4.4 Asymmetrical spasm in an 8-month-old child with symptomatic West syndrome. Courtesy of Dr F. Vigevano.

the asymmetric (or asynchronous) behavioral spasms, the maximal (or leading) EEG discharge was contralateral in 60%, ipsilateral in 4% and symmetric in 36%. Of the asymmetric (or asynchronous) EEG discharges, the maximal (or leading) behavior was contralateral in 52%, ipsilateral in 3% and symmetric in 45%.

It should be emphasized that, even in cases of diffuse pathology, ictal paroxysmal fast activity tends to be posteriorly predominant; therefore, if it occurs focally in the posterior region of one hemisphere (Altman and Shewmon, 1990), this fact, taken in isolation from other localizing information, should not be interpreted as indicating focal pathology restricted to that area. On the other hand, it would probably constitute a strong indicator of at least the *laterality* of pathology, although we have come across exceptions even to this rule, when one hemisphere was so abnormal that it could not participate in the generation of generalized paroxysmal fast activity (creating the deceptive appearance that the better hemisphere, with the fast-activity discharge, was the epileptogenic one).

Typical behavioral asymmetries were flexion, extension or abduction of one arm more than the other, or flexion of the hip and knee on one side more than the other. The degree of asymmetry ranged from mild to marked, both within and across patients. Behavioral asymmetry was most likely to occur, and was also most pronounced, in patients with hemiparesis and/or lesions or interictal dysfunction involving primary sensorimotor cortex unilaterally. Of particular interest is the fact that the paretic side tended to be the one with the *stronger* spasm (associated with a predominantly or exclusively contralateral EEG discharge in the more abnormal hemisphere), contrary to what one might predict on the basis of a purely brainstem theory of "spasmogenesis" (Carrazana *et al.*, 1990; Hrachovy *et al.*, 1981; Kellaway *et al.*, 1983).

Asynchrony of spasms was relatively common in patients with agenesis of the corpus callosum, in which case there was about equal distribution of the leading side within a given patient. If the underlying etiology was a unilateral lesion, however, the distribution of leading side was strongly skewed in favor of the EEG discharges being ipsilateral, and body movements contralateral, to the lesion. Such asynchrony constitutes even stronger evidence than asymmetry in favor of a primary role for the cortex in the initiation of spasms, at least in this particular subpopulation of patients.

Finally, EEG asymmetries in the inter-spasm interval also occur and are of potential localizing value. The most common type consists of greater attenuation on the more pathologic side. On other occasions, when neither side is greatly attenuated, there may be a frequency asymmetry with greater polymorphic slowing on the more abnormal side.

The following cases are offered to illustrate some of these concepts. J.S. began having focal seizures at age 2 days and infantile spasms at 4 weeks, both remaining medically intractable. Magnetic resonance imaging (MRI) revealed cortical dysplasia in the left parieto-occipito-temporal area, which was also metabolically abnormal on PET scan. EEG/video monitoring at age 4 months captured many ictal episodes beginning with a focal electrographic seizure in the left occipital region (Fig. 4.5a), leading into a cluster of spasms beginning 100 s later. A typical spasm-associated discharge 3 min into the cluster is shown in Fig. 4.5b; note both the asynchrony of the burst (beginning in the left posterior region) and the asymmetry of the paroxysmal fast activity, which is almost exclusively confined to the left hemisphere and is maximal posteriorly. As the cluster evolved, the inter-spasm intervals on the right began to fill in with delta–theta background before those on the left, which remained asymmetrically attenuated for another 2 min, as exemplified in Fig. 4.5c, taken from 6 min 11 s into the cluster. Note the continued focality of the paroxysmal fast activity. Following surgical resection of the dysplastic cortex, J.S. has done extremely well in terms of both seizure control and development.

Around 3.5 months of age, N.A.F. began having staring episodes and right hemiclonic seizures, which evolved over another 2 months into medically intractable infantile spasms. An EEG around that time showed intermittent hypsarrhythmia and left hemispheric slowing. By the time she was referred for telemetry at age 9 months, she manifested a right hemiparesis and right visual field deficit, and both structural and functional neuroimaging revealed abnormality of the entire left hemisphere. Median nerve somatosensory evoked potentials showed unilateral absence of the left thalamocortical peak. Interictal EEG showed spiking predominantly at F3, decreased background beta activity throughout the left hemisphere and poor sleep spindle formation on the left. Figure 4.6 illustrates a typical spasm 1 min into a cluster. Note the marked left hemispheric attenuation during the inter-spasm intervals, as well as the left posterior paroxysmal fast activity preceding the spasm-associated slow wave. Her seizures disappeared and development began to improve following a left

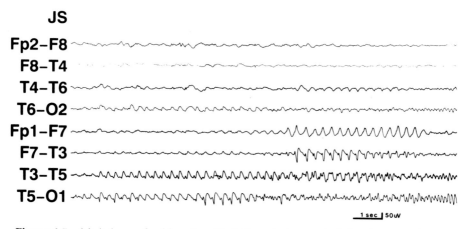

Figure 4.5 (a) A 4-month-old male with left posterior cortical dysplasia. A cluster of flexor spasms was "triggered" by this left occipital focal seizure, which began subclinically during sleep and then became associated with head and eye deviation to the left.

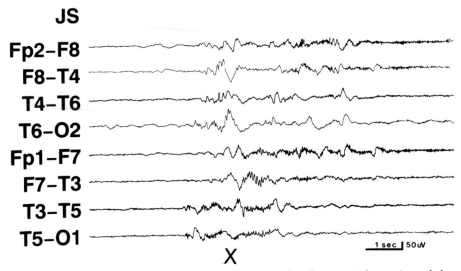

Figure 4.5 (b) Mild spasm ("X") from 3 min into the cluster, with tensing of the extremities and transient eye deviation to the right. The EEG discharge begins a fraction of a second earlier in the left posterior region, and the ictal fast activity is virtually confined to the left hemisphere.

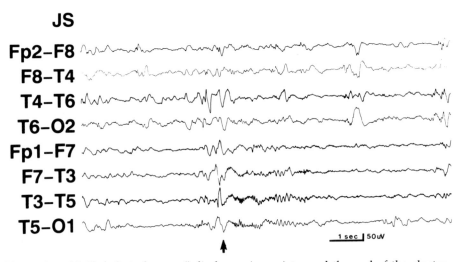

Figure 4.5 (c) "Subclinical spasm" discharge (arrow) toward the end of the cluster, illustrating unilateral attenuation of inter-spasm intervals over the left hemisphere and ictal fast activity still confined to the left hemisphere, maximal posteriorly.

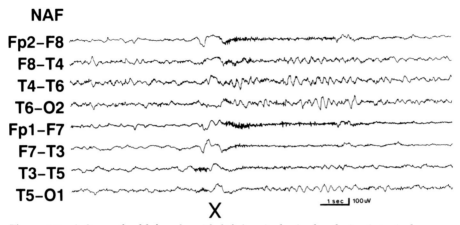

NAF

Fp2–F8

F8–T4

T4–T6

T6–O2

Fp1–F7

F7–T3

T3–T5

T5–O1

X

1 sec   100 µV

Figure 4.6 A 9-month-old female with left hemispheric dysplasia. A typical spasm ("X") from 1 min into a cluster, characterized by hip and knee flexion and upward eye deviation. EEG reveals marked left hemispheric attenuation during inter-spasm intervals and the left posterior paroxysmal fast activity preceding the spasm-associated slow wave (which in the life-sized tracing is easily distinguished from the muscle artifact that follows the spasm).

hemispherectomy. Histopathologic examination diagnosed diffuse hemispheric cortical dysplasia and neuronal heterotopias in the white matter.

Postinfantile Spasms

The final variation on the ictal theme is the occurrence of "infantile spasms" in older children. The spasm literature traditionally declares the upper limit for age of onset to be around 18 months (Holmes, 1987; Kellaway *et al.*, 1983; Weinmann, 1988) and the upper limit for age of occurrence to be around 2 years (Holmes, 1987). It is well known, however, that many cases of West syndrome evolve with age into the Lennox-Gastaut syndrome (Brown and Livingston, 1985; Lombroso, 1983a; Meencke, 1985; Weinmann, 1988), and some investigators have suggested that the infantile spasms of the former and the drop attacks of the latter are essentially the same basic pathophysiological entity (Egli *et al.*, 1985; Ikeno *et al.*, 1985; Donat and Wright, 1991d).

In addition, we have come across several cases of older children without Lennox-Gastaut syndrome who experienced seizures that seemed both behaviorally and electrographically indistinguishable from clusters of infantile spasms. The notion of "noninfantile infantile spasms" is even more oxymoronic than that of "subclinical spasms", and there ought to be a term such as "juvenile spasms", or more generically "epileptic spasms", reserved for such cases. This is not to imply, of course, that the concept of *West syndrome* should also be extended, because the similarity is confined to the electroclinical phenomenology of the spasms, not to the entire clinical context. Similar cases

(a)

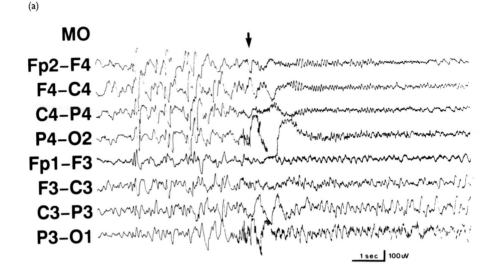

(b)

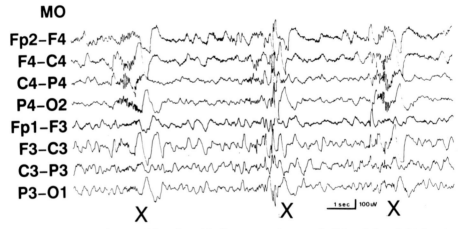

Figure 4.7 (a) A 3-year-old male with Rasmussen's encephalitis of the right hemisphere. A cluster of spasms was initiated by this hemitonic seizure (arrow) involving a "fencing" posture and head deviation toward the left, with a brief hemiclonic phase immediately before the spasms started. (b) A series of flexor spasms ("X") involving all four extremities, from 1 min into the cluster. Note the marked asymmetry of ictal fast activity and inter-spasm attenuation over the right hemisphere.

have also been reported by Gobbi *et al.* (1987, 1989, 1991a) with ages up to young adulthood.

M.O., for example, began having left focal motor seizures and progressive left hemiparesis at around 2 years of age. Within a few months the seizure type changed to repetitive head drops, and later to hemitonic seizures lasting 20–30 s followed by a cluster of generalized spasms. By age 3 years 4 months, when he was referred to us for evaluation, he had a moderate left hemiparesis. MRI was unremarkable, but PET showed diffuse right hemispheric hypometabolism. Interictal EEG showed right hemispheric slowing and frequent spiking, with unilateral right-sided absence of posterior dominant rhythm and sleep spindles. A typical seizure onset is shown in Fig. 4.7a, with right hemispheric fast activity associated with left hemitonic posturing. This lasted 23 s, and only 4 s later the spasm cluster began. Figure 4.7b illustrates a typical spasm discharge about 1 min into the cluster, not at all unlike the previously illustrated asymmetrical discharges, with greater paroxysmal fast activity and inter-spasm attenuation over the affected hemisphere. Following right hemispherectomy, M.O. has remained seizure-free. Pathologic examination diagnosed Rasmussen's encephalitis.

M.S. began having seizures at age 3–6 weeks and soon afterwards began having infantile spasms. An early EEG showed hypsarrhythmia and he was treated with adrenocorticotrophic hormone (ACTH) and later with a variety of antiepileptic drugs without success. He became severely developmentally delayed with spastic quadriparesis. Work-up prior to referral had suggested no particular etiology; MRI, PET and interictal EEG showed generalized atrophy,

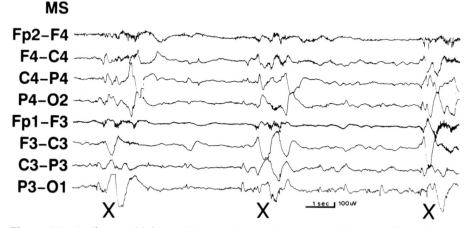

Figure 4.8   A 4½-year-old boy with spastic quadriparesis and intractable infantile spasms of unknown etiology. A series of violent spasms ("X") with bilateral arm abduction and extension, leg extension, eye deviation, grimacing and grunting. EEG shows essentially bilaterally symmetrical discharges consisting of high-amplitude slow waves with superimposed movement artifact over the left side of the head, and diffuse attenuation between spasms.

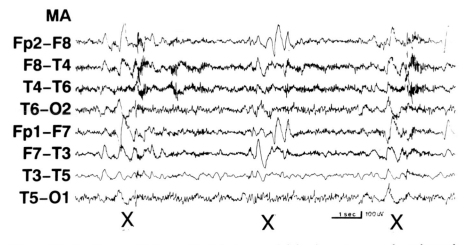

MA

Figure 4.9 An 8-year-old boy with left temporal lobe harartoma and prolonged clusters of spasms characterized by symmetrical arm abduction and neck and trunk flexion ("X"), with preserved consciousness in between. Ictal EEG consists of bursts of high-amplitude generalized slow waves.

diffuse hypometabolism, and generalized slowing and epileptiform discharges, respectively. EEG/video recording at age 4.5 years captured clusters of unusually violent, symmetrical flexion spasms of the entire body, associated with the characteristic ictal EEG pattern illustrated in Fig. 4.8. (Needless to say, he was not considered a surgical candidate.)

The oldest case of "juvenile spasms" that we have seen was 8 years old at the time of recording. M.A. began having brief staring spells at 1.5 years of age, which changed to more overt complex partial seizures with automatisms just before 4 years. At age 4.5 years, a left temporal lobe lesion was identified on contrast-enhanced MRI. Around the same time, the seizure type changed to clusters of transient symmetrical arm abduction and neck and trunk flexion, repeating every 4–8 s for up to 15 min at a time. At age 7.5 years, surgical excision of the lesion was performed, followed 2 months later by removal of residual left mesial temporal tissue on account of continued seizures. Histopathologic diagnosis was hamartoma.

For the next 3 months he was seizure-free but then experienced a recurrence of the same type of spasm clusters as before, although of lesser intensity. A follow-up EEG/video recording was performed at 8 years of age. The typical ictal EEG pattern is illustrated in Fig. 4.9: a 1 s burst of high-amplitude generalized slowing with each spasm, and disappearance of the usual background abnormalities (left hemispheric slowing and epileptiform discharges) between spasms. Interestingly, during these long clusters he was able to carry on conversations, count and read, although during phases of peak intensity of the spasms, his speed would decrease noticeably. Unfortunately, he continues to experience frequent seizures and is not considered a candidate for more extensive resection because, among other reasons, Wada testing demonstrated left hemisphere dominance for language.

CONCLUSION

The spectrum of infantile-spasm phenomenology is considerably broader than the traditional literature suggests. Undoubtedly, greater awareness of the possible variations on the theme will lead to more accurate diagnosis. In particular, consistent asymmetry and/or asynchrony of the ictal behavior and/ or associated ictal EEG discharge may constitute important supporting evidence for a lateralized or localized underlying etiology.

5

Other Types of Seizures

P. PLOUIN, O. DULAC

Infantile spasms (IS) are defined as the combination of epileptic spasms (ES) and diffuse spike activity occurring in infancy. Other types of seizures may precede and/or accompany ES, or may even follow them in the course of epilepsy. In this chapter, we focus on seizures preceding or accompanying ES.

Other types of seizure associated with ES have been clinically recognized for some time. Over the last decade, however, the development of long-term video/EEG monitoring and ambulatory EEG monitoring, as well as an increased interest in epileptic disorders of infants, have led to a better understanding of these seizures and their various etiologies.

Clinically, two situations seem to occur. In the first, other seizures are the first manifestation of epilepsy with ES occurring later; the most probable diagnosis in such cases is brain malformative syndrome or antenatal encephalopathy. In the second situation, other types of seizures are associated with acute insults (anoxic–ischemic encephalopathy, stroke, bacterial meningitis, head trauma, intoxication, etc.), sometimes including status epilepticus in the neonatal period or in early infancy. Then, following a possible seizure-free interval, ES occur. In the first situation, other seizures and ES belong to the same epileptic condition, probably age-dependent. In the second situation, ES may be considered the delayed epileptic consequence of the earlier brain damage. This dichotomy between the two situations has been clearly demonstrated by Velez *et al.* (1990), with differences in prognostic outcome.

Different types of seizures have been reported in association with ES: partial seizures (PS), myoclonic, tonic, tonic–clonic, akinetic, hemiconvulsive and even atypical absence seizures (Lacy and Penry, 1976, p. 169). Partial seizures co-existing with ES have long been recognized (Kellaway, 1959; Fukuyama, 1960; Jeavons and Bower, 1964, p. 82; Lacy and Penry, 1976; Bear *et al.*, 1982; Lombroso, 1982).

PARTIAL SEIZURES

Let us first focus on the difficulty distinguishing simple PS from complex PS in infancy. The loss of consciousness may be impossible to assess, even with video tape, so let us consider PS as a single entity without any difference concerning the patient's responsiveness. Partial seizures have been reported clinically in Aicardi syndrome, occurring from the neonatal period and preceding ES (Chevrie and Aicardi, 1984). Chevrie and Aicardi noted PS in half their patients. No precise clinical description was available before PS were recorded on EEG and videotaped.

A clinical description was first made by Bour *et al.* (1986), who recorded PS in seven of their eight patients, two of whom had also presented with generalized clonic seizures. Partial seizures began between 6 days and $2\frac{1}{2}$ months of age (mean = 2.1 months). Most of these PS were hemiclonic or hemitonic: hemitonic seizures were accompanied by apnea and cyanosis in two cases, by flush face in one case and by laughter in another; hemiclonic seizures were associated with chewing in two cases. In five patients, Bour *et al.* recorded PS immediately followed by a cluster of spasms, the cluster involving as many as 40 consecutive spasms.

Partial seizures have been reported in other etiologies of infantile spasms: tuberous sclerosis (Dulac *et al.*, 1984), agyria–pachygyria (Dulac *et al.*, 1983a), naevus linearis sebaceus (Vigevano *et al.*, 1984) and hemimegalencephaly (Paladin *et al.*, 1989). In 1984, Dalla Bernardina *et al.* called attention to the association of ES and PS as a frequent indication of a malformative etiology.

In 1988, Yamamoto *et al.* described four cases of infants with IS presenting with PS evolving to ES. These cases were documented by EEG video-telemetry recordings and the clinical analysis of PS was precisely related: "eye opening, side-to-side head shaking, and flush face" with a right or left occipital ictal discharge in case 1 with severe brain atrophy; "cessation of activity and grimacing that looked like laughter" with a left temporal ictal discharge in case 2 with tuberous sclerosis; "staring, increased limb tone, vomiting and oral automatism" corresponding to a left temporal ictal discharge in case 3 with brain atrophy; "cessation of activity and staring and clung to her mother as if threatened" with a left frontal ictal discharge in case 4 with a severe encephalopathy. In 1990, Chugani *et al.* reported partial seizures evolving to ES in three of four patients who they operated upon. In 1991, Donat and Wright reported the same pattern in infants with CNS malformations.

In 1993, Carrazana *et al.* reported 16 more infants presenting with the same pattern of facilitation of ES by PS. All cases were either symptomatic ($n = 13$) or cryptogenic ($n = 3$). In seven cases, PS developed 1–8 months before ES. The authors give a precise electroclinical description of all PS recorded. In order of prevalence, they found eye and head deviation ($n = 10$), localized clonus ($n = 10$) tonic posturing of the limb ($n = 6$) and facial twitching ($n = 5$). Blank staring, opisthotonos and other symptoms were less frequent.

The electroclinical analysis of PS demonstrates a good relation between the topography of the EEG discharges and the first clinical symptom of the seizure. Infants present with all kinds of PS – frontal, central, temporal and occipital – and the semiology is similar to that found in older children, except for subjective symptoms which cannot be reported at such an early age. In the patients of Carrazana *et al.* (1993), there was an excellent relation between the ictal onset of PS and the location of the structural abnormality (neuro-imaging) in 12 cases. This had been reported earlier in patients with Aicardi syndrome by Bour *et al.* (1986) who, using a CT scan, found an asymmetry in five cases with PS starting on the side of the smaller hemisphere.

The ictal EEG pattern of PS has been studied in some depth by Bour *et al.* (1986), who described a stereotypical pattern: diffuse flattening of the background activity, unilateral alpha rhythms, rhythmic theta, spikes or spikes and waves, inconstant unilateral alpha rhythm, possibly followed by a cluster of spasms. These seizures lasted between 20 s and 2 min. Yamamoto *et al.* (1988) reported various EEG patterns in their four cases: unilateral or diffuse flattening followed by theta or delta rhythmic waves. Carrazana *et al.* (1993) found the same features: alpha, theta or delta rhythmic waves, sometimes intermingled, possibly preceded by uni- or bilateral flattening. Among the patients of this last series, the underlying disorders in symptomatic cases were dysplastic abnormalities ($n = 8$), phakomatoses ($n = 3$), acquired encephaloclastic lesions ($n = 2$) and nonketotic hyperglycinemia ($n = 1$). It appears that the combination of PS and ES is probably age-dependent and not strictly related to a defined cortical lesion, although this pattern seems to result more frequently from brain malformation.

The association of ES and PS has also been reported by Lortie *et al.* (1993a) in a population of infants with occipital seizures. In evaluating 12 infants with occipital seizures associated with a demonstrable lesion on neuroradiology and/or occipital EEG focus, they found that ES were present in seven cases, both symmetrical and asymmetrical. Epileptic spasms preceded PS in the course of epilepsy ($n = 3$), started at about the same time ($n = 2$) or followed PS ($n = 2$). Once more, the relationship between ES and PS was present in patients with a lesional etiology.

In a prospective study of infants with ES, Plouin *et al.* (1993) performed 24 h ambulatory EEG monitoring in 74 patients. They recorded PS in 31 infants (51% of symptomatic cases, 33% of cryptogenic cases). In 14 patients, PS were immediately followed by a cluster of spasms consisting of a single ictal event. In a given patient, this sequence could be the only type of ictal event, or could be associated with clusters of spasms, or with isolated PS. Patients with a combination of PS and ES in a single ictal event were symptomatic ($n = 10$), including 2 cases with tuberous sclerosis, 1 with lissencephaly and 1 with hemimegalencephaly; the last 4 cases were cryptogenic, all with an unfavorable outcome. The analysis of interictal EEG background activity and of EEG activity between spasms led to the conclusion that the association of an asymmetrical EEG hypsarrhythmic interictal pattern, PS and lack of recurrence of hypsarrhythmia between spasms in a given cluster were due to symptomatic factors or to cryptogenic IS with a poor prognosis (Dulac *et al.*, 1986a). Chiron *et al.* (1991) reported that in patients with tuberous sclerosis treated by vigabatrin, there could be an increase in PS, although the ES stopped.

Regarding the localization of unilateral PS associated with ES, it would

Table 5.1 EEG localization of partial seizures

Study	Frontal	Rolandic	Temporal	Occipital	Hemispheric
Yamamoto *et al.* (1988)	1		2	1	
Carrazana *et al.* (1993)	2	5	3	4	2
Plouin *et al.* (1993)	4	8	8	4	7
Total	7	13	13	9	7

appear that most of these are rolandic and temporal. Occipital seizures have been noted in nine cases, and frontal ones in only seven cases (Table 5.1).

All these findings show that the association of ES and PS is probably more frequent than reported. When long-term video/EEG monitoring or ambulatory EEG monitoring is performed, the probability of recording these two events increases. The importance of this association is clear regarding the etiology as most cases are symptomatic, but it is particularly important in patients with negative MRI because it allows the prediction of a poor prognosis for both psychomotor development and epilepsy, and is a major indication for functional imaging which often reveals areas of hypometabolism.

OTHER SEIZURES

Seizures other than PS associated with ES were reported for the first time in 1955 by Druckman and Chao. Few details are available about such seizures. Velez *et al.* (1990) noted that generalized seizures could precede ES. Plouin *et al.* (1993) reported generalized seizures immediately followed or not by a cluster of spasms in a few cryptogenic cases. There is no precise clinical description of these seizures, since they were recorded during ambulatory EEG. Lortie *et al.* (1993a), in their series of infants with an occipital epilepsy, reported one case with generalized tonic seizures at the onset of epilepsy at the age of 2 months, preceding spasms and PS. That case was cryptogenic. In six other cases presenting with ES, two had generalized seizures, but they followed ES in the course of epilepsy. There is at present no clear explanation of the co-existence of other types of clonic or tonic generalized seizures with ES.

Regarding myoclonic seizures (MS), the situation is more complicated. Since the publication of *L'Encephalopathie Myoclonique infantile avec Hypsarythmie (Syndrome de West)* by Gastaut *et al.* (1964b), it has been clearly demonstrated that the electroclinical presentation of the two phenomena is different: a myoclonic jerk is a very brief muscular contraction preceded by a burst of polyspikes or polyspikes and waves, whereas a spasm is a short tonic contraction accompanied by generalized low-amplitude fast activity or by a generalized high-amplitude slow wave (Kellaway *et al.*, 1979).

Nevertheless, Dulac *et al.* (1993b) reported four families with infants presenting with ES and MS. Among the 13 siblings of these four families, 8 were affected (6 boys and 2 girls). Four patients had other seizure types before spasms (focal alternating clonic seizures or erratic myoclonic jerks). All patients had erratic myoclonus of the face and extremities, beginning either before or soon after the onset of spasms, and persisting throughout the follow-up period. Progressive microcephaly from 3 to 6 months of life was the second major feature. Neuroradiological investigations showed progressive brain atrophy in all cases from age 6 to 8 months. Biochemical and histological investigations remained negative. This condition may result from an inborn error of metabolism, although those presently identified could be excluded.

Donat and Wright (1992) reported an association of MS and ES in 11% of their video/EEG documented patients with West syndrome. They noted that ES occurred in waking, were usually serial and associated with the typical ictal pattern, although MS could occur either in waking or during sleep, usually singly and associated with multiple spikes and waves. However, one patient presented with MS during sleep that on awakening showed a progression through transitional forms both clinically and by ictal EEG into a series of ES and then back into MS. They concluded that there may be a close relationship between the mechanisms that generate MS and ES.

Classically myoclonic jerks may or may not be epileptic. In the reports we have analyzed, myoclonic jerks were considered to be epileptic because they were correlated with a generalized spike wave discharge. Nevertheless, infants with ES may present with numerous nonepileptic myoclonic jerks if drowsy, or during treatment with hydrocortisone or vigabatrin. In our experience with systematic EMG recording of deltoid muscle in infants with IS, nonepileptic myoclonic jerks are frequent.

Tonic seizures have also been reported in association with ES, but without any video/EEG data. The distinction between "short" tonic seizures and "long" spasms is often not clear: there is no precise definition concerning the duration of the tonic contraction in both ES and tonic seizures. In some infants, a tonic seizure may introduce the cluster of spasms; in others, tonic seizures are single, independent epileptic events.

Atypical absence seizures have been reported but none have been recorded. These seizures are more likely to be complex PS, true absences being very rare in the first year of life.

As an illustration, we have chosen an infant with agyria–pachygyria, recorded at the age of 5 months, before any treatment. On a single 3 h video-polygraphic recording, the infant exhibited a cluster of spasms preceded by PS (Fig. 5.1), PS (mostly on the right but also on the left hemisphere) (Figs 5.2–5.4), PS with contralateral clonic jerks (Fig. 5.5), myoclonic fits with brief polyspike bursts (Fig. 5.5), bilateral tonic seizures (Fig. 5.6) and a cluster of long spasms (Fig. 5.7). This shows how useful it is to have long-term recordings with surface EMG of the deltoid in infants with IS.

CONCLUSION

A high proportion of patients with ES exhibit other seizure types (particularly PS) that are usually overlooked clinically and by short EEG recordings. Partial seizures in patients with ES are likely to contribute to etiologic diagnosis, prognostic evaluation and choice of treatment (medical and surgical). Other seizure types are observed only in patients with unfavorable outcome, mainly related to the presence of focal cortical lesions. This is particularly true when a cluster of spasms is initiated by PS. However, this combination may be observed in patients with diffuse abnormalities (e.g. Aicardi syndrome, lissencephaly). The association between erratic myoclonus and ES is probably related to an unknown inborn error of metabolism, often indicating a poor neurological outcome.

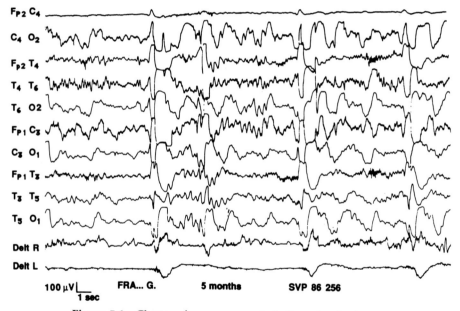

Figure 5.1 Cluster of spasms recorded after a focal seizure.

(a)

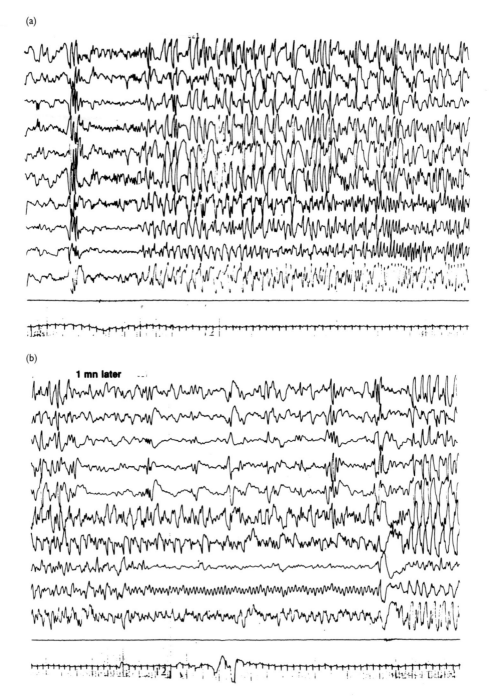

(b)

1 mn later

Figure 5.2   Subclinical left rolandic ictal discharge (a) evolving to the left temporal area with a different ictal pattern 1 min later (b).

(a)

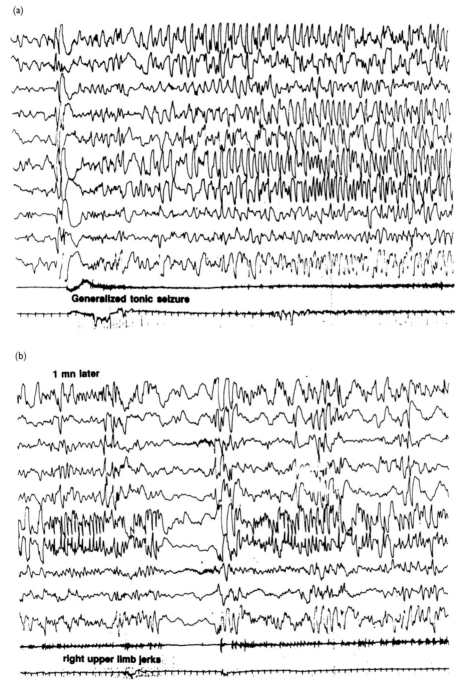

Generalized tonic seizure

(b)

1 mn later

right upper limb jerks

Figure 5.3 (a) Partial seizure initiated by a generalized polyspike burst with brief tonic contraction of the limbs followed by left rolandic theta activity. (b) Then, 1 min later, the ictal discharge is fragmented with rhythmic clonic movements of the right upper limb.

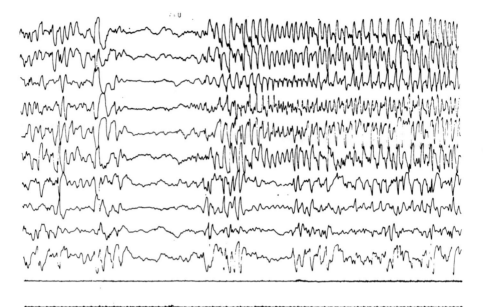

Figure 5.4   Right hemispheric ictal discharge without any clonic movement.

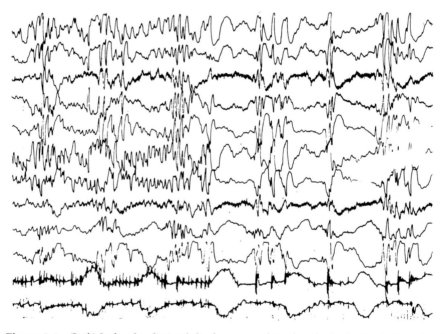

Figure 5.5   (Left) Left rolandic ictal discharge combined with rhythmic clonic jerks of both upper limbs most marked on the right side. (Right) Independent myoclonic jerks (more marked on the right) combined with brief generalized polyspike bursts.

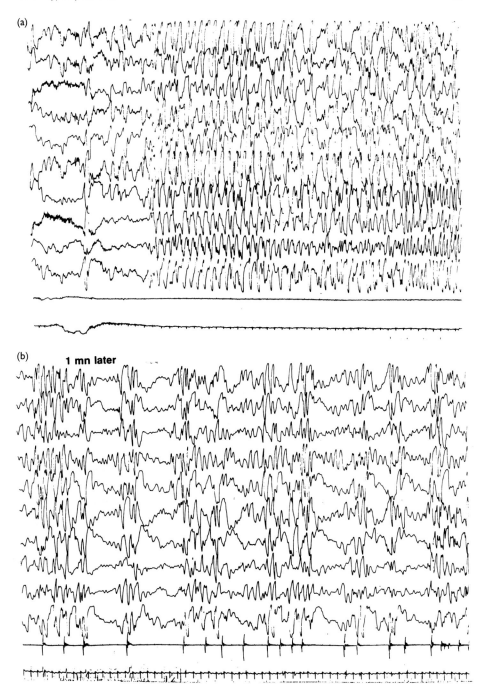

Figure 5.6 (a) Bilateral subclinical ictal discharge more marked on the left hemisphere. (b) Then, 1 min later, fragmented activity with bursts of slow waves and polyspikes and arrhythmic myoclonic jerks of the right upper limb.

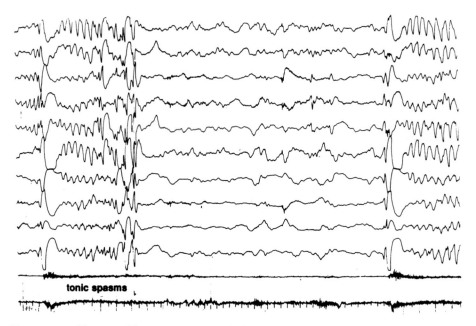

Figure 5.7 Cluster of long spasms, each beginning with a high-amplitude slow complex followed by rhythmic slow waves and polyspikes, lasting 6 s.

6

Interictal EEG: Variations and Pitfalls

B. DALLA BERNARDINA, K. WATANABE

The most common, although not the sole, EEG finding in patients with epileptic spasms (ES) is hypsarrhythmia (Lacy and Penry, 1976), which was defined by Gibbs and Gibbs (1952) as:

> random high voltage slow waves and spikes. These spikes vary from moment to moment, both in duration and location. At times they appear to be focal, and a few seconds later they seem to originate from multiple foci. Occasionally, the spike discharge becomes generalized, but it never appears as a rhythmically repetitive and highly organized pattern that could be confused with a discharge of the petit mal variant type. The abnormality is almost continuous, and in most cases it shows as clearly in the waking as in the sleeping record. It is referred to as hypsarrhythmia.

The above prototypic pattern is usually seen only in the early stage of the disorder and most often in younger infants, and there is a tendency for this pattern to evolve with time so that the anarchic and chaotic characteristics give way to a more organized pattern (Hrachovy and Frost, 1989a). Those who adhere rigidly to the original definition have called any variation of the prototypic pattern "modified hypsarrhythmia". But this term is also imprecise, because different workers appear to use it differently.

Gastaut *et al.* (1964b) classified hypsarrhythmia into "typical" and "atypical" cases, the latter into five main categories (Table 6.1), and they stated that typical hypsarrhythmia comprises 63%. Hrachovy *et al.* (1984) reviewed 290 24-h polygraphic records of 67 patients with infantile spasms (IS) aged 1–43 months, and described five varieties of modified hypsarrhythmia (Table 6.1), but did not

Table 1.1   Atypical or modified hypsarrhythmia

Gastaut *et al.* (1970)	Hrachovy *et al.* (1984)
Fragmented awake	With increased interhemispheric synchronization
Excessive slowing	Asymmetrical
Rapid activity	With a consistent focus
Asymmetrical	With voltage attenuation
With a focus	With high voltage slow activity

63

mention the distribution of each pattern among all records. They stated that more than one of the above variations might be seen at the same time in the EEGs of patients with IS.

These definitions of hypsarrhythmia and its variants are somewhat ambiguous, especially concerning the extent of its variability. Indeed, both incidental functional features (i.e. stage of evolution, vigilance, treatment and age) and structural features may contribute to the modification of the characteristics of the tracing. The clinical implications of each of these causes of modifications are, however, different in terms of outcome and therapeutic decisions. It is therefore important to determine which modifications relate to functional changes, and which ones relate to etiology and structural changes. This is difficult for a number of reasons: some authors use the terms hypsarrhythmia and IS interchangeably; most studies lack follow-up of electroclinical characteristics, including ictal and interictal features; and studies usually fail to link given electroclinical patterns to specific etiology and/or outcome. On the other hand, it is still to be determined whether hypsarrhythmia consists of an interictal or ictal tracing. There is a need to clarify these ambiguities in order to improve diagnostic work-up, prognostic evaluation and therapeutic strategies.

VARIATIONS OF HYPSARRHYTHMIA OF FUNCTIONAL ORIGIN

Qualitative Studies

Influence of States of Wakefulness and Sleep

It seems generally accepted that typical hypsarrhythmia occurs during wakefulness, and sleep causes fragmentation or a grouping of the continuous hypsarrhythmic pattern (Gastaut et al., 1964b; Hrachovy et al., 1984). But occasionally hypsarrhythmia may become more apparent or evident only during sleep, even when the awake EEG is normal (Jeavons, 1985). During rapid eye movement (REM) sleep, there is a marked reduction or total disappearance of hypsarrhythmia, occasionally leaving focal spikes or sharp waves (Gastaut et al., 1964b; Iwase and Watanabe, 1972; Hrachovy et al., 1981). Another interesting finding observed by Iwase and Watanabe (1972) during REM sleep was the periodic appearance of diffuse 14–19 Hz fast wave bursts in 12 of 34 cases (35%) studied polygraphically. In two of these subjects, the fast wave bursts persisted until clinical attack of ES finally occurred in association with the same type of fast wave bursts and the patients awoke. A striking similarity between the fast wave burst during REM sleep and ictal EEG of ES led us to postulate that the same neurophysiological mechanisms might be involved in REM sleep and attacks of ES, and pontine reticular formation might be responsible for these attacks. Exactly the same phenomenon was reported by Hrachovy et al. (1984).

There is a marked reduction or disappearance of hypsarrhythmia immediately after arousal from non-REM (NREM) sleep, which may last from a few seconds to many minutes (Hrachovy *et al.*, 1984).

Changes in Hypsarrhythmia with Age

Hypsarrhythmia undergoes a gradual change with age, becoming less disorganized with greater interhemispheric synchronization (Lacy and Penry, 1976; Hrachovy *et al.*, 1984). A long-term follow-up study of patients with IS disclosed that 50% of patients had normal EEGs, 46% focal or other abnormalities, and 4% continued to have hypsarrhythmia (Jeavons *et al.*, 1970). In a follow-up study beyond 11 years of age, hypsarrhythmia transformed most frequently to focal or multifocal discharges, and next most frequently to generalized spike waves although clinically tonic seizures were the most frequently observed seizure type (Negoro *et al.*, 1983; Watanabe *et al.*, 1987a,b). During the transitional stages from West syndrome to Lennox-Gastaut syndrome (LGS), modified hypsarrhythmia with increased interhemispheric synchronization or disorganized slow spike waves occurs (Ohtsuka *et al.*, 1989). But these patterns may also occur in cases without transition to LGS. It is rather difficult to determine the degree of interhemispheric synchronization by which we define paroxysmal abnormalities as either modified hypsarrhythmia or disorganized slow spike waves. An EEG shown to be modified hypsarrhythmia by Westmoreland and Gomez (1987) displayed spike waves too well organized to be categorized, in our opinion, as modified hypsarrhythmia.

Interictal EEG of Patients with Active IS

There have been no clinically based studies of EEG findings at the onset or at the initial active stage of IS, because most studies have concerned only patients who had both IS and hypsarrhythmia, or patients with IS at various stages of the disorder (Lacy and Penry, 1976). Thus, only about 60% of patients were reported to have true or modified hypsarrhythmia (Lacy and Penry , 1976). In a study of EEG features until the onset of IS (Watanabe *et al.*, 1973, 1987a,b), a few patients showed only focal spikes in NREM sleep at the onset of IS, although hypsarrhythmia was a predominant EEG finding in most cases.

Quantitative Study

In order to clarify the scope of interictal paroxysmal EEG abnormalities in IS, Watanabe *et al.* (1993) studied the EEG features of 82 infants aged 2–30 months before receiving treatment for IS. Isolated spasms were allowed to be present but patients having tonic seizures were excluded. The spasms exhibited by the patients in this study consisted of a more or less generalized tonic contraction of brief duration associated with ictal EEG discharges, mainly consisting of synchronization or high-voltage slow wave transient with or without super-imposed fast activity.

Interictal paroxysmal EEG abnormalities were analyzed in terms of type, continuity, interhemispheric synchrony, topography and wave component in each state of wakefulness and sleep. Each 20 s epoch of the whole record was scored as one of the items in each category and the most predominant was taken to represent a given state. Stage 4 sleep was often difficult to assess and was not analyzed.

Modified hypsarrhythmia in this study refers to variations described by Hrachovy et al. (1984).

1. *Type of paroxysmal discharges*. Hypsarrhythmia (typical or modified) was more frequently seen in NREM sleep (86% in stage 1 and 99% in stage 2/3) than in wakefulness (64%) or arousal (54%), whereas focal or multifocal spikes occurred more frequently in wakefulness than in NREM sleep. In a few cases, there were no spikes at all in wakefulness, stage 1 sleep or arousal. In REM sleep, hypsarrhythmia was not observed and there were focal or multifocal spikes, or no spikes at all. Fast wave bursts as mentioned above occurred periodically in 16 of 32 cases (50%) in which REM stage was recorded.

The change with age was clear only in wakefulness. Hypsarrhythmia was least frequent after 1 year of age only in wakefulness. No changes with age were observed during sleep.

2. *Continuity of paroxysmal discharges*. Continuity was assessed by measuring the duration of a burst of paroxysmal discharges. When there were long and short bursts in an epoch, they were scored as longer bursts. Almost continuous patterns were most frequent in wakefulness and stage 1 sleep and decreased during stages 2 and 3, whereas episodic patterns were least frequent in wakefulness and increased with advancing sleep stage. Suppression-burst patterns occurred only in stages 2 and 3 at 6 months or less. There was no change in continuity with age.

3. *Interhemispheric synchrony of paroxysmal discharges*. Almost asynchronous discharges are similar to those seen in typical hypsarrhythmia and almost synchronous pseudorhythmic ones to those typically seen in LGS. Between these two extremes, slightly increased and moderately increased synchrony were scored. Almost asynchronous patterns were least frequent in wakeful-ness, and increased with advancing sleep stage. Moderately increased synch-rony was more often seen in wakefulness and decreased with increasing sleep stage. An increase in almost asynchronous patterns with advancing sleep stage was only evident before 1 year of age. A reduction in moderately increased synchrony with advancing sleep stage was only observed after 1 year of age. Slightly increased synchrony increased during stages 2 and 3 after 1 year of age. This may be due to the sum of two factors: an increase in asynchrony with advancing sleep stage and an increase in synchrony with increasing age.

4. *Topography of paroxysmal discharges*. There was no definite topographic dominance of paroxysmal discharges in most cases. This may be an overesti-

mate because EEG recordings with a gain of 100 μV/1 cm might have obscured focal accentuation. Posterior dominance was next frequent, but anterior dominance was rare and observed only after 1 year of age. No topographic dominance was more frequent in stages 2 and 3 than in wakefulness, but this was due to the presence of more focal spikes in this state.

5. *Wave component.* The wave component did not change with state or age.

VARIATIONS OF HYPSARRHYTHMIA OF STRUCTURAL ORIGIN

Quantified analysis of the characteristics of hypsarrhythmia has failed to demonstrate significant differences according to various etiologies (Watanabe *et al.*, 1993). However, several characteristics have been reported to be indicative of symptomatic rather than idiopathic cases:

- asymmetric hypsarrhythmia (Lombroso, 1983a; Hrachovy *et al.*, 1984; Watanabe *et al.*, 1993);
- predominance of focal slow activity (Parmeggiani *et al.*, 1990);
- persistence of focal spikes following intravenous diazepam administration (Dulac *et al.*, 1993a).

When considering the whole EEG pattern and the way it builds up, specific characteristics are apparent which help to distinguish symptomatic from idiopathic cases. In addition, particular aspects are correlated to specific etiologies and a predictable outcome (Dalla Bernardina, 1992).

Metabolic Diseases

In metabolic diseases, the interictal pattern is only rarely – if ever – very transiently hypsarrhythmic. Most often the picture associates multifocal abnormalities with complex bursts of spikes, sharp waves and slow waves, separated by random episodes of EEG flattening. When a more structured hypsarrhythmic pattern appears, the patient has already been suffering from various types of seizures and other neurological symptoms for a long period. In fact, picture at onset is usually that of a condition called either early epileptic myoclonic the encephalopathy (Dalla Bernardina *et al.*, 1983, 1992a,b, 1993) or early myoclonic encephalopathy (Aicardi, 1992).

This condition is characterized by massive flattening of background activity, with superimposed polymorphous bursts of slow spike waves that are often asynchronous on both hemispheres. The tracing is only slightly modified by sleep. Polygraphic records show the co-existence of subcontinuous jerks, related or not to EEG paroxysms, and of frequent and erratic partial seizures. Concomitantly, neurological impairment worsens progressively over a period of months, at which point EEG polygraphic records show subcontinuous and asynchronous suppression bursts, especially during sleep (Fig. 6.1a,b). Partial seizures and myoclonia persist, and repetitive symmetric extensor spasms with opisthotonos appear.

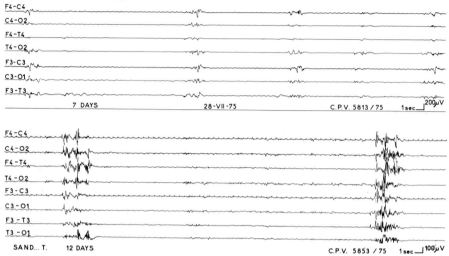

Figure 6.1(a) A newborn suffering from a nonketotic hyperglycinemic encephalopathy. It is possible to see periodic bilateral bursts of paroxysmal activity during very low background activity.

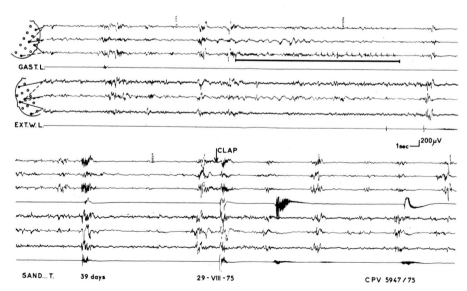

Figure 6.1(b) Co-existence of bilateral spasms, induced myoclonia and subclinical partial seizures.

This electroclinical picture characterizes most cases of nonketotic hypergly-cinemia and Menkes disease patients (Dalla Bernardina *et al.*, 1979, 1983). A similar picture may be observed in some cases of Alpers disease (Boyde *et al.*, 1986). Therefore, the subcontinuous diffuse discharges mimicking hypsarr-hythmia are constantly associated with more or less bilateral myoclonus, and this apparently interical pattern consists in fact of a myoclonic status.

In other instances, patients exhibit no paroxysmal EEG abnormalities. It is only later during follow-up that multifocal spikes, diffuse bursts of poorly organized paroxysms mixed with fast polyspikes, become evident when background activity and neurological condition are severely impaired. The spasms are associated with other partial or generalized seizures, and they are mostly tonic, rarely occurring in clusters. From the onset, these patients constantly have audiogenic jerks associated with doubtful EEG modifications. A similar picture has been reported in patients with biotinidase deficiency (Colamaria *et al.*, 1989).

Brain Malformations

Relatively specific interictal EEG patterns occur in diffuse malformations such as Aicardi syndrome, lissencephaly and hemimegalencephaly (see Chapter 15). Therefore, critical dysplasias (CD) share specific electroclinical features (Dalla Bernardina, 1993):

1. The hypsarrhythmic pattern occurs in a cortex producing abnormal background activity. The resulting pattern is a mixture of very high-amplitude paroxysmal abnormalities with unusually high-amplitude ($>150\,\mu$V), fast (>15 Hz) activity. In diffuse CD like lissencephaly, this pattern appears between 4 and 6 months of life, is slightly modified by sleep, and persists for several years. In holoprosencephaly, it is present from birth (Fig. 6.2) and tends to disappear with increasing age (Watanabe, 1976; Dalla Bernardina *et al.*, 1992a,b, 1993). There is no relationship between this more or less continuous interictal pattern, the presence or absence of spasms, and the response to treatment. In unilateral or focal CD, the hypsarrhythmic pattern is unilateral like in hemimegalence-phaly, or clearly asymmetric, and often associated with more or less focal, unusually fast activity.

2. The interictal awake EEG is often characterized by focal or multifocal paroxysmal abnormalities, and it is only during slow wave sleep that the picture becomes more hypsarrhythmic (Dalla Bernardina *et al.*, 1993).

3. In the majority of cases, the hypsarrhythmic pattern appears in the context of a particular EEG pattern, already recognizable from the neonatal period. This particular pattern consists of an association of delta–theta sharp waves and sequences of unusually fast activity, either alternating or inter-mingled (Dalla Bernardina *et al.*, 1993). A similar pattern is recognizable from the first days of life. The early electroclinical pattern of Aicardi syndrome is

particularly demonstrative (Fig. 6.3a,b). The spasms are almost always preceded by focal discharges that are frequently subclinical, appearing very early in life, often long before the appearance of hypsarrhythmia. A particular ictal event consists of a focal discharge followed by pseudoperiodic diffuse slow waves associated with a brief, fast activity discharge combined with more or less evident spasms (Fig. 6.4a–e). This ictal event was first described by Dalla Bernardina *et al.* (1984), and it strongly suggests malformation, as confirmed in later case reports (Yamamoto *et al.*, 1988; Carrazana *et al.*, 1993). Such ictal discharges may remain without clinical expression, particularly during sleep (see Chapter 4). In rare cases, this pseudoperiodic slow wave pattern may involve only one hemisphere. In other cases, the ictal event consists of repetitive "dystonic movements involving one arm and the neck with eye deviation". This type of seizure, suggestive of an abrupt and dystonic postural adjustment, is associated with a brief sequence of fast activity on EEG. Their epileptic nature usually remains unrecognized, also because of the major behavioral disturbances that are often combined with their occurrence. Hypsarrhythmia typically disappears between consecutive events of this periodic manifestation, which may be clinical or subclinical.

4. Two other features are the asynchrony and rhythmicity of both the ictal and interictal patterns. Asynchrony is particularly evident in Aicardi syndrome. It is probably not only due to callosal agenesis, but also related to age. It is most evident in cases of focal or multifocal CD (Dalla Bernardina *et al.*, 1993). Rhythmicity is most evident when CD is more diffuse, and it is particularly evident in holoprosencephaly (Watanabe *et al.*, 1976; Dalla Bernardina *et al.*, 1993). It must be pointed out that in most cases rhythmicity is not associated with hypsarrhythmia. The seizure type remains stereotyped throughout evolution.

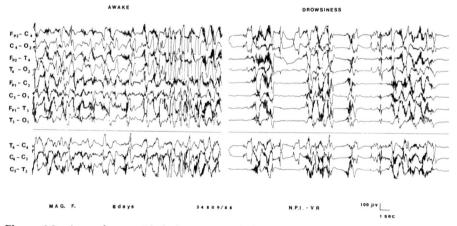

Figure 6.2 A newborn with holoprosencephaly. Note the unusual continuous sequence of pseudorhythmic fast polyspikes followed by a slow wave of very high amplitude when awake and during sleep.

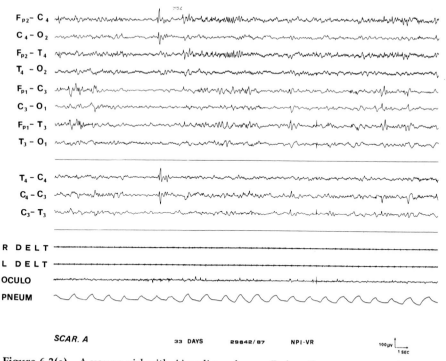

Figure 6.3(a) A young girl with Aicardi syndrome. Before the appearance of spasms, there is a peculiar sequence of asynchronous theta waves mixed with unusually fast activity, asynchronous discharges of both hemispheres and a brief subclinical right frontotemporal seizure.

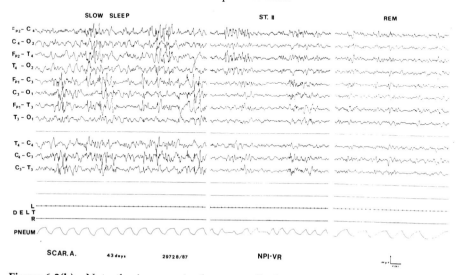

Figure 6.3(b) Note the increase in the unusually larger asynchronous theta waves during slow sleep and the presence of independent multifocal slow waves during REM sleep.

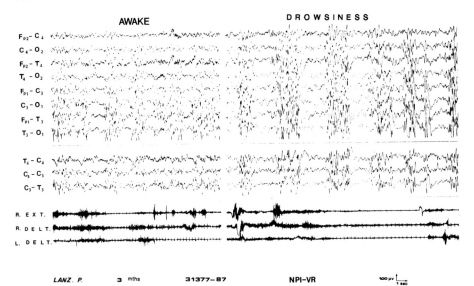

Figure 6.4(a) A young girl with focal left frontoparietal pachygyria. Note that the unilateral hypsarrhythmic pattern seen during wakefulness diffuses during sleep.

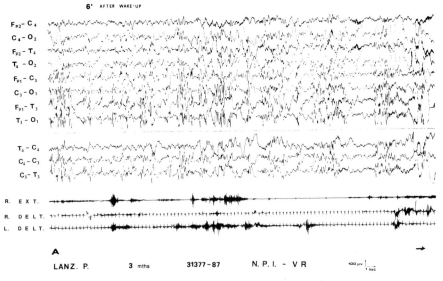

Figure 6.4(b) Upon waking, unilateral hypsarrhythmia reappears.

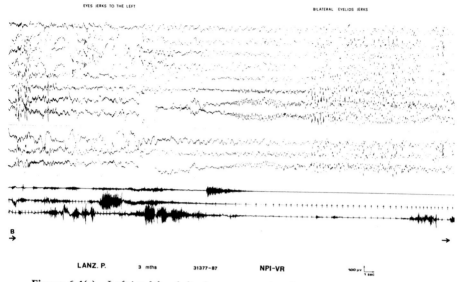

Figure 6.4(c) Left ictal focal discharges associated with bilateral eyelid jerks.

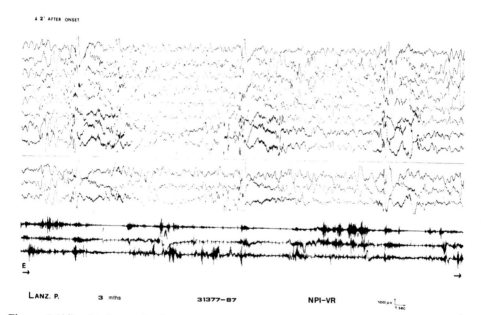

Figure 6.4(d) At the end of the partial seizure, bilateral spasms appear and the hypsarrhythmic pattern disappears.

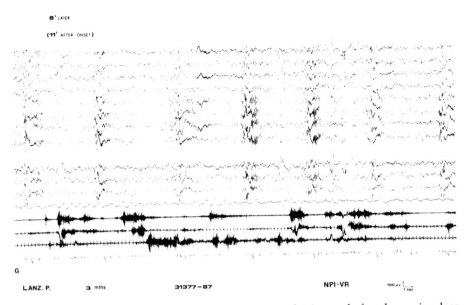

Figure 6.4(e)   The periodic spasms persist for several minutes before becoming less clinically evident. The ictal event is constituted by bilateral fast activity discharges which predominate on the left hemisphere.

Clastic Forms

Well-defined electroclinical patterns are rare in clastic disorders, since this group is heterogeneous, resulting from a great variety of pre-, peri- and post-natal diseases. The only relatively homogeneous pattern is that of posterior porencephaly. In such cases, asymmetry of background activity with focal slow waves and spikes over the temporo-occipital region of the abnormal hemisphere is evident before the occurrence of hypsarrhythmia. When it occurs, the latter is unilateral or asymmetrical, and the pattern is more diffuse only during sleep. We would like to stress that in many cases the pseudo-hypsarrhythmic pattern is purely the result of a recording artifact. In fact, using a sufficient number of electrodes, it becomes evident that the paroxysms are more strictly localized to the posterior region. Moreover, polygraphic records frequently permit the recognition of brief focal seizures occurring either before the appearance of spasms or between them. These seizures consist of focal flattening with a superimposed low-amplitude, fast rhythm associated with a fleeting deviation of the eyes.

On the other hand, it is important to note that porencephalic lesions due to prenatal insult may co-exist with CD. In such cases, the electroclinical pattern may be more complex, since both fast rhythms and pseudoperiodic spasms may co-exist. This picture is a good indication of the mixed (clastic–malformative) etiological condition produced by some infectious fetopathies.

Considering the clastic conditions as a whole, common features include:

- more or less severe background impairment with frequent asymmetries, both when awake and during sleep;
- focal or multifocal paroxysmal abnormalities, often varying in morphology because of fluctuating slow abnormalities;
- during sleep, paroxysmal abnormalities increase greatly, consisting of fast spikes or polyspikes.

In summary, hypsarrhythmia in clastic disorders consists of a transient phenomenon in the course of multifocal epilepsy, and even during this period of generalization it is still possible to recognize multiple focal and polymorphous abnormalities. Ictal events recur when awake and during sleep. They frequently have a tonic component combined with a low-amplitude, fast discharge (Fig. 6.5a,b). During the course of a single recording, they may be unilateral or bilateral, and interrupt only transiently the hypsarrhythmic pattern. There are frequent episodes of status epilepticus. Many patients exhibit both massive epileptic myoclonia and/or nonepileptic, spontaneous or provoked "spasms".

Cryptogenic and Idiopathic Cases

These must be considered in the end, since their recognition requires the prior exclusion of features suggestive of symptomatic etiology. Patients without evidence of symptomatic etiology but with poor outcome probably harbor undisclosed brain lesions, and are therefore called "cryptogenic". On the other hand, lack of evidence of cortical involvement combined with a favorable outcome define idiopathic IS. Such a diagnosis can only be suspected when the following characteristics are met (Dulac *et al.*, 1986a, 1993a; Dalla Bernardina *et al.*, 1992a,b; see also Chapter 21):

1. Hypsarrhythmia consists of a typical diffuse bilateral pattern that is continuous when awake, more or less fragmented during slow sleep, and disappears during REM sleep.
2. Between spasms of a cluster, the interictal activity recurs (Fig. 6.6a,b).
3. Following intravenous benzodiazepine and/or steroid treatment, the interictal abnormalities disappear, leaving no focal abnormalities.
4. In some cases at the very beginning, hypsarrhythmia is not completely structured, giving the impression of a fragmented pattern. In such conditions, bilateral physiological background activity, and well-defined physiological rhythms during sleep, are recognizable between the bursts.
5. Ictal events are electrochemical, bilateral, symmetric and synchronous, separated by hypsarrhythmia even within a cluster (Fig. 6.7a,b).
6. Although there may be moderate neuropsychological impairment, it does not comprise focal deficits.

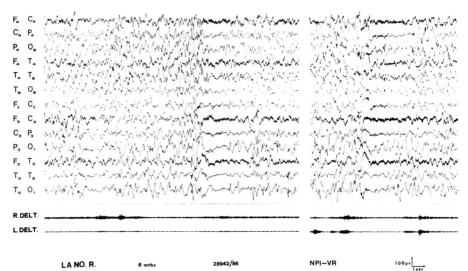

Figure 6.5(a) A young boy with a tetraparetic palsy following a severe neonatal anoxo-ischemic insult, and suffering from frequent spasms and tonic seizures since the age of 4 months. On a poorly organized background activity, frequent multifocal paroxysmal abnormalities may be seen, often diffusing on both hemispheres and interrupted by subclinical seizures consisting of brief bilateral discharges of small amplitude and fast activity.

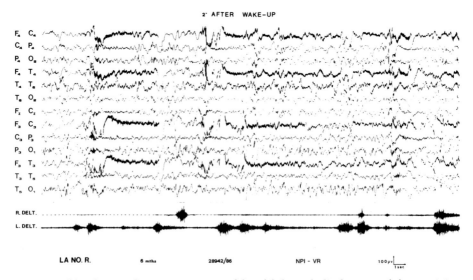

Figure 6.5(b) On awakening, a series of brief bilateral discharges of fast activity modify only partially the interictal paroxysmal abnormalities. Spasms with the EEG ictal events are difficult to recognize because of the presence of subcontinuous nonepileptic abnormal movements.

A last question that applies in particular to patients with cryptogenic or idiopathic IS is whether hypsarrhythmia consists of an ictal or an interictal phenomenon. It is most unlikely that the spasms can by themselves account for the neuropsychological impairment that occurs suddenly in previously normal infants. Furthermore, the same type and frequency of spasms fail to produce similar abrupt and homogenous neuropsychological impairment in symptomatic cases without true continuous hypsarrhythmia. This strong link between true hypsarrhythmia and neuropsychological impairment is strongly suggestive of a continuous ictal event. Therefore, in cryptogenic and idiopathic cases, the first target of treatment should be hypsarrhythmia, not the spasms.

In conclusion, although the characteristics of hypsarrhythmia alone are not helpful from the diagnostic and therapeutic points of view because of their great variability, analysis of the various interictal patterns combined with that of other features that define the electroclinical pattern contribute to a correct diagnostic work-up and therapeutic decision in a number of cases (Dalla Bernardina *et al.*, 1992; see also Tables 6.1–6.3 and Chapter 13).

DIFFERENTIAL DIAGNOSIS

The EEG in some conditions bears a resemblance to the early picture of Angelman syndrome, Down syndrome, postanoxic–ischemic encephalopathy and hypsarrhythmia without seizures.

1. *The early picture of Angelman syndrome.* The initial picture has been reported as being that of West syndrome (Jeavons *et al.*, 1964), mainly because the EEG picture has been frequently interpreted as that of hypsarrhythmia. In fact, from the first months of life, and often before the appearance of any clinically recognized seizure, the EEG is grossly abnormal (Matsumoto *et al.*, 1992; Sugimoto *et al.*, 1992). A well-organized background activity is difficult to recognize, because of the presence of subcontinuous rhythmic (5–6 Hz) theta activity. This activity is relatively monomorphous and predominates at the centroparietal regions. More diffuse bursts of high-amplitude delta waves are frequently associated, giving the impression of a hypsarrhythmic pattern. In addition to this polymorphous and subcontinuous pattern, frequent sequences of sharp 3–4 Hz waves with superimposed spikes producing unusual spike waves mainly involve the parietal regions, both synchronously and asynchronously. They are frequently induced by eye closure. They may remain focal or produce a diffuse burst suggesting an atypical absence. The electromyographic recording permits the recognition of the presence of subcontinuous myoclonus and frequent brief massive myoclonic or tonic spasms. The spasms are never related to a significant EEG modification. The myoclonic jerks may be either erratic and asynchronous without a recognizable relationship with the EEG pattern, or more rhythmic and synchronous and strictly related to the rhythmic burst of theta activity. The electroclinical pattern (Fig. 6.8) therefore appears to

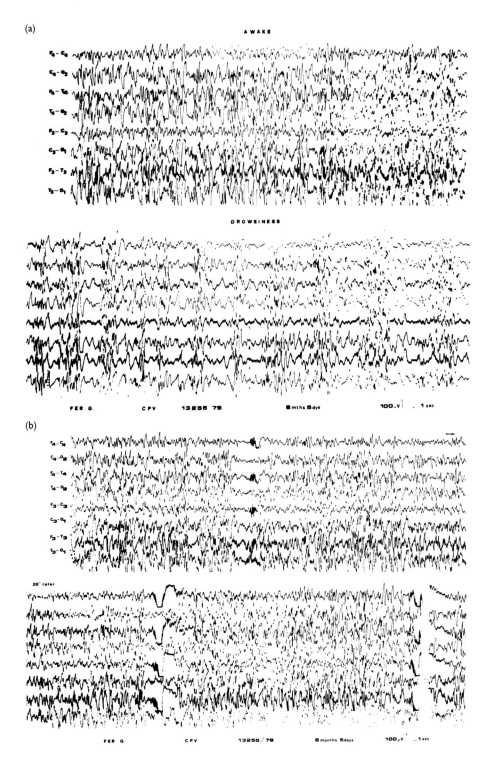

be very similar to that described as "myoclonic status in fixed encephalopathies" by Dalla Bernardina *et al.* (1992c). Recognition of this picture suggests that the clinical picture of ataxia and jerking movements characteristic of Angelman syndrome are at least in part of an epileptic nature. It also explains why they can be improved by antiepileptic treatment such as ethosuximide.

The abnormalities observed in the awake state become continuous during drowsiness and during the whole period of slow sleep of the first cycle. During REM, diffuse discharges disappear, whereas focal birolandic spikes appear. In contrast, during the second cycle of sleep, the picture is dramatically different, with a marked reduction in diffuse abnormalities, and the appearance of well-defined physiological rhythms like spindles that were unrecognizable during the first cycle. During evolution, clinically more evident, usually clonic seizures may appear. According to yet unpublished personal data, patients with 4p-syndrome exhibit similar characteristics.

2. *Down syndrome.* Several reports mention West syndrome as a relatively frequent manifestation in patients with Down syndrome not having suffered from any ischemic insult (Pollack *et al.*, 1978; Guerrini *et al.*, 1979; Dalla Bernardina, 1992). Indeed, typical hypsarrhythmia was exhibited by five of seven Down syndrome patients. However, other patients may exhibit a pseudo-hypsarrhythmic pattern in the second year of life resulting from frequent bursts of diffuse spike waves with an evident fast polyspikes component, and the ictal manifestations consist of massive jerks more than of true epileptic spasms (see Chapter 20).

3. *Postanoxic–ischemic encephalopathy.* Infants who have suffered from anoxia–ischemia (i.e. near drowning or complications of anesthesia) exhibit paroxysmal abnormalities consisting of long-lasting bursts of suppression, and ictal events are massive myoclonus eventually becoming associated with action myoclonus (Pampiglione, 1963).

4. *Hyposarrhythmia without seizures.* These always result from a clastic etiology. It is first necessary to exclude any subclinical seizures by means of long-duration polygraphic recording. In such patients, the hypsarrhythmic pattern has the same significance as that of other conditions with a transient increase in spike activity, such as "continuous spike waves during slow sleep" observed in the course of partial epilepsy in older children (Patry *et al.*, 1971; Dalla Bernardina *et al.*, 1992b). This type of tracing is age-related, it disappears spontaneously, and following its disappearance the patient remains with focal or multifocal paroxysms.

Figure 6.6(a)   A normally developing young boy suffering from a series of bilateral spasms which appeared 20 days earlier. Upon awakening, there was a true bilateral and continuous hypsarrhythmic pattern which was fragmented during sleep.

Figure 6.6(b)   Between the spasms characterized by a brief bilateral discharge of very small amplitude and fast activity, it is possible to note the persistence of a true hypsarrhythmic pattern.

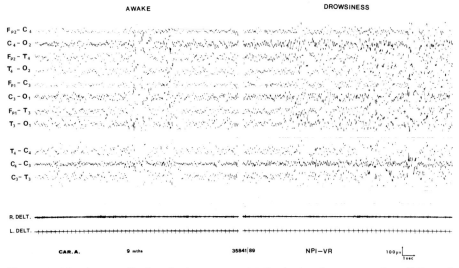

Figure 6.7(a)   A normally developing young girl displaying frequent series of bilateral spasms which appeared some days before. On a recognizable bilateral rhythmic background activity, brief discharges of diffuse slow-amplitude spike waves can be seen, leading to a pseudo-hypsarrhythmic pattern only briefly.

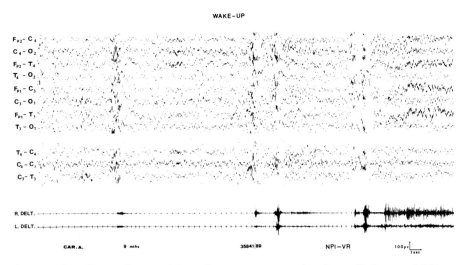

Figure 6.7(b)   On awakening, bilateral spasms appear related to a discharge of diffuse polyspike waves. To the right, between the spasms, note the presence of the background activity.

In summary, interictal EEG varies from one patient to another and within a given patient, and age, stage of sleep–wake cycle and etiology contribute to its characterization. Hypsarrhythmia is but one of the EEG patterns that can be encountered in patients with IS, and must be distinguished from secondary generalized paroxysmal activity.

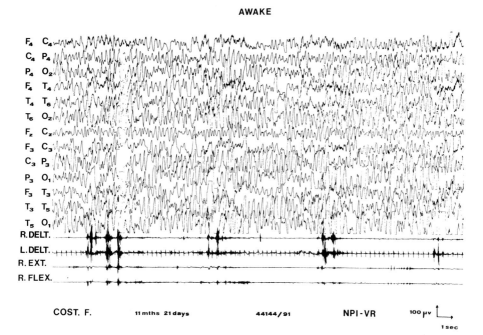

Figure 6.8 A young boy with Angelman syndrome. Note the continuous slow waves with superimposed spikes predominating in the posterior regions mimicking a hypsarrhythmic pattern. The EMG polygraphic record shows the subcontinuous erratic myoclonic jerks mixed with other abnormal movements.

7

Neuropsychological Aspects

I. JAMBAQUÉ

Mental deterioration is classically described as one major component of the West syndrome triad (Gastaut *et al.*, 1964b; Jeavons and Bower, 1974). More specifically, it is characterized by a loss of psychomotor abilities, social interactions and interest in one's surroundings.

Children with infantile spasms (IS) have in general poor intellectual development. Approximately 80% of them have significant cognitive impairment, often complicated by emotional–behavioral disturbances (Lacy and Penry, 1976). However, mental retardation is not constant (Sorel, 1972) and some

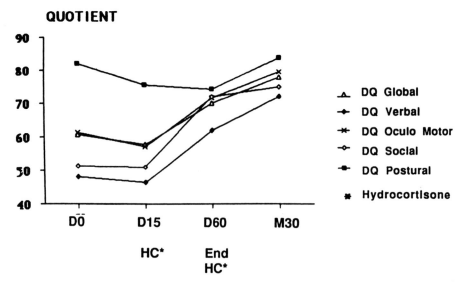

Figure 7.1 Follow-up developmental quotient in patients with West syndrome treated for 2 weeks with hydrocortisone 15 mg/kg followed by a 2 week decrement. Note that the subquotients are correlated during follow-up and that steroid treatment increases the cognitive disorders transiently.

patients may have normal cognitive development after a history of IS. Thus, there is great variability in cognitive outcome, which reflects the heterogeneity of the etiologies, and therefore the diversity of brain abnormalities. Some etiologies and/or demonstrable lesions may indicate a more severe prognosis than others. This is well established for tuberous sclerosis (Riikonen and Amnell, 1981). Other factors, including delay in diagnosis, EEG characteristics and evolution of the epilepsy, may also predict cognitive outcome. Normal development prior to the onset of spasms is often considered to be a favorable predicting factor but is often difficult to assess when patients are less than 3–4 months old. Together, these predicting factors are only moderately reliable. Recent studies indicate that neuropsychological status observed in patients at the onset of the epileptic syndrome is a complementary and useful predicting factor (Jambaqué *et al.*, 1989; Guzzetta *et al.*, 1993).

MENTAL DETERIORATION

Illingworth (1955) first described in detail the regression of mentation in infants with an onset of IS between 4 and 8 months. He observed that behavioral regression consisted of a loss of motor control (head, sitting position) and a reduction in social interactions. Sometimes these infants no longer reached for objects, smiled or tracked visually. Eventually they appeared to be blind.

Mental deterioration often occurs at the onset of the first spasms, and occasionally follows or even precedes them (Gastaut *et al.*, 1964b; Jeavons and Bower, 1964). The deterioration progresses rapidly over a period of 3–5 weeks. When mental retardation is present before the onset of spasms, mental regression is more difficult to assess. The severity of mental delay and deterioration is undoubtedly related to the nature of the underlying neurological disorder. However, some children do not present with mental regression or may even continue to develop normally despite the occurrence of IS.

Neuropsychological studies have shown hypotonia, poor smiling, loss of intentional grasping, passivity in front of the mirror, lack of eye contact and loss of ocular tracking, in the acute phase of IS (Dongier *et al.*, 1964; Jambaqué *et al.*, 1989). Regression of vocal production and the absence of any reaction to voices and/or nonverbal auditory stimuli are often present. Although most patients have global mental regression, the severity and the spectrum of neuropsychological impairment may differ among patients.

Based on an indifference to one's surroundings often observed in these infants, several authors have stressed the association between early signs of autism and IS, the latter possibly representing an acquired and sometimes reversible autistic state (Taft and Cohen, 1971; Sauvage, 1984). During IS, infants often exhibit secondary stereotypies like hand flapping and head banging. Visual inattention appears to be an important factor in the general disorganization of patients' interpersonal relationships at the onset of IS (Jambaqué *et al.*, 1993). The infants do not turn their head towards visual stimuli and lack visual contact. They no longer take any notice of people and they fail to smile and are unable to recognize familiar faces. The absence of visual contact is thus associated with an ability to produce and maintain interpersonal contact.

STEROID TREATMENT

Although steroid therapy plays a major part in the treatment of IS (see Chapter 22), its effect on mental development is still debated (Jeavons *et al.*, 1973). During the acute phase, steroid therapy is often associated with a marked worsening of the mental regression. Prospective neuropsychological studies have shown deterioration of cognitive functions after only 2 weeks of steroid treatment, and subsequent improvement over a longer period after withdrawal of steroids (Dongier *et al.*, 1964; Jambaqué *et al.*, 1989). Some of these neuropsychological manifestations appear to correspond with the usual side-effects of steroids, and include irritability, insomnia and apathy. Stereotypies can appear transiently or, if already present, can be exaggerated during this period.

It remains unclear whether the cognitive worsening associated with steroid therapy reflects reversible brain shrinkage, which is a constant feature on CT scan (Ito *et al.*, 1983; Langenstein *et al.*, 1979), or decreased metabolic activity of the brain, expressed by decreased blood flow (Chiron *et al.*, 1993). In addition, steroids may interfere with the mineralocorticoid and glucocorticoid receptors of the brain (Joels and de Kloet, 1992). The hippocampus is a major neural target tissue for steroids and chronic glucocorticoid administration could worsen hippocampal damage in the aftermath of seizures (Sapolsky, 1987). Glucocorticoid-receptor activation and the resultant increased calcium influx may result in impairment of function and eventually neural loss (Joels and de Kloet, 1992). Whether patients are likely to benefit more from high or low doses of steroids remains unanswered (see Chapter 22).

RECOVERY OF COGNITIVE FUNCTIONS

Neuropsychological evaluation at the onset of spasms provides useful information. Prospective studies have shown a significant correlation between developmental quotients at onset of spasms and at 3 years of age (Dongier *et al.*, 1964; Jambaqué *et al.*, 1989; Guzzetta *et al.*, 1993). The best clinical indexes are visual tracking and reaction to sensory stimuli, rather than the less specific features such as muscle tone.

A small number of patients (5%) with probable idiopathic West syndrome (see Chapter 20) recover completely (Dulac *et al.*, 1986a, 1993a; Vigevano *et al.*, 1993). In a series of 12 cases followed to the age of 7–11 years, none showed a relapse to seizures and all had normal IQ with normal academic achievement (Dulac *et al.*, 1993a). The main characteristics of this subgroup was normal development prior to the first spasms (including the ability to reach for objects) and no major deterioration at the onset of the disease. In particular, none of the infants who recovered completely showed significant loss of the visual or auditory senses.

There is general agreement among researchers that mental outcome is much better in cryptogenic than in symptomatic IS. It has been found that 31% (Lombroso, 1983a) to 56% (Lerman and Kivity, 1982) of patients with cryptogenic IS (or idiopathic IS, since both were usually combined in older series in which the distinction between idiopathic and cryptogenic IS was not made) achieve a normal outcome, compared with 0% (Chevrie and Aicardi, 1971) to 14% (Lombroso, 1983a) of those with symptomatic IS. Infants with cryptogenic IS may have no reaction to auditory stimuli during the acute phase, but they do not show major visual deterioration. Later, these children can have a normal IQ even though they have persistent temporal lobe epilepsy (Dulac *et al.*, 1993a). On the other hand, patients with cryptogenic IS and more marked mental regression frequently suffer from severe cognitive sequelae.

Patients with symptomatic IS usually have a poor prognosis. For example, mental retardation and behavioral disorders occur in most patients with tuberous sclerosis and IS, particularly when they have many major cortical tubers. However, a small number of patients with the same disease may not experience mental retardation (Jambaqué *et al.*, 1991). Generally, these patients have a single cortical tuber, shown by magnetic resonance imaging (MRI), and their seizures are rapidly controlled by therapy. Similarly, IS are often easily controlled by steroids with no relapse by patients with neurofibromatosis type 1, whose mental outcome is thereafter favorable (Motte *et al.*, 1993).

The persistence of secondary generalized seizures is indicative of a worse mental outcome in patients with IS, regardless of the etiology. Therapies aimed at controlling these secondary epilepsies are thus urgently needed. Most patients with tuberous sclerosis who exhibit severe mental retardation and autistic manifestations continue to experience generalized seizures (Yamamoto *et al.*, 1987; Jambaqué *et al.*, 1991). The recent demonstration that the outcome of patients with tuberous sclerosis and IS can be markedly improved when their epilepsy is controlled (Chiron *et al.*, 1990a) offers hope.

LONG-TERM SEQUELAE

Mental retardation is observed in 71–81% of patients with IS, and is severe in more than half of them (Aicardi, 1986a; Favata *et al.*, 1987). Psychiatric disorders were diagnosed in 28% of cases in one series, in which autism and hyperkinesia were equally represented (Riikonen and Amnell, 1981).

Although most children have long-term sequelae after IS, neuropsychological outcome is more variable than expected. Many patients have global mental retardation, but others have more specific cognitive deficits. Whether global or selective, the mental regression observed in these patients at the onset of IS includes deterioration of neurosensorial functions (particularly *visual*) and the appearance of indifferent behavior. After IS, some children may have retarded speech in particular, whereas others may have defective visuospatial skills. Interestingly, the most frequent impairments observed are disorders of visuo-motor coordination, dyspraxia, piecemeal vision, space orientation and object recognition impairment, all of which are known to be sequelae of cortical blindness. Functional neuroimaging may demonstrate the involvement of specific areas, which appear to correlate with the type of observed neuropsychological deficits. When hypoperfusion is in the parieto-occipital areas, visuaspatial deficits are mainly observed (Dulac *et al.*, 1987a; Chugani *et al.*, 1990; Jambaqué *et al.*, 1993).

A number of patients remain autistic after IS, from 13% in cryptogenic IS (Riikonen and Amnell, 1981) to 58% in tuberous sclerosis (Hunt and Dennis, 1987). In tuberous sclerosis, most autistic children appear to have multiple, large bifrontal and posterior tubers on MRI and intractable seizures after IS (Jambaqué *et al.*, 1991). Autism may persist even when the epilepsy is controlled, particularly in cryptogenic IS. In these cases, autistic behavior is associated with mental retardation which worsens during the second year of life. SPECT studies show hypoperfusion in the frontal lobes and in the posterior regions (Chiron *et al.*, 1993). It is striking to note that autistic behavior worsens at the age at which the frontal areas involved would normally mature.

MECHANISMS OF COGNITIVE TROUBLES

Although IS are often associated with cognitive dysfunction, it is clear that this part of the triad is not constant. A small percentage of infants with IS have no major mental deterioration during the acute phase of epilepsy and achieve full recovery of cognitive function (Dulac *et al.*, 1993a). For those patients, it is tempting to think that the paroxysmal activity is the main component involved in their cognitive deterioration. Reversibility of the epilepsy accounts for full recovery of cognitive function.

On the other hand, mental retardation is clearly present before the first seizures in a number of patients for whom the occurrence of generalized epilepsy is an additional factor in their mental regression. In such cases, mechanisms combine to impair cognitive function: the first consists of brain lesions expressed by pre-existing mental retardation, and the second is transitory, consisting of major and diffuse paroxysmal activity. The type of selective cognitive dysfuction is correlated with the topography of brain involvement (Jambaqué *et al.*, 1993). However, many infants have multiple brain lesions and therefore global cognitive dysfunction.

Patients who have minor or moderate visual/auditory dysfunction generally have a favorable prognosis and this may include a number of infants with symptomatic IS. Conversely, patients with early severe central visual disturbances are at risk of developing mental retardation, including autistic features and dyspraxic disorders. In these infants, visual dysfunction mimics cortical blindness and its association with social unresponsiveness can appear as autism.

In addition, patients with pre-existing mental retardation may be particularly sensitive to the negative effects of steroids on cognitive function.

NEUROPSYCHOLOGICAL ASSESSMENT

Early assessment of neuropsychological prognosis can guide rehabilitation. Given the important prognostic value of pre-existing mental impairment, it is crucial to determine whether visual tracking and voluntary grasping are acquired prior to the first spasms. Several standardized scales can be used to assess the developmental status of infants according to different functions: gross and fine motor activity, eye–hand coordination, vocalization, problem solving, imitation, comprehension, and social interaction (Molfese, 1992). More specific cognitive assessment may, however, be required to identify infants with mild to moderate impairments. Subtle changes are frequently harder to detect in early life, particularly those involving visual or auditory function. Finally, it is our experience that the early identification of visual impairment may guide early and efficacious neuropsychological rehabilitation.

8

Differential Diagnosis

N. FEJERMAN

The frequent misdiagnosis of epileptic seizures has in general been due to overdiagnosis, namely labelling as epileptic various paroxysmal or episodic symptoms which are not epileptic in nature (Jeavons, 1985; Fejerman and Medina, 1986; Aicardi, 1986a). From the clinical point of view, the diagnosis of epileptic spasms in older children (Gobbi *et al.*, 1987) remains problematic, as illustrated by the persistent confusion with tics when the symptoms are first encountered. At present, pediatricians still consider infantile spasms (IS) as a syndrome, in combination with diffuse EEG interictal paroxysmal activity. In fact, the EEG is so often the major tool in the diagnosis that the patient is considered as having "hypsarrhythmia" when he or she has IS, but the ictal event is hardly ever mentioned. Difficulties with diagnosis also occur in patients who do not exhibit the various interictal EEG abnormalities described in Chapter 6. The latter may appear a few days later, usually within less than 2 weeks, and often initially during sleep. Therefore, if there is any doubt, a second EEG recording should be performed 2 weeks later both during sleep and wakefulness.

A significant number of younger children with IS are diagnosed as having *colic* (Fejerman, 1972). In addition, the differential diagnosis of IS encompasses a wide range of nonepileptic conditions and a few epileptic seizures and syndromes occurring in infancy (see Tables 8.1 and 8.2). The most difficult differential diagnosis involves atypical cases, with early or late onset, with spasms restricted to upward eye movements, and cases of severe spasticity. In the following, we will first differentiate between IS and nonepileptic events, and then differentiate between IS and various other epileptic syndromes.

NONEPILEPTIC PAROXYSMAL DISORDERS OR EPISODIC SYMPTOMS WITH ONSET DURING THE FIRST YEAR OF LIFE (TABLE 8.1)

Benign Neonatal Sleep Myoclonus

Myoclonic jerks are typically seen in the distal portions of limbs and disappear when the baby awakes. The jerks may start in one limb or bilaterally and persist

Table 8.1   Differential diagnosis of infantile spasms: Nonepileptic paroxysmal disorders or episodic symtoms with onset during the first year of life

1. Abdominal pain (colic)
2. Benign neonatal sleep myoclonus
3. Hyperekplexia
4. Sandifer syndrome
5. Early breath-holding spells and syncopal attacks
6. Adverse reactions or intolerance to exogenous agents
7. Paroxysmal dystonia and choreoathetosis (paroxysmal torticollis, benign infantile dystonia)
8. Increased Moro reflex and attacks of opisthotonos
9. Self-gratification or masturbation-like episodes
10. Benign paroxysmal tonic upward gaze
11. Shuddering attacks
12. Benign myoclonus of early infancy (or benign nonepileptic infantile spasms)

in a rhythmic fashion for a few minutes to half an hour (Fejerman, 1991a,b). The onset is typically in the first days or weeks of life and the intensity decreases progressively until around 6 months of age (Coulter and Allen, 1982). In several reported series, with a follow-up of only a few years, neurological status and EEG have remained normal (Coulter and Allen, 1982; Blennow, 1985; Resnick *et al.*, 1986; Tardieu *et al.*, 1986). More recently, a patient was described who exhibited both sleep myoclonus and myoclonic–astatic epilepsy at the age of 3 years, but EEG and CT scan had been abnormal in the neonatal period (Nolte, 1989).

Hyperekplexia

Hyperekplexia is a rare disease that is often confused with epilepsy in the first year of life. Both major and minor variants of hyperekplexia or "startle disease" have been reported. Most cases have a familial incidence with autosomic transmission, which is either dominant (Suhren *et al.*, 1966; Andermann *et al.*, 1980) or recessive (Saenz-Lope *et al.*, 1984). Other cases are sporadic (Gastaut and Villeneuve, 1967). The disease was recently shown to be linked to the short arm of chromosome 5 (Rayn *et al.*, 1992).

The most clearly described cases involve infants presenting since birth with marked muscular hypertonia and severe jerks induced by sound or tactile stimuli. Tonic and clonic generalized attacks with cyanosis occur during sleep. These cases are usually misdiagnosed as spastic quadriparesis with stimulus-sensitive myoclonic epilepsy, and it is easy to consider artifacts in the EEG as abnormal discharges. We have noted that touching the dorsum of the nose elicits, more easily than other parts of the body, symmetrical myoclonic jerking of the four limbs. Hypertonia without pyramidal signs decreases with time. Affected children walk at 2–3 years of age and generally present with mild mental retardation. Clonazepam is the drug of choice, clearly reducing the paroxysmal episodes that occur during sleep, and drop attacks due to stimulus-induced myoclonus (Fejerman and Medina, 1988).

"Minor" and atypical cases may lack early hypertonia or a clear response to tactile stimuli, as recently seen in two cases. One was a 2-month-old girl with startle reactions to sound but no tactile stimulus-induced myoclonus, who had unusual brief tonic generalized fits during sleep. Physical and EEG examinations were normal. She showed an excellent response to clonazepam. The other case was a boy with normal cognitive development and muscle tone, who showed stimulus-induced myoclonus at 6 months of age. This consisted of flexion of the head with extension and elevation of the upper limbs after a sudden unexpected noise. Incidentally, this child did not respond to clonazepam but his startles were completely controlled by piracetam (Obeso *et al.*, 1986; Fejerman, 1991b).

The disease usually improves, although occasionally a baby may die from cardiopulmonary arrest during an episode occurring in sleep. This type of attack can be stopped by forced flexion of the head and legs, as described by Vigevano *et al.* (1989a).

Sandifer Syndrome

Sandifer syndrome occurs in infants below 6 months of age. Patients exhibit, usually after a meal, brief tonic contractions of the upper limbs with contortions of the neck, and head tilting. Gastro-esophageal reflux is usually severe, and may be associated with hiatus hernia (Werlin *et al.*, 1980). The symptoms may appear in normal babies, but also in children with cerebral palsy (Stephenson, 1990). Evidence of gastrointestinal reflux and normal EEG are not sufficient to confirm the diagnosis, unless a favorable outcome follows specific treatment by posture and thickening of food.

Early Breath-holding Spells and Syncopal Attacks

It may be difficult to recognize atypical breath-holding spells with generalized tonic spasms when the triggering or provoking cause is not obvious. Anoxic episodes or syncopal attacks in early infancy may also be misleading. In a study of clinical features of anoxic episodes with EEG flattening induced by ocular compression in 100 children, "stiffening", "brief tonic flexion of upper limbs" and "jerks that are more in the nature of spasms than myoclonic phenomena" were found in 60–70% of cases (Stephenson, 1990).

Adverse Reactions or Intolerance

Adverse reactions or intolerance to various exogenous agents have been reported in infants with symptoms such as dystonic posturing, shuddering, tonic spells and myoclonic jerks. Drug ingestion should be investigated through precise inquiry. Metoclopramide and carbamazepine were prescribed for several patients (Gatrad, 1976; Pellock, 1987), and other drugs like prochlor-perazine, droperidol and trimeprazine have been reported in single cases (Stephenson, 1990). Intolerance to the ingestion of food additives has also been incriminated as a cause of shuddering attacks in infants (Reif-Lehrer and Stemmerman, 1975).

Paroxysmal Dystonia and Choreoathetosis

Classical paroxysmal choreoathetosis of Mount and Reback and paroxysmal kinesigenic choreoathetosis are rare familial conditions which usually com-mence after the first year of life (Lance, 1977; Tibbles and Barnes 1980). However, transient dystonic posturing has been reported in the first year of life in otherwise normal babies, under the heading "benign infantile dystonia" (Willemse, 1986; Deonna et al., 1991). In addition, nine patients with a negative family history were reported to have fits usually lasting several minutes, occurring from once a month to several times a day, and characterized by opisthotonos, symmetric and asymmetric hypertonia of the upper limbs without any disturbance of consciousness. Age of onset was between 3 and 5 months (Angelini et al., 1988). The duration of these attacks, like those of "benign childhood paroxysmal torticollis" (Deonna and Martin, 1981), is clearly different from that of epileptic spasms (ES).

Increased Moro Reflex and Opisthotonos

Increased Moro reflex and opisthotonos mimicking epileptic spasms may occur in patients with spastic tetraparesis, particularly due to severe leukoma-lacia. In these patients, EEG abnormalities with spikes and slow waves may be recorded, mainly involving posterior areas of the brain, even in nonepileptic patients. Unless the ictal event is actually recorded, it is most difficult to distinguish this condition from IS due to post-ischemic encephalopathy.

Self-gratification or Masturbation-like Episodes

In rare but very striking cases, an infant girl is referred because of brief episodes of eye staring with adducted thighs, sometimes with rhythmic contractions of the lower limbs and trunk. One should consider self-gratification and mastur-bation despite the child's young age (Fejerman and Medina 1986; Stephenson, 1990).

Benign Paroxysmal Tonic Upward Gaze

Benign paroxysmal tonic upward gaze occurs between 6 and 20 months of age in previously healthy infants (Echenne and Rivier, 1992). Tonic upward gaze occurs in clusters, every 2–8 s over a period of several minutes. During the episode, consciousness is preserved and tracking objects downwards pro-duces vertical nystagmus. During the attacks, EEG is normal. The frequency of the episodes decreases progressively and they disappear after 1–2 years. A single familial case with dominant transmission has been reported (Campistol et al., 1993).

Shuddering Attacks

Shuddering attacks were reported in children as an early manifestation of essential tremor (Vanasse et al., 1976). Three of six cases started with "attacks of stiffening" around 4–6 months of age, and the episodes became recognizable as shuddering attacks between 1 and 4 years of age. Similar spells occurred several times a day in neurologically normal children with normal EEG (Holmes and Russman, 1986). Except in cases clearly associated with familial essential tremor, I believe that most patients reported to have "shuddering attacks" with onset in the first year of life have in fact "benign myoclonus of early infancy" (Fejerman, 1977).

Benign Myoclonus of Early Infancy

Benign myoclonus of early infancy (BMEI) or benign nonepileptic infantile spasms has strikingly similar clinical features to IS. It is also the most challenging diagnostic alternative in the hands of child neurologists. I have found it to be 10–20 times less frequent than IS. This incidence probably includes cases otherwise diagnosed as "idiopathic shuddering attacks" during the first year of life (Holmes and Russman, 1986).

In 1976, Fejerman presented as "benign myoclonus of early infancy" 10 infants with fits resembling ES, but with clinical, EEG and evolutionary features allowing clear differential diagnosis with IS (Fejerman, 1977; Fejerman and Medina, 1977). These cases were later included in another report (Lombroso and Fejerman, 1977), and eight new cases were added (Fejerman, 1980, 1984). The follow-up of the 18 cases in this series ranged between 9 and 21 years (Fejerman, 1991a,b). Since 1980, we have treated an approximately similar number of additional cases who are not included in the present report but who showed similar clinical and evolutionary patterns.

The differential diagnosis of IS and BMEI is shown in Table 8.2. Several brief series of BMEI have been reported recently (Gobbi et al., 1982; Giraud, 1982; Dravet et al., 1986; Beltramino, 1987), stressing the importance of the differential diagnosis of BMEI and IS, which is highlighted by the proposal to name this syndrome "benign nonepileptic infantile spasms" (Dravet et al., 1986).

Three cases in one series were diagnosed as IS, although EEG abnormalities were not present (Sorel, 1978) and the diagnosis of BMEI was reached retrospectively. All cases were referred because of repeated jerks of the neck and upper limb muscles, producing abrupt flexion or rotation of the head and extension with abduction of the limbs. In nine patients these jerks were repeated in series and in another nine they were described as "shuddering attacks of head and shoulders sometimes extending to the upper limbs". In several cases, shuddering or abrupt tremor alternated with definite myoclonic jerks. Consciousness was not affected during the fits, not even in a baby who had repeated myoclonus over a period of 30 min. Myoclonus was only seen during the waking state, and especially when the infant was most alert, such as during meals or when playing with her parents. During the first weeks or months, the jerks appeared several times a day. Age of onset ranged between 4 and 9 months, similar to that of IS. Neurological examination was normal in all cases and repeated EEGs during waking and sleep showed no abnormalities. Extensive laboratory work-up disclosed no metabolic or imaging abnormalities. Most of the children had cognitive maturation that was even advanced for their age, and of their 36 parents, 21 were educated to university level, including eight psychologists and six physicians.

Only three patients received ACTH according to the initial diagnosis of IS, but thereafter most of the patients received no medication. The frequency of fits tended to increase initially, but diminished after several months. Most of the children were free of attacks during the second year of life, and only in two patients were sporadic myoclonic jerks seen in the third year. None of the patients showed any type of seizures thereafter. Speech and intellectual development were both normal in all cases and six children showed hyperkinetic behavior.

The etiopathogenic mechanisms of these jerks are not clear at present. A hereditary trait has recently been suggested (Galletti *et al.*, 1989), but the three cases from the same family started with jerks during the first and second months of life, which is much earlier than the rest of the cases in the series.

In summary, after reviewing this list of rare – or maybe not so rare – nonepileptic conditions, it is possible to state that any motor fit of tonic posturing or myoclonic episode occurring in children during the first year of

Table 8.2 Differential diagnosis of cryptogenic infantile spasms and benign myoclonus of early infancy

Similarities		
Age of onset 4–9 months		
Normal development (until onset)		
Myoclonic or brief tonic contractions in neck, shoulders and upper limbs		
Occurring in series		
Several fits per day		
Differences	*West syndrome*	*Benign myoclonus*
Seizures	During waking and during sleep	During waking (exceptional during sleep)
EEG	Always abnormal almost always hypsarrhythmia	Always normal
Psychomotor retardation	In all nontreated and many treated cases	Never

life, while asleep, awake or both, especially if repeated in series, should initially be considered in the differential diagnosis of IS. Usually, a careful history, followed if possible by direct or video observation of the fits, will be enough to confirm or not a diagnosis of IS, remembering that in very rare cases of IS, interictal EEG is normal at onset and the diagnosis is delayed by 1–2 weeks until abnormalities appear, at least during sleep.

OTHER EPILEPTIC SEIZURES OR SYNDROMES WITH ONSET DURING THE FIRST YEAR OF LIFE (TABLE 8.3)

Infantile spasms is not the only epileptic syndrome with onset during the first year of life, and differential diagnosis within epilepsies is important (Table 8.3). Large series of patients with epilepsy at this age have been reported and in general prognosis is not very good, even in syndromes other than progressive encephalopathies and epileptic encephalopathies (Chevrie and Aicardi, 1978; Matsumoto *et al.*, 1983; Cavazzuti *et al.*, 1984).

Progressive encephalopathies presenting with epileptic seizures in infancy may be due to metabolic diseases or to structural abnormalities (Fejerman, 1991a,b). Most of these conditions exhibit myoclonic seizures together with other types of epileptic fits, and have therefore also been labelled "progressive myoclonic epilepsies" (Marseille Consensus Group, 1990). Some of these progressive encephalopathies may show clinical and EEG features of IS (Fejerman, 1991a,b).

We include under the term "epileptic encephalopathy" any condition – even in the absence of progressive metabolic and/or structural brain abnormalities – displaying extremely abnormal brain electrical activity (e.g. a burst–suppresion pattern and hypsarrhythmia), which may not only be the cause of seizures but also interfere with cognitive functions, leading to the arrest or regression of intelligence or behavior. Epileptic encephalopathies in early infancy include "early myoclonic encephalopathy" (EME), "early infantile epileptic encephalo-pathy with suppression burst" (EIEE) and IS. In the last revised classification of epilepsies and syndromes (1989), EME and the EIEE were considered to be among the symptomatic generalized syndromes of nonspecific etiology, whereas other epileptic encephalopathies were included within the cryptoge-nic or symptomatic forms.

Table 8.3 Differential diagnosis of infantile spasms: Other epileptic seizures or syndromes with onset during the first year of life

1.	Early myoclonic encephalopathy
2.	Early infantile epileptic encephalopathy
3.	Benign myoclonic epilepsy of infancy
4.	Cryptogenic or symptomatic myoclonic–atonic–astatic epilepsies
5.	Early-onset Lennox-Gastaut syndrome
6.	Partial seizures mimicking asymmetric infantile spasms

Early Myoclonic Encephalopathy

Most cases begin during the first month of life, with erratic, partial myoclonus involving the face or limbs, associated with massive myoclonus and partial seizures. During both wakefulness and sleep, the EEG shows bursts of irregular spikes and slow waves separated by periods of flattening of the tracing, called the "burst-suppression" pattern (Figs 8.1 and 8.2). According to Aicardi (1984), after the first 3 months brief tonic seizures or spasms may appear and the burst–suppression pattern tends to be replaced by atypical hypsarrhythmia, blurring the boundaries with IS. Severe neurological damage is always present and a significant number of patients die before 2 years of age. The etiology appears in the main to consist of inborn errors of metabolism, including glycine encephalopathy (Dalla Bernardina *et al.*, 1979, 1983). Some authors have also reported EME to result from neuronal migration disorders or other nonprogressive structural brain abnormalities (Aicardi, 1984; Aicardi and Gomez, 1989). However, in a recent series of 23 cases of early infantile epileptic syndromes with burst–suppression, not one case of neuronal migration disorder was associated with the typical picture of EME (Schlumberger *et al.*, 1992), and one-third of the patients could not be classified in either of the two presently identified epileptic syndromes with a burst-suppression pattern.

Early Infantile Epileptic Encephalopathy

Early infantile epileptic encephalopathy was described by Ohtahara *et al.* (1976). Its main features are: onset within the first days or weeks of life

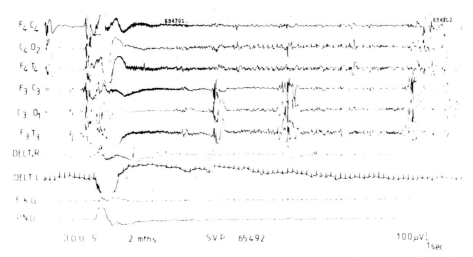

Figure 8.1 A 2-month-old infant who, at 2 weeks of age, developed massive and erratic myoclonus, axial hypotonia and trismus, and died at 8 months. EEG shows asynergy with focal discharges.

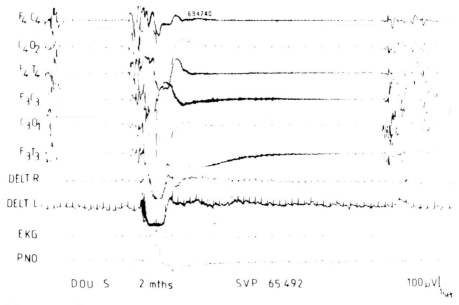

Figure 8.2 The same infant as in Fig. 8.1. The EEG shows asynergy with a suppression–burst pattern and massive myoclonus.

(Ohtahara *et al.*, 1987); associated tonic spasms with a burst–suppression pattern on both the waking and sleeping EEG (Fig. 8.3); its frequent evolution to West syndrome (WS) with intractable seizures; and severe psychomotor retardation. Various malformations including Aicardi's malformation, hemi-megalencephaly (see Chapter 15) and olivary-dentate dysplasia (Robain and Dulac, 1992) have been reported.

In one series of 14 cases, cerebral atrophy or porencephaly were reported in 8 cases, Aicardi syndrome in 2, subacute diffuse encephalopathy in 1 and unknown etiology in 3 (Ohtahara *et al.*, 1987). These authors insist on differentiating EIEE from EME on the basis of absence of myoclonia, a more typical EEG and the presence of cerebral abnormalities before onset of seizures. Other authors consider that EIEE is more likely to be an early form of IS (Fejerman and Medina, 1986; Lombroso, 1982). In either case, we must acknowledge Ohtahara's concept of "age-dependent epileptic encephalopathy" (Ohtahara *et al.*, 1987; Ohtsuka *et al.*, 1986), which notes that the same variety of etiologic agents will give rise to different epileptic syndromes according to the age at which the seizures appear and EEG abnormalities. In this series, 9 of the 14 cases evolved to WS and of 88 patients with WS, 27 went on to develop Lennox-Gastaut syndrome.

Benign Myoclonic Epilepsy in Infancy

Besides the epileptic encephalopathies with myoclonic components appearing in early infancy, there are idiopathic, cryptogenic and symptomatic epilepsies

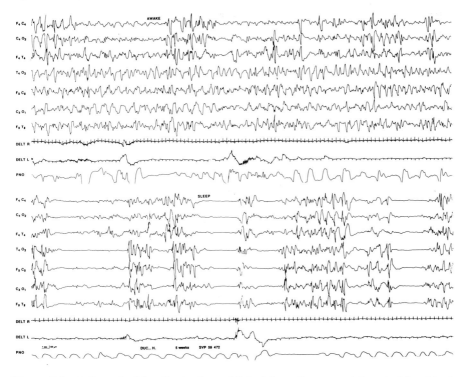

Figure 8.3 A 5-week-old patient who exhibited from the neonatal period focal tonic seizures with secondary generalization. Note the suppression–burst pattern during sleep. Neuropathology disclosed olivary-dentate dysplasia (Robain and Dulac, 1992).

with early onset which must be considered in the differential diagnosis of IS. Benign myoclonic epilepsy of infancy has its onset during the first year of life. The seizures are brief myoclonic jerks, usually with head drop. Ictal EEG shows spike-wave or polyspike-wave discharges, which are activated in the early stages of sleep. The interictal waking EEG may be normal. Seizures are usually controlled with valproate, but some patients in the initial series manifested behavioral or learning disorders at school age (Dravet and Bureau, 1981; Dalla Bernardina *et al.*, 1983).

Cryptogenic or Symptomatic Myoclonic–Atonic–Astatic Epilepsies

A definite group of patients with normal cognitive development until onset of myoclonic seizures between 1 and 10 years of age has been recognized by several authors (Doose *et al.*, 1970; Aicardi and Chevrie, 1971; Loiseau *et al.*, 1974; Jeavons, 1977; Aicardi, 1981; Lombroso, 1982). The fits are described as brief myoclonic jerks, usually axial or bilateral, in the face, neck or limbs, which may cause axial anteflexion ranging from a slight flexion of the head to a sudden fall to the floor. Interictal EEG shows generalized spike waves and polyspike waves, and often 4–7 Hz high-amplitude slow-wave activity. The combination of generalized seizures with axial flexion and major diffuse EEG paroxysmal activity may be confused with rare cases of late-onset WS, beginning in the second or third year of life.

Early-onset Lennox-Gastaut Syndrome (LGS)

Even though LGS starts in the vast majority of cases between 1 and 7 years of age (Aicardi, 1986b), early-onset cases are seen occasionally. Since tonic seizures are a usual manifestation, it may not be easy to differentiate between early LGS and late WS, in particular because the early cases also tend to show less typical EEG abnormalities. Of course, differentiation is easier after recognizing an association with atonic seizures and atypical absences. In any case, one would not be able to distinguish the prognostic differences between late WS and early LGS. Furthermore, as a whole, infantile epilepsies other than WS and LGS share a poor prognosis, since in one series only 22% of the affected infants showed normal intellectual development after more than 1 year of follow-up (Aicardi, 1981).

Partial Seizures Mimicking Asymmetric Epileptic Spasms

The relationship between partial seizures and ES has only recently been studied, even though "other seizures" were always recognized in patients with IS (Jeavons and Bower, 1964; Lacey and Penry, 1976). Sometimes partial seizures may mimic asymmetric ES. In fact, unilateral ES were seen in 6% of cases in one series (Lombroso, 1983a) and we also had several cases with unilateral hypsarrhythmia (Fejerman and Medina, 1986). However, it was noted that ES were the initial clinical ictal pattern in 3 of 40 children with partial epilepsy beginning before 3 years of age (Dravet *et al.*, 1989). According to these authors, even though their three patients had ES as presenting symptoms, they were classified as belonging to partial epilepsy on account of a typical partial EEG pattern. However, this is not a differential diagnosis but a nosological issue, since there is growing evidence that some ictal patterns in patients with ES combine a focal discharge and a cluster of spasms that may be asymmetrical (Bour, 1986; Carrazana *et al.*, 1990) and a number of patients with IS may develop partial epilepsy.

The differential diagnosis of the hypsarrhythmic pattern is considered in Chapter 6.

9

Neuropathological Studies

O. ROBAIN, H.V. VINTERS

INTRODUCTION

The specific clinical aspects of infantile spasms (IS) have long been recognized and have become more clearly defined since the first description of the syndrome in 1841 (West, 1841). Neuropathological descriptions of the entity have been plentiful and have emphasized the heterogeneous morphologic substrates of IS. Jellinger (1987) reviewed 214 necropsy cases, including 50 brains of afflicted children that he had examined personally. Whereas brain structural correlates of IS had, until recently, been ascertained largely by necropsy studies, the increasing use of extensive cortical resections (carried out after meticulous neuroimaging and electrophysiological investigations) to treat intractable IS has rendered fresh brain tissue available to morphologists, biochemists and even neurophysiologists for novel investigations pertinent to the pathogenesis of this tragic disorder (Chugani *et al.*, 1993; Vinters *et al.*, 1992, 1993b). Nevertheless, the difficulties in classification that are evident from a clinical and electroencephalographic (EEG) point of view also frequently apply to a consideration of the neuropathological findings.

The neuropathologist who attempts to understand how a given lesion of the central nervous system (CNS) produces repetitive spasms encounters several difficulties. The first of these results from a relative paucity of detailed clinical and EEG data often found in the presentation of neuropathological case reports. For instance, there is frequently confusion between IS and other epileptic syndromes of infancy such as neonatal myoclonic encephalopathy or early infantile epileptic encephalopathy. The second difficulty results from the marked heterogeneity (especially from a pathologic perspective) of reported cases. The variability of CNS lesions that can produce IS is easily apparent upon even a cursory review of the reports by Bignami *et al.* (1964), Christensen and Melchior (1960), Harris and Pampiglione (1962), Jellinger (1970, 1987), Marciniak *et al.* (1971), Meencke and Gerhard (1985), Morimatsu and Sato (1983), Okuyama (1965), Pfeiffer (1963), Palm *et al.* (1986), Paludan (1961), Riikonen (1982) and Radermaker *et al.* (1964). The list of morphological lesions associated with IS increases substantially when one considers the many patients who have had neuroimaging studies but no neuropathological assessment.

A reasonable neuropathological classification scheme – especially one based on pathophysiological mechanisms – is thus difficult to conceptualize. For example, although the brainstem may play a significant role in generating or sustaining seizure activity within the CNS, lesions associated with IS are usually localized to the cerebral hemispheres. A simplistic but functional categorization of CNS lesions seen in IS could be given as: (a) diffuse cerebral lesions, (b) focal cerebral lesions and (c) cases in which there is no evidence of major neuropathological change in the brain. Group (c) is taken, for the present, to include the minimal neuronal cytoarchitectural lesions of questionable significance that are described under the label "microdysgenesis" (Meencke and Janz, 1984). An important caveat pertinent to the issue of "causality" versus "association" needs to be emphasized: although we will detail below the evidence that certain structural anomalies of the brain are often seen in infants with IS, the exact pathway(s) by which these abnormalities produce a given seizure disorder (e.g. at the level of the individual neuron, neurotransmitter molecule, cell membrane, etc.) is/are almost never known (Vinters *et al.*, 1993a).

DIFFUSE CEREBRAL LESIONS

Nearly all cerebral lesions that result from extensive brain damage *in utero* or in the perinatal period have been reported as "causes" of IS, as have cerebral malformations that may result from anoxic–ischemic insults to the embryo or fetus early in gestational life – the issue is complicated by our lack of understanding of the precise etiology of many malformations of the CNS (Friede, 1989). Furthermore, morphological distinctions cannot always be made accurately among the observed lesions, for example hemimegalencephaly may show components of agyria–pachygyria and/or polymicrogyria (see below; De Rosa *et al.*, 1992). It is, however, worth emphasizing three major disorders of the central neuraxis that are strongly associated with IS:

Agyria–Pachygyria/Lissencephaly

This complex malformation of the cortical mantle has been described as a "cause" of IS by many authors, including Bignami *et al.* (1964), Bordarier *et al.* (1986), Crome (1956) Dhellemmes *et al.* (1988), Dulac *et al.* (1983a, 1987c), Goutières and Aicardi (1971), Harris and Pampiglione (1962), Jellinger (1987), Meencke and Gerhard (1985), Riikonen (1982) and Wenderowich and Sokolansky (1934). Infantile spasms may occur in as many as 75% of infants with agyria–pachygyria. Among four patients with this malformation examined at necropsy by one of us (O.R.), all of the affected infants had exhibited IS.

Excellent reviews of the genetic and clinicopathological features of this disorder (with or without IS), including the results of neuroimaging studies, have recently been published (Aicardi, 1991b; Barkovich *et al.*, 1991; Dobyns *et al.*, 1984).

In the most severe manifestation of this disorder, agyria, there is a complete absence of secondary sulci or gyri, the cortical ribbon is enlarged and considerably widened, and the cortical network of neurons is markedly disorganized (Druckman *et al.*, 1959; Stewart *et al.*, 1975). Horizontal neuronal lamination is often nonexistent (Fig. 9.1). Golgi impregnation demonstrates many inverted large pyramidal neurons in the superficial zones of the cortical ribbon (Robain and Deonna, 1983; Bordarier *et al.*, 1986). The malformation is thought to result

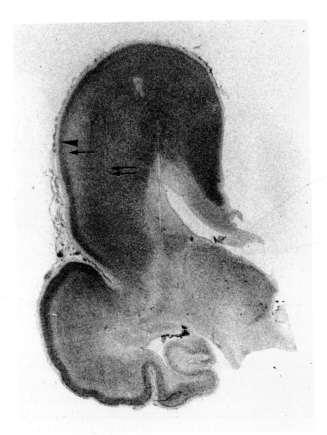

Figure 9.1 Agyria. A four-layered aspect with a molecular layer, a dense cellular external part (arrowhead), a sparse cellular layer (arrow), and a very large fourth layer corresponding to the neurons which have not completed their migration (double arrow). Note the lack of differentiation of the cortex into different areas. Magnification ×1.70.

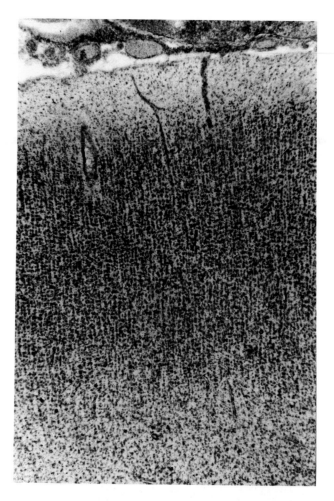

Figure 9.2   Agyria: external part of the cortex. The radial arrangement of the neurons is clearly visible but there is a complete disappearance of horizontal organization. Note the lack of differentiation of the cortical neurons which have in this whole area the same size and the same shape. Magnification ×170.

from a gross disturbance of neuronal or neuroblast (neuronal precursor) migration from the germinal matrix region, which begins early in development of the cerebral hemispheres (before the 16th postconceptual week). In major forms of the malformation, there is no differentiation into specific cortical areas (Fig. 9.2).

The Aicardi Syndrome

This syndrome is strongly associated with IS. In a review of the literature by Chevrie and Aicardi (1986a), 151 of 184 afflicted patients (~80%) exhibited IS, and in the large majority of children, IS onset was before the age of 3 months. Neuropathological documentation of Aicardi syndrome is still incomplete – its anatomical aspects have been reviewed by Billette de Villemeur *et al.* (1992). It has three major components: (1) agenesis of the corpus callosum, (2) periventricular nodular heterotopias and (3) diffuse dysgenesis of the cortex (Fig. 9.3). It is sometimes labelled "microgyria", since there is a more or less extensive folding of the gyri (Fig. 9.4). In essentially all cases studied histologically (Billette de Villemeur *et al.*, 1992; de Jong *et al.*, 1976; Ferrer *et al.*, 1986), there has been complete loss of horizontal lamination of the cortex, each type of neuron

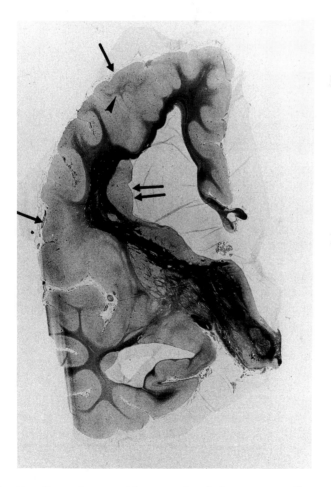

Figure 9.3 Aicardi syndrome with agenesis of the corpus callosum, microgyric appearance of the cortex (arrows) and periventricular heterotopias (double arrow). Note the macrogyric aspect of the microgyric areas due to the fusion of adjacent molecular layers. Thin myelinated strands into the cortex (arrowhead) indicate the complexity of the architecture of this malformed cortex. Magnification ×1.70.

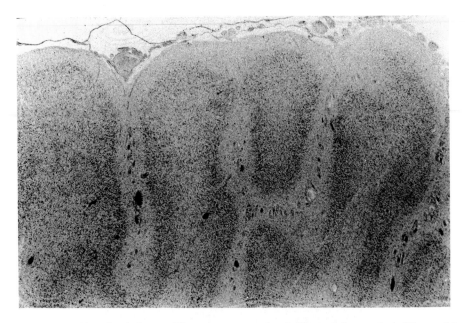

Figure 9.4   Aicardi syndrome. There is an excessive folding of the cortical ribbon with fusion of adjacent molecular layers. Note the complete lack of horizontal organization of the neurons. Magnification ×64.

(large pyramids, small pyramids and granule cells) being found to be scattered without apparent order throughout the expanse of the cortical ribbon. This component of the malformation almost certainly results from a neuronal migration disorder (NMD), as evidenced also by the presence of frequent ectopic neurons in the subcortical white matter. The result is a complete lack of differentiation of malformed cortical areas. Indeed, the malformed cortex does not vary significantly from one area to another.

Hemimegalencephaly

Although (by definition) this involves only one cerebral hemisphere (Fig. 9.5), hemimegalencephaly (HME) should be included in the group of diffuse cortical malformations. The malformation often results in IS (Tjiam *et al.*, 1978) that may occur very early in life, sometimes during the first postnatal week. The neuropathological manifestations of the disorder, as identified in autopsy material (Robain *et al.*, 1988), include disappearance of the horizontal laminations of the cortex, which lack differentiation. The cortex in HME is thickened and contains many giant neurons up to 60–80 μm in diameter, scattered throughout the cortical ribbon (Bignami *et al.*, 1968). In addition, all of the cases observed by one of us (O.R.) exhibited many neuronal heteropias in the subcortical regions (e.g. white matter), the components of which also included

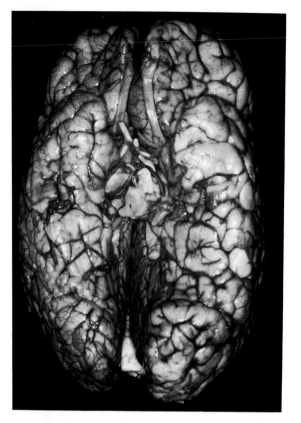

Figure 9.5 Hemimegalencephaly: diffuse hypertrophy of the left hemisphere. Note the macrogyric aspect particularly visible in the temporal lobe.

giant neurons (Fig. 9.6). Abnormal, frequently enlarged and multinucleated glial cells, and bundles of glial fibers sometimes merging with otherwise typical Rosenthal fibers, have also been reported (Robain *et al.*, 1989) (Fig. 9.7). These components of the malformation closely resemble (qualitatively if not always topographically) changes seen in the cortical tubers of patients with Bourneville's tuberous sclerosis, and in cortical resection specimens (lobectomies) from older epileptic patients who show "focal cortical dysplasia" on neuropathological assessment (Taylor *et al.*, 1971).

We have also studied three examples of HME causing intractable seizures (including IS) that were treated by hemispherectomy (De Rosa *et al.*, 1992) using immunohistochemical, ultrastructural and morphometric techniques. Severe disorganization of the cortical ribbon (cortical dysplasia), was seen in all cases and included lesions best characterized as hemilissencephaly and polymicrogyria (PMG). Cortical abnormalities and heterotopic neurons, as described above, were seen. Immunohistochemical analysis demonstrated

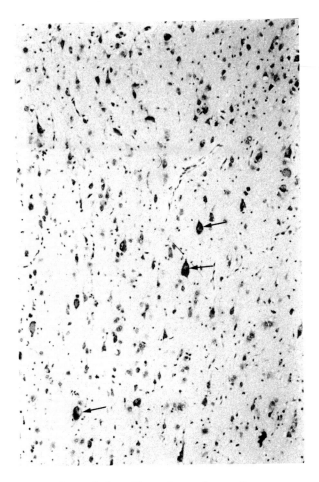

Figure 9.6 Hemimegalencephaly. Giant hyperchromatic neurons are scattered throughout the subcortical white matter (arrows). Magnification ×160.

cellular colocalization of the astrocytic markers glial fibrillary acidic protein (GFAP) and vimentin in one case of hemilissencephaly. Morphometric data indicated significant increases (over autopsy controls) in neuronal profile area in all examples of HME. Neuronal cell density was significantly increased above controls in one patient. Ultrastructural study of brain tissue from one patient showed neural processes and cytoplasm to contain abundant electron-dense paracrystalline inclusions resembling Rosenthal fibers, as well as dense accumulations of neurofilaments and irregularly spaced nonmembrane-bound electron-dense structures that could not be further characterized (De Rosa *et al.*, 1992). We concluded that HME results from severe cortical dysplasia/disorganization that may be caused by one or more of several insults in the developing brain, and reflects abnormal or altered signals that regulate cortical morphogenesis.

Miscellaneous

Many types of brain malformation other than those highlighted above may result in IS. Among other forms of cortical dysplasia (using the broadest definition of this term) that may be responsible, PMG was described by Bamburg and Matthes (1959), Billette de Villemeur *et al.* (1992), Christensen and Melchior (1960), Jellinger (1970), Kramer (1953) and Meencke and Gerhard (1985). This malformation, usually bilateral and often in the territories of supply of large cerebral vessels (e.g. the middle cerebral arteries), may involve the cortex to varying degrees (Friede, 1989). From a neuropathological viewpoint, PMG is not a homogeneous lesion. In some instances, there is no horizontal stratification of neurons (unlayered PMG). This type of cortical dysplasia

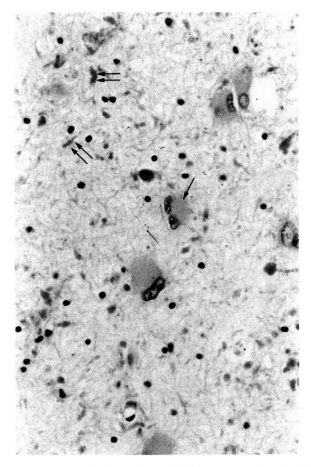

Figure 9.7 Hemimegalencephaly. Subcortical white matter showing large glial cells sometimes binucleated (arrow) and many Rosenthal fibers (double arrows). Magnification ×320.

seems often to be associated with agenesis of the corpus callosum and frequently produces IS (Billette de Villemeur *et al.*, 1992). In such patients, the cortex histologically resembles that seen in Aicardi syndrome (see above). In other examples of PMG, horizontal neuronal lamination remains visible. Most typically, this presents to the pathologist as a four-layered cortex with an acellular midcortical zone (Fig. 9.8). Many investigators consider this malformation to be post-migratory (McBride and Kemper, 1982; Richman *et al.*, 1974; Williams, 1976) or conclude that it has occurred at a late stage of neuronal migration, that is, at a point in time when it cannot fully prevent the normal disposition of neurons in the various cortical layers (Dvorak *et al.*, 1978; Humphreys *et al.*, 1991). This second variant or type of PMG may occur in isolation or at the border zone of an injured area of neocortex, either circumscribed (as in porencephaly) or extensive (hydranencephaly). Both types of destructive lesion can also produce IS (Christensen and Melchior, 1960; Cusmai *et al.*, 1988; Neville, 1972; Yakovlev and Wadsworth, 1946).

Destructive cortico-subcortical lesions occurring at later time points in the course of neocortical development have been mentioned as causes of IS, the most typical being multicystic encephalomalacia, which some authors describe as cystic gliotic encephalopathy (Harris and Pampiglione, 1962; Martin *et al.*, 1961). Several other abnormalities, constituting a heterogeneous group of disorders, have been implicated as causes of IS. Entities on the list include major cerebral malformations such as holoprosencephaly and arhinencephaly

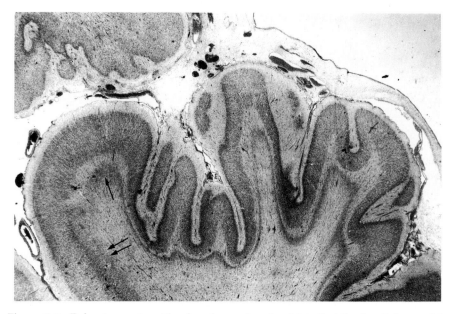

Figure 9.8 Polymicrogyria with a four-layered cortex. Note that the fourth layer of the microgyric cortex (arrow) is in continuity with the sixth layer of the normal adjacent cortex (double arrow). Magnification ×16.

(Jellinger, 1970; Kotte and Künze, 1971; Robain and Gorce, 1972), and lipidoses and leukodystrophies, for example Krabbe's disease (globoid cell leukodystrophy). Obviously, lesions encountered in the CNS of patients with IS are not always restricted to the cortex – indeed, they have been reported in the white matter, the most frequently quoted is the periventricular leukomalacia (Bignami *et al.*, 1966). In this case, the infarcts are mainly located at the ventricular corners and along the occipital horns inducing a destruction of the pyramidal tracts and of the visual radiations. Metabolic brain abnormalities such as phenylketonuria, a disease which primarily involves CNS myelin (Malamud, 1966) have also been noted.

FOCAL AND MULTIFOCAL LESIONS

Many types of focal and multifocal brain lesion have been reported in association with IS. These include infectious disorders caused by parasites (e.g. toxoplasmosis; Riikonen, 1982) and viruses (e.g. cytomegalovirus, CMV; Dumermuth, 1966; Christensen and Melchior, 1960), and metabolic diseases such as Leigh syndrome, in which the neuropathological changes consist of bilateral and symmetrical necrosis in the basal ganglia and brainstem (Kamoshita *et al.*, 1970). We shall emphasize three main types of structural abnormality: (1) focal cortical dysplasia, an example of a group of lesions that is essentially restricted to the cortex and may produce either IS or focal epilepsy in older patients; (2) tuberous sclerosis, an example of a neurocutaneous disorder (phakomatosis) with multifocal brain lesions as well as visceral anomalies and tumors that plays a major part in the occurrence of symptomatic IS, and (3) brainstem lesions, which are discussed because of the suspected pathophysiological role this region of the CNS may play in IS.

Focal Cortical Dysplasia (FCD)

This abnormality was first described in elegant detail by Taylor *et al.* (1971) as an apparent cause of focal epilepsy in patients who had undergone cortical resection, usually a lobectomy, to treat an intractable seizure disorder. Subsequent clinicopathological descriptions followed this theme (Moreland *et al.*, 1988). Generalized cortical dysplasia (CD) may appear morphologically as a diffusely thickened cerebral cortex (Marchal *et al.*, 1989). It has now become possible to identify CD and closely related cortical malformations (e.g. hemimegalencephaly) using high-resolution imaging techniques, such as magnetic resonance imaging (MRI) (Farrell *et al.*, 1992; Palmini *et al.*, 1991a,b; Barkovich and Chuang, 1990; Kuzniecky *et al.*, 1991a; Kazee *et al.*, 1991). Cortical dysplasia may be associated with IS, and some cases can be effectively treated by surgical resection of the affected cortex (Farrell *et al.*, 1992). This has also been the experience of one of the authors (O.R.). FCD may be the result of abnormal migration of neuronal precursors from the germinal matrix to cortex (Rakic,

1988b), so that many authors describe this group of entities by the term "neuronal migration disorders" (NMD) (Barth, 1987; Palmini et al., 1991a,b).

Despite some variation among cases, the histopathological aspects of CD are characteristic, and include widening of the gyri (macrogyria), which is sometimes visible on the pial surface before a specimen is cut, but almost invariably becomes apparent on the cut surface of the specimen or in appropriately stained whole mounts (Fig. 9.9). This abnormal region of cortex is usually firm to palpation, and both in texture and gross appearance resembles a tuber of tuberous sclerosis. Histologically, three main types of abnormality are noted by light microscopy:

Disorganization of the Neuronal Cytoarchitecture

This is a constant feature, though it may be present in only a restricted zone of cortex. The cortical ribbon is thickened and horizontal lamination has disappeared or is at best difficult to define clearly, but the organization of neurons into vertical columns is, for the most part, preserved. The cortex–white matter junction is blurred and there are usually numerous single neurons (or heterotopic collections of neurons) in the subcortical white matter. In many cases, there may be giant neurons (up to 60–80 μm in diameter) similar to those encountered in HME (Robain et al., 1988) scattered throughout the thickness of the cortical ribbon.

Anomalies of the Glia

Anomalies of the glia (especially astrocytes) first described by Taylor et al. (1971) have been re-emphasized by Farrell et al. (1992). In the experience of one of us (O.R.), they occur in approximately half of affected patients. In the most characteristic cases, they include the presence of very large cells (up to 80 μm in diameter) which are often bi- or multinucleated. Some of the cells have eccentric nuclei and abundant glassy or hyaline cytoplasm, and resemble the "balloon cells" which are a common (essentially defining) feature of the tubers of tuberous sclerosis (Farrell et al., 1992). The cells are variably immunoreactive with antibodies to GFAP. By ultrastructural examination, they contain numer-

---

Figure 9.9 (A) Two slices of fixed brain (surgical specimen) from a patient with multiple foci of cortical dysplasia (CD). Whereas the cortex–white matter junction is clearly demarcated throughout much of the specimen, two gyri on the right (arrow) show macrogyria with loss of the cortex–white matter demarcation. Microscopic sections showed severe CD with neuronal disorganization and "balloon cells". (B) Magnified view of another slice from the same specimen shows most of the cortex–white matter junction to be indistinct. (C) Whole mount (stained with Kluver-Barrera technique) shows relatively preserved cortex to the right of the micrograph, but an indistinct junction to the left, with linear extension of "fingers" of white matter into the cortex, and a jagged appearance to the cortex–white matter junction (panel C is from a different patient).

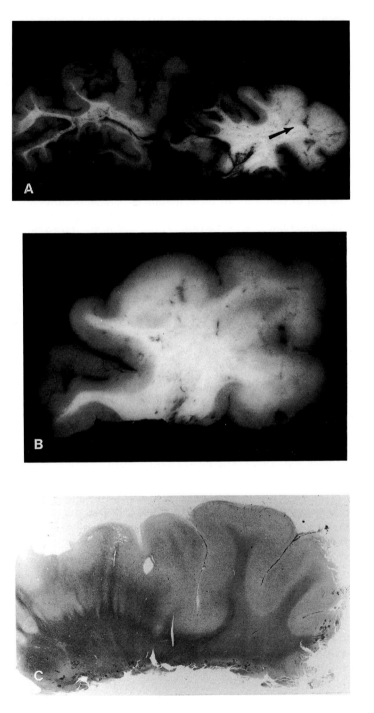

Figure 9.9

ous cytoplasmic filaments which may be grouped into bundles (Farrell *et al.*, 1992), and elongated structures resembling Rosenthal fibers may be seen.

In the experience of one of us (H.V.V.), severe degrees of CD with neuronal disorganization, marked widening of the cortical ribbon, neuronal cytomegaly and secondary cytoskeletal neuronal disorganization may be seen in the total absence of atypical balloon-type astrocytes.

Calcifications

Numerous calcifications may be seen in the abnormal cortex, either as perivascular concretions or as small free calcospherites of small diameter, measuring less than 100 μm in diameter in most instances. These regions of dystrophic calcification have been less commonly observed in the experience of one of us (H.V.V.). However, when present, they may rarely be detectable *in vivo* by computerized tomographic (CT) scan.

This type of CD is thought to originate prior to the end of the period of neuronal/neuroblast migration to the neocortex, that is, before the 20th week of gestation. It is associated with an abnormal distribution of catecholaminergic and serotoninergic nerve terminals (Trottier *et al.*, 1992).

Tuberous Sclerosis – Bourneville's Disease

This phakomatosis may be responsible for as many as 25% of cases of IS (Huttenlocher, 1985; Gomez, 1979). Its neuropathological aspects are well known (for a review, see Bender and Yunis, 1980). In three cases reviewed by one of us (O.R.), the findings were similar to those noted in the classic descriptions (Thibault and Manuelidis, 1970; Ribadeau Dumas *et al.*, 1973; Probst and Ohnacker, 1977). The most characteristic cerebral feature of tuberous sclerosis is the presence of cortical tubers, restricted zones of abnormal cortex that are almost undistinguishable (out of context) from foci of CD (see above). The tubers manifest as severe disorganization of the cortical cytoarchitecture, sometimes with giant neurons containing heterogeneous cytoskeletal abnormalities (Hirano *et al.*, 1968) that may include neurofibrillary tangle-like structures and granulovacuolar degeneration, and variably subtle to overwhelming infiltration among the neurons by large plump cells that are essentially identical to the "balloon cells" described above as occurring in CD. These cells have some features of astrocytes, since they are variably immunoreactive with anti-GFAP, but they may represent undifferentiated or "dedifferentiated" neurectodermal cell types. Even by ultrastructural examination, it may be difficult to determine with certainty whether the cytoplasmic filaments are glial or neurofilamentous in nature (Bender and Yunis, 1980). A further similarity between tuberous sclerosis and CD is that both types of lesion may be multifocal. However, in tuberous sclerosis there are associated subependymal giant cell astrocytomas, periventricular "candle gutterings", and visceral abnormalities that are in general not present in individuals with "simple" CD (Critchley and Earl, 1932).

Lesions of the Brainstem

Structural abnormalities of the brainstem, particularly the tegmentum of the pons, have been studied in several cases of IS (Sinton and Patterson, 1962; Morimatsu and Sato, 1983; Satoh *et al.*, 1984; Tominaga *et al.*, 1986). In most instances, these lesions are seen in association with abnormalities of the neocortex, basal ganglia and/or cerebellum. It is not always straightforward to determine the exact cause of such multifocal lesions. Some are clearly sequelae of anoxic–ischemic brain injury (i.e. are "post-anoxic"; Sinton and Patterson, 1962), whereas others are reminiscent of neuropathological changes noted in association with subacute necrotizing encephalomyelopathy (Leigh disease) (Kamoshita *et al.*, 1970; Richter, 1957).

Findings in Surgically Resected Cortical Tissue

For several decades, surgical resection of cerebral cortex thought to be the focus of seizures (including IS) has been successfully carried out in epileptic children. Such corticectomies are gaining acceptance as one therapeutic modality that can be used to treat drug-resistant intractable epilepsy in the infantile and pediatric age group. As neuropathologists, we have the opportunity of examining intriguing and unique structural lesions at a time (in the child's development) when they are, presumably, relatively unaffected by secondary neuropathological change that can result from a longstanding seizure disorder. These specimens can also be studied using intracellular neuronal recordings, allowing for previously undreamed of opportunities to potentially establish structure–function correlations (Vinters *et al.*, 1993a).

Of 13 children who initially underwent corticectomy (including hemispherectomy) for IS at the UCLA Medical Center (Vinters *et al.*, 1992), 12 had structural lesions that could be classified as malformative/hamartomatous or destructive. The malformative lesions affected cortex and white matter, and frequently resembled CD as described above, with significant abnormalities of lamination of the neocortex, with or without the presence of "balloon cells" resembling gemistocytic astrocytes. Immunohistochemical findings on the specimens suggested the local proliferation of primitive or multipotential neuroectodermal cells as one substrate for the seizure disorder. Similarities of the dysplastic lesions to tubers of tuberous sclerosis were described above. Similar neuropathological change was identified in corticectomy specimens from older patients (Farrell *et al.*, 1992), with the additional findings of Ramussen encephalitis (Vinters *et al.*, 1993c) and Sturge-Weber-Dimitri syndrome (encephalotrigeminal angiomatosis) noted in the latter group.

We have further been intrigued by the cytoskeletal abnormalities that are found almost universally in the neuronal cytoplasm of patients with severe

CD, whether in infants with IS or older patients (Duong *et al.*, in press). We have compared the cytoskeletal abnormalities of cortical neurons in human CD (Fig. 9.10) with the neurofibrillary tangles (NFTs) seen in cortical neurons of patients with Alzheimer disease using immunohistochemical methodology, incorporating antibodies directed against high or medium molecular weight neurofilament epitopes, phosphorylated or nonphosphorylated forms of neurofilament proteins, ubiquitin, the microtubule-associated protein tau, and paired helical filaments (PHF), the latter an immunohistochemical and ultra-structural defining feature of Alzheimer disease NFT. A strong abnormal increase in immunoreactivity to the medium and high molecular weight neurofilament epitopes was seen in hypertrophic neurons of cortex with CD. The neurofilamentous accumulations in cell bodies of CD could also be immunostained with antibodies to phosphorylated and nonphosphorylated neurofilament epitopes, ubiquitin and tau, but were not immunoreactive with anti-PHF. The results suggest that the cytoskeletal abnormalities observed in CD neurons may result at least in part from alterations in either the level of expression, phosphorylation state or transport of cytoskeletal components (Duong *et al.*, 1993). Of course, the role of the cytoskeletal anomalies in producing or sustaining a seizure disorder and/or mental retardation in a given patient are unclear, but certainly worthy of further investigation.

MINIMAL CORTICAL LESIONS

Frequently, neuroradiological investigations (including functional imaging studies) in IS fail to disclose any significant (or at least radiographically detectable) abnormality, though there are clear-cut clinical and characteristic electroencephalographic indications of the disorder in symptomatic individuals. Minimal histological abnormalities have been reported in some of these cases. Meencke and Janz (1984) have described such minor abnormalities under the label "microdysgenesis". This descriptive term includes: (1) accumulation of neurons in the molecular layer of the neocortex, (2) ectopic neurons in the leptomeninges, (3) accentuation of the columnar disposition of cortical neurons, and (4) increase in the number (frequency) of ectopic neurons in the subcortical white matter. These findings have been reported in both idiopathic generalized epilepsy (Meencke and Janz, 1984) and in IS (Meencke and Gerhard, 1985). The significance of the lesions, however, has been questioned by several authors (e.g. Lyon and Gastaut, 1985).

PATHOPHYSIOLOGICAL CONSIDERATIONS

The obvious goal of describing the neuropathological findings in brain tissue from patients with IS is to try to gain an understanding of the pathogenesis, or at least the pathophysiology, of the disorder – indeed, this is one of the

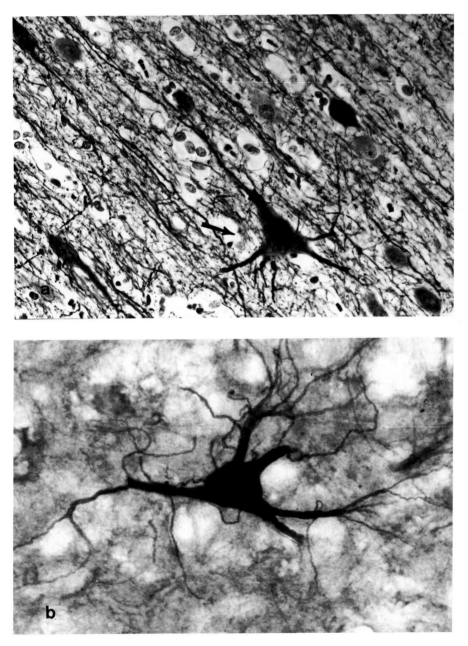

Figure 9.10 Cytoskeletal abnormalities in cortical resection specimens. (A) A 3.5-month-old child with HME. The Bielschowsky-stained section shows darkly stained neurons (arrow) containing neurofilamentous disorganization. (B) Section of cortex from the same patient immunoreacted with anti-SMI 32 (against nonphosphorylated neurofilament). Note the dense staining of neuronal cytoplasm and several cell processes. Magnification ×430 for (A) and (B).

fundamental goals of any neuropathologist who devotes him or herself to a study of the morphological substrates of epilepsy (Vinters *et al.*, 1993a; Lennox, 1966). No simple pathological interpretation of IS, especially with respect to causality or pathogenesis, can be inferred from the various lesions of the CNS that we have reviewed above. What is the relationship between the neuropathological lesions and the clinical and electrophysiological aspects of IS? It has been postulated that subcortical structures are the site of origin of IS (Hrachovy and Frost, 1989a; Martin *et al.*, 1961). However, this hypothesis correlates only weakly with neuroanatomical findings. There remain very few puzzling cases in which lesions have been encountered primarily or exclusively in the brainstem. As noted throughout this chapter, in most instances the structural abnormality resides in the hemispheric cortex, either focally or diffusely. This finding leads to the following conclusion: subcortical structures may be involved in the production of IS, but the "triggering area" is most likely to be cortical. This hypothesis is not incompatible with the suspected role of the brainstem: inactivation of the cholinergic systems can be correlated with the rare cases in which lesions are found in the brainstem. On the other hand, the transient increase of activity of serotoninergic and noradrenergic systems, seen in the more numerous cases in which the brainstem is preserved, suggest activation of neurons of the median raphe nuclei and the locus ceruleus, respectively.

If we consider that the "triggering" site for spasms is the neocortex, it remains difficult to comprehend why both diffuse and focal lesions are capable of producing the same types of seizure (i.e. IS), although we know that lesions of the cortex may produce focal seizures in infancy, just as they do in childhood and adulthood. Indeed, whatever their basic underlying mechanism, spasms are completely different from the localized discharge of an assembly of neurons that is generally thought to result in a focal seizure. Nevertheless, IS may occur as the result of a "zone of cortical abnormality".

It may be postulated that the immaturity of the cortex is necessary to produce a spasm with transient and diffuse suppression of cortical electrical activity, instead of a focal or generalized tonic–clonic seizure discharge. The correlation of maturation of the cortex and evolution of IS becomes clearer when one observes that after months or years, IS evolves into focal or multifocal (generalized) epilepsy. As illustrated above, the main cortical neuropathological findings in patients with IS consist of either extensive unifocal, multifocal or diffuse dysplasia or brain damage, with or without an associated metabolic abnormality. Whatever the precise patter of neurophysiological disorganization, the hypsarrhythmic pattern is diffuse, involving the entire cortex. Focal or diffuse brain metabolic abnormalities may be detected by positron emission tomographic (PET) scanning (Chugani *et al.*, 1984, 1993).

Another curious question arises: Why do spasms subside over time in certain patients but not others? It is conceivable that at the onset of IS, the cortex is incompletely differentiated into specific areas. Although the delineation of cortical "specialization" seems to be determined very early and already exists at the level of the ventricular zone (Rakic, 1988a; Dehay *et al.*, 1991), cortical development is a long-lasting phenomenon. Globally, it progresses from back to front and finds its macroscopic expression in the appearance of gyri. In the malformations that are most commonly associated with protracted spasms, the gyri are either completely or mostly lacking (lissencephaly, pachygyria, agyria) or extensively abnormal (Aicardi syndrome). With either maformation, the cortical areas do not become differentiated, and (remarkably) infantile spasms tend to be the most refractory and last for the longest period of time.

The occurrence of spasms for a more restricted period in more or less focal cortical lesions is more complex and difficult to interpret. The reason(s) why, during the first year of life, focal or multifocal cerebral lesions are more likely to produce diffuse neurophysiological disorganization (presumably leading to "electrophysiological chaos") remains unknown. What is the role played by diffuse synaptogenesis that will later selectively regress (Becker, 1991), as reported for instance in the occipital cortex (Blue and Parnavelas, 1983; Vrensen *et al.*, 1977)? In addition, the number of interhemispheric axon fibers has been followed throughout early life in cats and has been shown to be redundant during the first stages of development, decreasing by 60% subsequently (Berbel and Innocenti, 1988).

CONCLUSIONS

Infantile spasms can be observed in a variety of clinicopathological settings, including those that result in focal, multifocal or diffuse brain lesions. Cortical abnormalities are observed in the majority of cases that come to necropsy or surgery, or are examined by high-resolution neuroradiographic imaging methodologies. The spasms occur for a relatively restricted time period, usually limited to the first year of life. The appearance of spasms seems to be related to an absence of differentiation of the cortex into specific or specialized areas, a change that is particularly prominent and significant in diffuse neocortical malformations such as those that occur in agyria–pachygyria–lissencephaly, Aicardi syndrome or HME – these three malformations are remarkably able to "induce" spasms, though IS can be present in infants with a large variety of structural brain abnormalities.

10

Structural Imaging: CT and MRI

C. DIEBLER, O. DULAC

Infantile spasms (IS) is an age-related epilepsy syndrome that is the result of various causes. Neuroradiological investigations represent a key stage in the search of an etiology. They may reveal focal or even diffuse cerebral lesions. In determining a precise etiology, they help to give a prognosis and to orient the therapeutic approach, since some patients need specific drug treatments, whereas others may be candidates for early surgery.

Some brain lesions may be missed by computed tomography (CT) and magnetic resonance imaging (MRI) and only be disclosed by functional imaging. The neuropediatrician and neuroradiologist are thus frequently confronted with the problem of when to go beyond CT and MRI with functional imaging in order to disclose focal lesions amenable to surgery.

Neuroradiological investigation of structural lesions in IS is based primarily on findings from CT scans and MRI. In over one-third of infants with IS, the history and clinical examination provide the etiological diagnosis (Diebler and Dulac, 1987). In another 15% of cases, CT scan shows easily identifiable malformative, destructive or space-occupying lesions. Other cases exhibit nonspecific CT abnormalities, mainly consisting of focal or diffuse atrophy (Diebler and Dulac, 1987). Overall, the incidence of abnormalities on CT scan ranges from 61% (Diebler and Dulac, 1987) to 90% (Ludwig, 1987). A recent analysis of the value of CT in IS from our own series of 364 patients revealed abnormalities in 57.42% (Table 10.1). In all these cases, MRI was useful in determining more precisely the type or extent of the lesions, and about 10% of the cases with normal CT scan exhibited an abnormal MRI, mainly consisting of cortical dysplasia (Van Bogaert et al., 1993).

TECHNICAL CONSIDERATIONS

When interpreting CT and especially MRI images in children with IS, one must consider normal changes in the brain's appearance due to maturation which

Table 10.1 CT findings among 364 patients with infantile spasms

	n	%
Normal	155	42.58
Diffuse atrophy	79	21.70
Tuberous sclerosis	38	10.44
Porencephaly	29	7.96
Leukomalacia	11	3.02
Hemimegalencephaly	8	2.20
Agyria	8	2.20
Aicardi syndrome	8	2.20
Focal atrophy	7	1.92
Focal dysplasia	4	1.09
Multicystic leucomalacia	3	0.82
Callosal agenesis	2	0.55
Leukodystrophy	2	0.55
Hydrocephaly	2	0.55
Bilateral porencephaly	1	0.27
Laminar heterotopia	1	0.27
Holoprosencephaly	1	0.27
Growing porencephaly	1	0.27
Microcephaly	1	0.27
Angioma	1	0.27
Microgyria	1	0.27
Leigh syndrome	1	0.27

are particularly marked in the first months of life, and nonspecific changes induced by some drugs.

Myelin Maturation on MRI Images (Valk and Knaap, 1989)

The typical age of onset of IS is at about 3–5 months of age, when dramatic maturational changes in myelination lead to a modification of the white matter signal on MRI; this maturation has a different time course in the different regions of the brain.

At birth, myelination can be seen in the posterior limb of the internal capsule, with extension to the globus pallidus and thalamus. From this newborn pattern, myelination progresses in the direction of the sensory cortex and the occipital lobes. From the third and fourth months myelination proceeds in the frontal direction, and from the fourth and fifth months in the temporal direction. The arcuate fibers are reached between the 12th and 14th months.

Unmyelinated white matter has a higher signal than the gray matter in T2 weighted images. With myelination, the signal of the white matter decreases to become progressively lower than that of the gray matter. At a transition period, the white matter can no longer be distinguished from the gray matter. The date of the transition period varies from 6 to 12 months (Dietrich *et al.*, 1988). The "isointense" pattern between white and gray matter is also dependent on the type of equipment, the field strength and values of TR and TE used (e.g. 3000/ 120, 2000/85, etc.) (Dietrich *et al.*, 1988).

Sometimes inversion-recovery sequences (2000/500, 1500/400, etc.) may help to better delineate the thickness of the cortex in infants aged about 1 year. These sequences with multiple thin slices allow three-dimensional reconstruction giving a cartography of the cerebral cortex.

The Effect of Steroids

Brain shrinkage may appear a few days after the commencement of steroid treatment. Langenstein *et al.* (1979) performed CT scans before, during and after ACTH treatment in IS patients and found the cerebral ventricles, sulci and cisterns to be enlarged during ACTH administration, resembling severe general cortical and subcortical atrophy. After discontinuation of ACTH, the appearance of the brain on CT returned more or less to that seen pretreatment. Similar findings were reported by Deonna and Voumard (1979). Satoh *et al.* (1982) found brain shrinkage in all IS patients studied with sequential CT scans (Fig. 10.1). This was particularly marked in the youngest patients, two of whom also had subdural effusions. Ito *et al.* (1983) showed in their 24 reported cases that brain shrinkage becomes apparent with steroid treatment regardless of the etiology of IS. The changes on CT were observed less than 1 week following commencement of treatment, and increased in severity as the number of ACTH injections increased. In four infants with ACTH treatment lasting for 2 months,

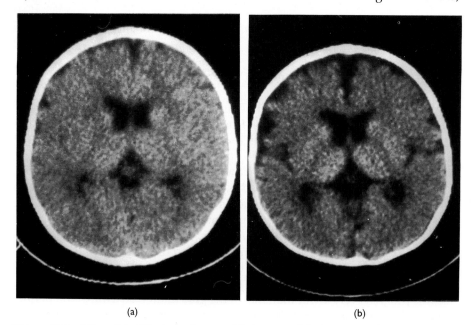

(a)   (b)

Figure 10.1 Idiopathic West syndrome. CT is normal before steroid treatment (a). After 1 month of treatment, the ventricles and cortical sulci are moderately enlarged (b).

the "cerebral atrophy" remained for 4–5 months after discontinuation of treatment. Furthermore, in one case, ACTH therapy was followed by hydrocephalus that required shunting (Ito *et al.*, 1983).

CAUSES USUALLY IDENTIFIED BEFORE RADIOLOGICAL INVESTIGATION

In a number of cases, neuroradiological investigation is performed after the etiological diagnosis of IS has been assessed on history, on clinical examination or on biochemical or virological studies. In such instances, it may help to determine the topography and extent of brain lesions.

Acute Prenatal Disorders

Extensive brain lesions due to acute vascular or infectious diseases are major causes of IS. A *twin pregnancy* may produce *multicystic encephalomalacia* (Fig. 10.2) as a consequence of intravascular coagulation produced by a macerated twin; or periventricular leukomalacia as a consequence of prematurity. In the latter case, the irregular and widened size of the posterior aspect of the lateral ventricles may be seen on CT, and MRI is useful for showing directly the ischemic areas in the periventricular white matter (Figs 10.3 and 10.4).

Infectious fetopathy due to *toxoplasmosis* (Christensen and Melchior, 1960; Diebler and Dulac, 1987) is easily recognized by the presence of periventricular calcifications in conjunction with hydrocephalus. In *rubella* fetopathy, the brain is usually small with occasional calcifications with areas of low density in the brain tissue (Riikonen, 1984a; Diebler and Dulac, 1987). In *cytomegalovirus* fetopathy, the brain is small, the calcifications are usually around the ventricles, and CT scan may show areas of low density and multiple porence-

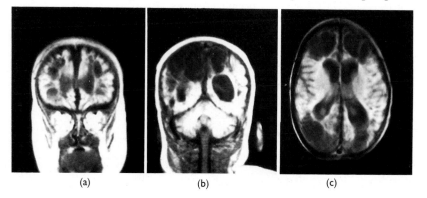

(a) (b) (c)

Figure 10.2   Twin pregnancy. Microcephaly and encephalopathy in 4-month-old with infantile spasms. MRI T1 frontal (a, b) and axial (c) views. Multiple intracerebral cysts predominating in the anterior and posterior regions. Enlargement of the ventricles and sulci.

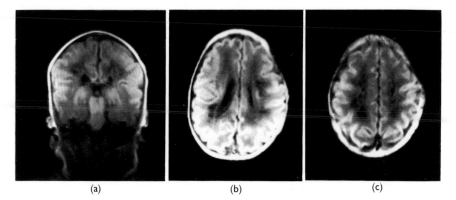

Figure 10.3 Prematurely born infant. Microcephaly and diplegia. MRI T1 frontal (a) and axial (b, c) views. Multiple small porencephalic cysts within the periventricular white matter. Abnormally low attenuation of the white matter.

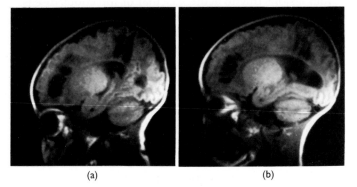

Figure 10.4 Prematurely born infant with IS from the age of 7 months. MRI T1 sagittal views. Large periventricular leukomalacias in the two frontal and the two parieto-occipital regions.

phaly. The problem of cytomegalovirus infection is noteworthy, since postnatal infection has long been thought to produce IS. It is now clear that it was a fortuitous association and that only prenatal cytomegalovirus infections are able to produce brain lesions causing IS (Midulla *et al.*, 1976). Infectious etiologies associated with IS are discussed in Chapter 19.

Neurocutaneous Syndromes

Most neurocutaneous syndromes with onset of epilepsy in the first year of life can produce IS (see also Chapters 16 and 17). The diagnosis is based on cutaneous findings. In Recklinghausen's neurofibromatosis, CT is usually normal (Huson *et al.*, 1988; Diebler and Dulac, 1987). MRI T2 weighted sequences may disclose areas of increased signal in the cerebral white matter or basal ganglia, but their significance remains unknown (Pognanno *et al.*, 1988;

Fig. 10.5). One case with hemimegalencephaly and spasms responded to steroid therapy (Cusmai *et al.*, 1990b).

In the Solomon syndrome, a midline linear nevus may be associated with hemimegalencephaly (Vigevano, 1984; Kurokawa *et al.*, 1981). In incontinentia pigmenti, multiple destructive lesions lead to atrophy and porencephaly (Avrahmi *et al.*, 1985).

Although rare, IS may occur in Sturge-Weber syndrome (Millichap *et al.*, 1962) in which CT and MRI demonstrate the angioma and associated ischemic lesions after contrast medium administration, as well as hypertrophy of the homolateral choroid plexus secondary to abnormal venous drainage (Diebler and Dulac, 1987; Enjolras and Riché 1990, Fig. 10.6).

The Ito syndrome may be associated with various types of brain malformations, including porencephaly, hemimegalencephaly (Ardinger and Bell, 1986), corpus callosum lipoma (Diebler and Dulac, 1990), heterotopias of the white matter (Rosenberg *et al.*, 1984) and agyria (personal series).

Bourneville's tuberous sclerosis is the most frequently encountered neurocutaneous syndrome that produces IS (see Chapter 16). Over half of patients with tuberous sclerosis and epilepsy develop IS (Dulac *et al.*, 1984). Subependymal nodules are present from birth, at which time they may be calcified, but generally they grow slightly and calcify further during the first few months of life. These nodules are not enhanced by contrast medium administration. The cortical areas of hypodensity on CT represent the major tubers that are more readily observed on MRI, where they appear as hyposignal areas in T1 and hypersignal areas in T2 weighted images (Figs 10.7 and 10.8). These hypersignal areas are particularly evident after 2 years of age and may not be visible at onset of IS because of inadequate myelination. Repitition of the examination

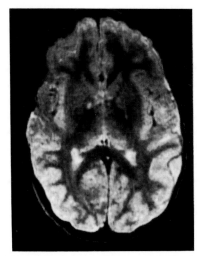

Figure 10.5 A 4-year-old boy with neurofibromatosis 1 who had recovered from IS with normal development. MRI T2 axial view shows a small area of hypersignal in the right basal ganglia region.

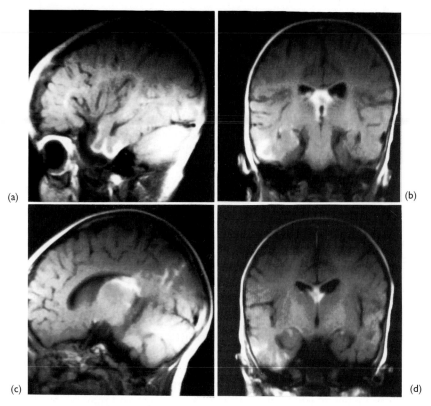

Figure 10.6   A 6-month-old girl with Sturge-Weber disease and infantile spasms. MRI T1 with contrast enhancement in the sagittal (a, c) and frontal (b, d) views shows multiple lesions of the cortical and leptomeningal regions in the temporal and parieto-occipital lobes. Enlargement of the central venous system (b, c, d) is secondary to abnormal venous drainage.

shows that there is no modification of the number, size and topography of the tubers, and that no new tubers appear with increasing age. The topography of the major tubers seems to have great prognostic value, since patients with posteriorly located tubers are the most likely to develop spasms; patients with additional tubers in anterior areas suffer a persistent generalized epilepsy with the characteristics of multifocal epilepsy or Lennox-Gastaut syndrome (Cusmai *et al.*, 1990a). In one series, three of five such patients had autistic features (Jambaqué *et al.*, 1991). Although intraventricular astrocytomas are never symptomatic in infancy, they may be observed from the first year on, showing clear contrast enhancement on MRI and on CT.

Inborn Errors of Metabolism

In contrast with the other causes, inborn errors of metabolism only occasionally produce IS, except for rare instances such as phenylketonuria. Although these

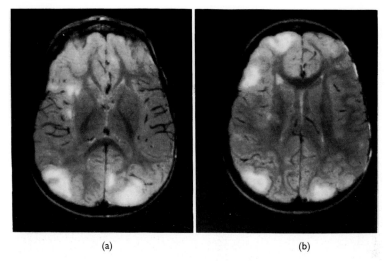

(a)   (b)

Figure 10.7 A 2-year-old boy with tuberous sclerosis and intractable infantile spasms. MRI T2 axial views show multiple tubers disseminated in both hemispheres both anteriorly and posteriorly.

disorders may show radiological abnormalities, their final diagnosis depends upon biochemical testing. In most instances, CT scan is normal or shows mild and nonspecific brain atrophy as in phenylketonuria (Diebler and Dulac, 1987), biotinidase deficiency (Colamaria *et al.*, 1989), pyridoxine-dependency (Jeavons and Bower, 1974), nonketotic hyperglycinemia (Dalla Bernardina *et al.*, 1979) and neonatal adrenoleukodystrophy (Aubourg *et al.*, 1986). In other cases, radiological findings may be somewhat more specific, and consist of low attenuation of the white matter as in Krabbe's disease (Jeshima *et al.*, 1983), orthochromatic leukodystrophy (Dabbagh and Swaiman, 1988; Fig. 10.9), pyruvate carboxylase deficiency and *N*-acetylaspartate aciduria (Rutledge *et al.*, 1986), or show symmetrical lesions in the basal ganglia as in Leigh's disease (Paltiel *et al.*, 1987; Fig. 10.10).

Perinatal Disorders

Although it used to be the typical and most frequent cause of IS, anoxic–ischemic encephalopathy in the full-term newborn has become much more rare as a cause of IS than premature delivery (see also Chapter 18).

After anoxia–ischemia in the full-term newborn, CT scan may demonstrate various types of lesions: single or multiple porencephalies (Fig. 10.11), severe cortical atrophy, or areas of widening of the depth of the sulci, a condition called "ulegyria". MRI shows more precisely the extent of the lesions, particularly when they involve the cortex, as in ulegyria; it also shows thinning of the corpus callosum, a consequence of focal or widespread necrosis of the cerebral cortex (Diebler and Dulac, 1990).

In prematurely born infants, anoxia typically produces periventricular leuco-

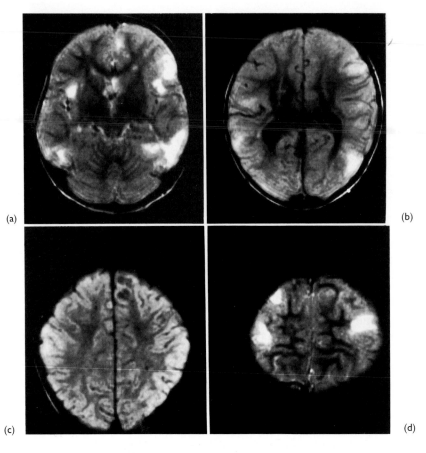

(a)   (b)

(c)   (d)

Figure 10.8 A 14-month-old girl with tuberous sclerosis and infantile spasms followed by intractable generalized seizures. MRI axial views T1 (a, d), proton density (b) and T1 (c). T1 and proton density images show the tubers as multiple areas with high signal. On T1 images, the tubers correspond to subcortical areas with hyposignal distending the overlying cortex, as in the left frontal regions of (c).

malacia, appearing on CT as an irregular widening of the lateral ventricles and on T1 weighted MRI sequences as periventricular areas with diminished signal. After the first year of life, these areas show an increased signal in T2 weighted sequences (Fig. 10.12).

Following severe neonatal hypoglycemia (Riikonen and Donner, 1979), CT scan may show nonspecific brain atrophy.

Postnatal Disorders

A number of postnatally acquired, usually bilateral, insults to the brain may also give rise to IS, some of which are reviewed here. Near drowning (Hrachovy *et al.*, 1987) and apparent life-threatening events (Aubourg *et al.*, 1985)

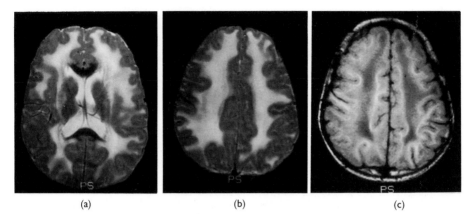

(a) (b) (c)

Figure 10.9 A 6-month-old girl with infantile spasms. Her brother developed genera-lized epilepsy at 3 years with the same MRI aspect. MRI T2 (a, b) and T1 (c) axial views. The white matter exhibits a diffuse hyposignal in T1 and hypersignal in T2, suggesting the diagnosis of leukodystrophy. Biochemical investigations were negative.

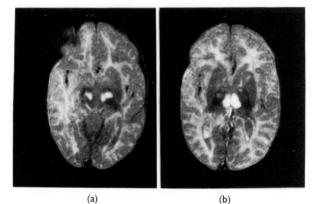

(a) (b)

Figure 10.10 A 5-month-old boy with progressive floppiness and infantile spasms. MRI T2 axial views. Bilateral grossly symmetrical lesions of the midbrain and of the thalamic regions, suggesting Leigh's disease.

are causes of anoxia–ischemia that are often overlooked as causes of IS. On CT and MRI, bilateral areas of hemispheric necrosis mainly involve the white matter at the junction of the sylvian and posterior cerebral arteries (Fig. 10.13).

Bacterial meningitis in the newborn period or in infancy produces focal or multifocal areas of hemispheric necrosis or brain atrophy due to arterial or venous infarcts or to brain abscess (Lombroso, 1983b; Diebler and Dulac, 1987). Herpetic encephalitis lesions mainly involve the temporal and eventually the frontal and parietal lobes, rarely the occipital lobes, with focal atrophy and calcifications. When restricted to the limbic system, the lesions are best seen on coronal MRI planes (Ohtaki *et al.*, 1987; Diebler and Dulac, 1990; Fig. 10.14). Subdural hematoma and other traumatic lesions of the newborn or infant

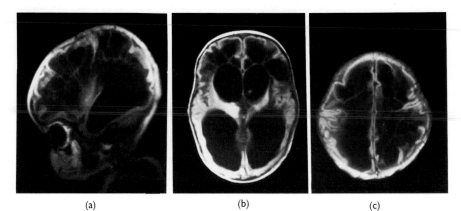

(a)   (b)   (c)

Figure 10.11   Full-term infant with severe perinatal anoxia, seizures in the first days of life and infantile spasms at the age of 3 months. MRI T1 (a) and axial (b, c) views showing clear enlargement of the ventricles and numerous confluent porencephalic cysts in the two cerebral hemispheres.

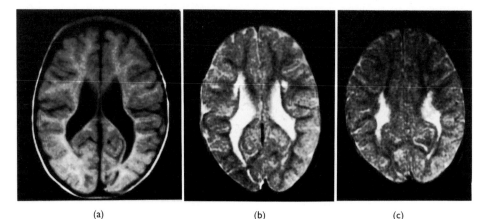

(a)   (b)   (c)

Figure 10.12   A prematurely born boy with infantile spasms overlooked until the age of 14 months. Diffuse leukomalacia predominating in the posterior regions, presenting on T1 weighted images (a), ventricular enlargement and, on T2 weighted images (b,c), clear hypersignal of the internal capsulae and in the posterior white matter.

produce brain atrophy or multiple porencephalic cysts (Millichap *et al.*, 1962; Diebler and Dulac, 1990).

Cases with Negative Investigation

In a number of cases, CT scan and MRI remain normal, although a precise cause of brain dysfunction is recognized, based on clinical, biochemical or cytogenetic data: trisomy 21, neurofibromatosis and phenylketonuria are three major examples.

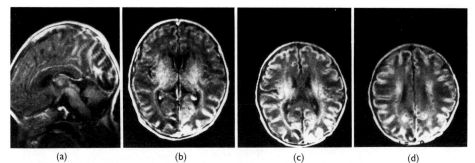

(a) (b) (c) (d)

Figure 10.13 A 4-month-old boy with sudden infant death syndrome and status epilepticus followed by infantile spasms. MRI T1 sagittal (a) and axial (b, c, d) views after the episode of status epilepticus showing diffuse necrosis of the subcortical white matter.

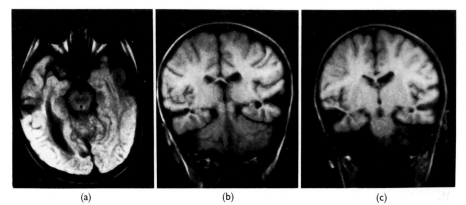

(a) (b) (c)

Figure 10.14 A 6-month-old boy with infantile spasms. History reveals vesicular rash in the first days of life. MRI T1 axial (a) and coronal (b, c) views. The bilateral destructive and atrophic lesions in the temporal lobes suggesting sequelae of neonatal herpetic encephalitis.

CAUSES IDENTIFIED BY NEURORADIOLOGICAL INVESTIGATIONS

Malformations

Identifiable malformations occur in 24% (Singer *et al.*, 1982) to 45% (Diebler and Dulac, 1987) of patients with IS. In callosal agenesis, there is dorsal displacement of the third ventricle and lateral displacement of the lateral ventricles; the frontal horns are stretched and narrow in contrast to the enlarged occipital horns. Callosal agenesis may be complete or partial, involving the posterior portion more frequently than the anterior portion; the diagnosis of partial callosal agenesis requires MRI confirmation with sagittal planes. The callosal agenesis which produces IS is usually associated with brain atrophy (Fig. 10.15; Diebler and Dulac, 1987). In other cases, it is associated with irregular lateral ventricles due to periventricular heterotopias, particularly in Aicardi syndrome, which occurs in girls and includes the presence of retinal

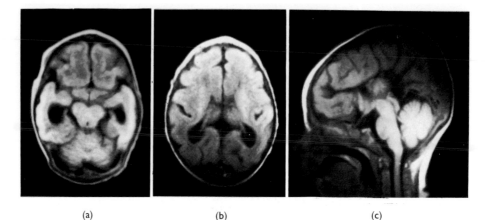

(a)   (b)   (c)

Figure 10.15 A 4-month-old boy with infantile spasms and without psychomotor development. MRI T1 axial (a, b) and sagittal (c) views show complete agenesis of the corpus callosum and diffuse pachygyria.

lacunae (Aicardi *et al.*, 1969). Such findings may not appear on neuroradiological investigations (Fig. 10.16). On the other hand, similar cases have been reported in girls who lacked fundoscopic abnormalities (Carrazana *et al.*, 1990; Yamagata *et al.*, 1990) and on rare occasions in males (Diebler and Dulac, 1990), although it remains controversial whether the latter belong to Aicardi syndrome (Aicardi, 1980). Therefore, the clinical spectrum of Aicardi's malformation seems to be wider than claimed (Chevrie and Aicardi, 1986b) prior to the advent of MRI.

In patients who exhibit IS, holoprosencephaly is occasionally predicted by facial abnormalities consisting of hypotelorism, hypoplastic philtrum or a facial cleft. Patients with IS more often have lobar or semi-lobar than alobar holoprosencephaly. In the alobar form, the third ventricle is rarely apparent, and it opens dorsally into a wide cavity corresponding to the fused lateral ventricles; the prosencephalon is placed anteriorly like a shell of cerebral tissue along the temporal and frontal vaults. In the semilobar form, the hemispheric tissue may be present posteriorly, and the small third ventricle opens into a horseshoe-like single lateral ventricle (Fig. 10.17). The diagnosis of lobar holoprosencephaly is more difficult: the interhemispheric fissure is present, the third ventricle is narrow and opens into the fused lateral ventricles; MRI shows that the frontal cortex is not interrupted at the midline, at the depth of the interhemispheric fissure.

The septal dysplasia which produces IS is most often associated with bilateral porencephaly bordered by heterotopias (Dekaban, 1965), and polymicrogyric cortical areas, a malformation also called "schizencephaly" (Yakovlev and Wadsworth, 1946; Fig. 10.18).

In agyria–pachygyria, which frequently presents with IS, CT scan shows that the cortex is smooth and abnormally thick. In rare cases, the four layers of cortex may be recognized around the shallow sylvian fissure between the

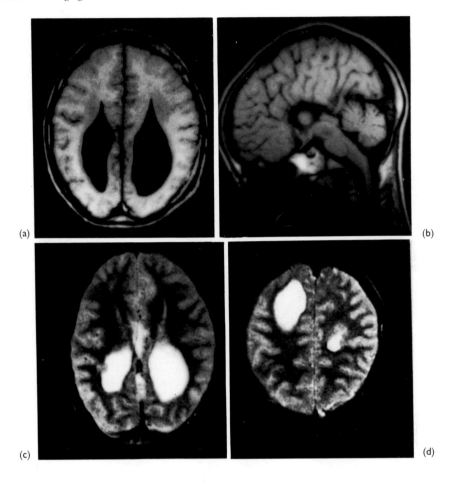

(a)   (b)   (c)   (d)

Figure 10.16 A 10-year-old girl with retinal lacunae and intractable infantile spasms due to Aicardi syndrome. MRI T1 axial (a), sagittal (b) and T2 axial (c, d) views showing complete agenesis of the corpus callosum and periventricular heterotopia (c, d).

hypoplastic frontal and temporal lobes. They consist of a thin, dense external layer followed successively, towards the lateral ventricles, by a thin layer of edematous density, a thick, dense layer which may correspond to the fourth layer on histologic examination, and a large layer of edematous density corresponding to the hypoplastic white matter (Fig. 10.19). In less severe forms, cerebral sulci are more numerous. Pachygyria usually involves the entire cortex (Fig. 10.15); however, it may be restricted to its anterior or posterior half. Laminar dysplasia, which may also be associated with IS, is a different form of the same migration disorder and both may be genetically linked (Pinard *et al.*, in press); it is easily recognized on MRI as a subcortical linear band of gray matter separated from the cortex by white matter (Marchal *et al.*, 1989). It may develop between two layers of white matter or along the walls of the lateral ventricles.

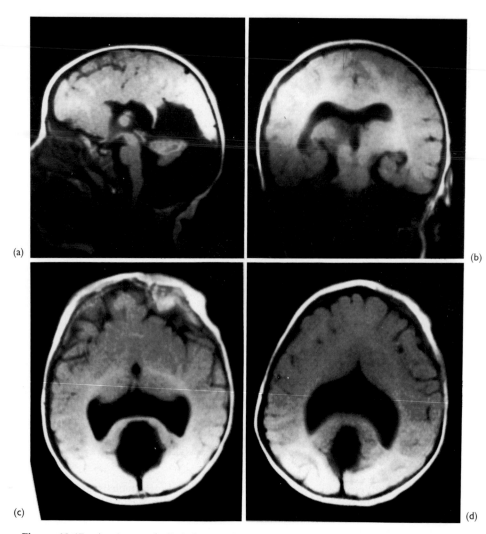

(a)

(b)

(c)

(d)

Figure 10.17 A microcephalic infant with major axial hypotonia, pyramidal signs and infantile spasms. MRI T1 sagittal (a), frontal (b) and axial (c, d) views show semilobar prosencephaly with fused frontal lobes, the third ventricle opening dorsally in a telencephalic single ventricle. The posterior interhemispheric fissure is visible. Cerebellar hypoplasia.

Radiological evidence of smooth cortex does not imply Bielschowsky's four-layered agyria–pachygyria. In Fukuyama and Walker-Warburg's malformation and in microgyria, the brain also exhibits a smooth cortical surface on gross examination. Thus, the typical EEG abnormalities consisting of high-amplitude discharges of fast activity (Dulac *et al.*, 1983a, Gastaut *et al.*, 1987), are useful to support the diagnosis of Bielschowsky's malformation when chromosome 17 appears normal on high-resolution techniques (Dobyns *et al.*, 1984).

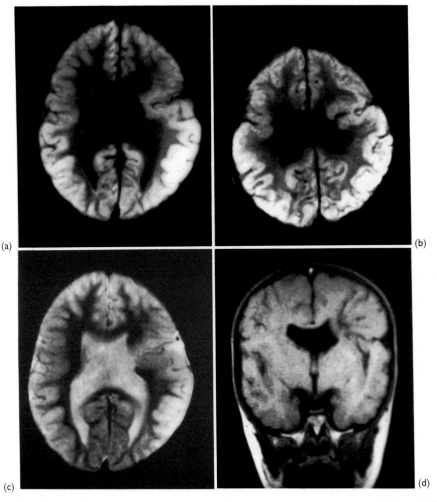

(a)   (b)

(c)   (d)

Figure 10.18 Right hemiparesis and prior infantile spasms in a 2-year-old boy. MRI proton density (a, b), T2 (c) and T1 (d) views show the absence of the septum pellucidum, a collapsed porus of the left sylvian region surrounded by cortical polymicrogyria.

Hemimegalencephaly may also produce IS together with a burst–suppression pattern on EEG (Paladin *et al.*, 1989). CT shows the enlargement of one hemisphere with apparent displacement of the midline and ipsilateral ventriculomegaly, thus differentiating the malformation from a tumor or from an eventual atrophy of the contralateral hemisphere. The density of the white matter may be decreased; the cortex is thickened with wide sulci and may show small diffuse calcifications. MRI shows clearly the thick cortex with shallow gyri and the abnormal white matter presenting an inreased signal on T2 weighted images (Figs 10.20 and 10.21). Heterotopias, calcifications (Kalifa

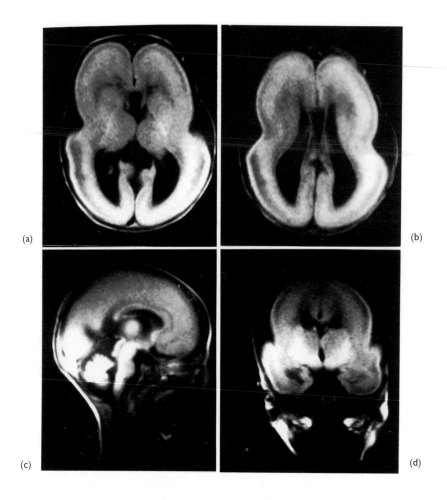

Figure 10.19 A 4-month-old girl with infantile spasms, microcephaly, facial dysmorphia and no psychomotor development. MRI T1 axial (a, b), sagittal (c) and frontal (d)
views show complete agyria with thick cortex, open sylvian fissure and moderate
enlargement of the ventricles.

et al., 1987) and vascular dysplasia (Araki *et al.*, 1987) may be observed within
the abnormal hemisphere. The cerebral dysplasia may involve the entire
hemisphere or be restricted to a part of it. Thus there seems to be a continuum
between hemimegalencephaly and focal cortical dysplasia.

Cortical dysplasia has long been overlooked as a cause of IS. It may be visible
on CT scan as an area of smooth and thick cortex overlying occasionally
hypodense white matter. When CT scan is normal, MRI with T2 weighted
sequences may show an asymmetry of the white matter in the involved lobe:
the limits between white and gray matter are poorly defined, and the white
matter signal is more intense than on the normal side (Van Bogaert *et al.*, 1993;

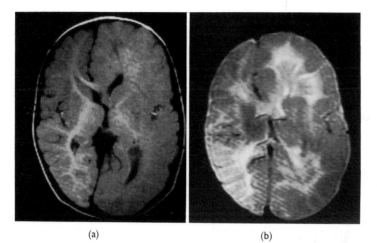

(a)　　　　　　　　　　(b)

Figure 10.20 A 5-month-old child with right upper-limb seizures from birth and infantile spasms from 6 weeks of age. MRI axial T1 (a) and T2 (b) views show left hemimegalencephaly of the whole hemisphere with thickening of the cortex, abnormal white matter and heterotopia within the white matter.

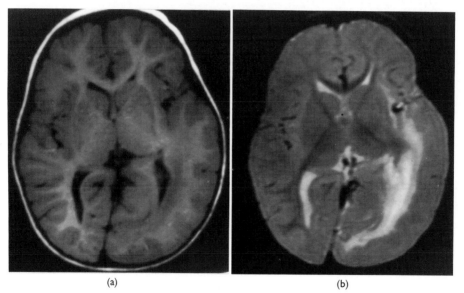

(a)　　　　　　　　　　(b)

Figure 10.21 A 15-month-old girl with infantile spasms from the age of 3 months. MRI axial T1 (a) and T2 (b) views show hemimegalencephaly of the posterior half of the left cerebral hemisphere with pachygyric, thick cortex and abnormal underlying white matter.

Figs 10.22, 10.23). However, a number of cortical dysplasias are overlooked by MRI, in which case functional imaging seems to be the most sensitive method of investigation (Chugani *et al.*, 1992, 1993).

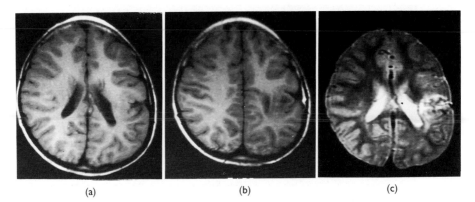

(a)   (b)   (c)

Figure 10.22 A 4-year-old girl with right focal seizures from day 5 of life, infantile spasms at 3 months, right hemiplegia and bilateral pyramidal signs. MRI axial T1 (a, b) and T2 (c) views show focal cortical dysplasia in the left sylvian region with thickening of the cortex showing hyposignal on T1 and hypersignal on T2 views.

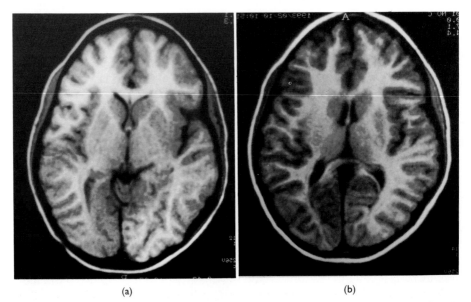

(a)   (b)

Figure 10.23 A 5-year-old girl with ictal nystagmus from 6 weeks of life, infantile spasms at 3 months and oculoclonic seizures at 5 months, following steroid treatment. MRI T1 axial views show thickening of the right temporo-occipital cortex, better analyzed on inversion recovery sequence.

In bilateral rolandic dysplasia, a rare cause of IS, CT scan shows bilateral symmetrical abnormalities with increased cortical thickening. MRI with sagittal sections shows that the sylvian fissure is abnormally oriented upward. The degree of perisylvian cortical abnormalities varies between patients (Kuzniecky *et al.*, 1989; 1991b).

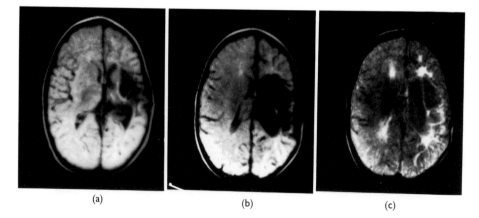

(a)   (b)   (c)

Figure 10.24 A 1-year-old girl prematurely born, with right hemiplegia and bilateral pyramidal signs. MRI T1 (a, b) and T2 (c) axial views show left hemiatrophy with large porencephalic cyst in the left sylvian region. T1 (c) reveals diffuse ischemic lesions in the white matter.

Only in one case has hamartoma of the tuber cinereum been reported to be associated with IS (Garcia Alvarez *et al.*, 1992). It consists of a mass located in the interpeduncular cistern between the internal carotids and the basilar artery in front of the pons, and is best seen on sagittal MRI planes (Diebler and Dulac, 1990).

Destructive Lesions

Infantile spasms are a usual expression of hydranencephaly. On CT, both lateral hemispheres are nearly completely destroyed and replaced by two large cysts separated by the intact falx. Small islands of cortex may be preserved in the temporal and occipital areas, but it is not always clear whether they are neurophysiologically connected to the subcortical structures (Neville, 1972). Multicystic encephalomalacia comprises multiple intracerebral cysts with diffuse cerebral atrophy (Jellinger, 1970; Diebler and Dulac, 1987).

Porencephalic cysts have a different appearance depending on whether they were formed during the second or the third trimester of pregnancy. Porencephaly originating in the second trimester involves the entire thickness of the cerebral mantle (Fig. 10.18). In some cases, the walls of the pre-existing cysts are joined; in such cases, a small ventricular diverticulum perpendicular to the ventricular wall with corresponding focal enlargement of the pericerebral spaces is an indirect sign of previous focal necrosis. Polymicrogyric cortex around the cyst appears on CT scan as a cortex of abnormal thickness and density. Porencephalic cysts developed in the third trimester or in the neonatal period do not necessarily involve the entire thickness of the cerebral mantle (Fig. 10.24). They may be limited to a circumscribed cortical or periventricular area, and sometimes they expand with dilatation of the ipsilateral ventricle and

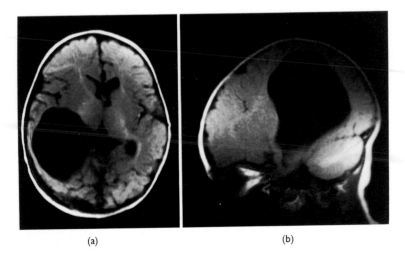

(a)   (b)

Figure 10.25   A 2-year-old boy who has recovered from West syndrome beginning at 5 months of age with left transient hemiparesis. MRI T1 axial (a) and sagittal (b) views show expanding porencephalic cyst of the right temporoparietal region communicating with the ventricular trigona.

Table 10.2   Focal brain lesions with infantile spasms Cusmai *et al.*, 1988)

	n	%
Porencephaly	15/17	88.2
Perinatal damage	11/15	73.3
Left hemisphere	12/15	80.0
Most of one hemisphere	7/15	46.7
Localized to rolandic or occipital	8/15	53.3
Frontal involvement with persistent epilepsy	5/6	83.3
Total	17/174	9.8

with contralateral displacement of the falx and sagittal sinus (Diebler and Dulac, 1987; Fig. 10.25).

In one series, 9.8% of patients with IS examined by CT scan had single focal lesions without microcephaly (Table 10.2). Most patients had suffered acute brain damage between 28 weeks of gestation and 3 months of postnatal life. Lesions were most frequently seen in the left hemisphere and in the parieto-occipital region (Cusmai *et al.*, 1988).

Leukodystrophy

This is a very rare radiological finding in patients with IS. The white matter is either normal or hypodense on CT scan and it gives a high-intensity signal on T2 weighted MRI sequences. Familial cases have been reported (Bignami *et al.*,

1966) and this was the case for one patient in our series (Fig. 10.9): the brother of this girl with IS had mild mental delay, macrocephaly and generalized tonic–clonic seizures beginning at 5 years; both siblings had leukodystrophy. In a mentally retarded patient with only microcephaly, there was an obvious delay of myelin maturation visible on MRI (Van Bogaert *et al.*, 1993), as occasionally seen in nonepileptic retarded patients.

MRI in patients with IS and normal CT scan may disclose a hypersignal of the white matter as shown in 9 of 13 patients in one series, 6 of whom suffered from severe mental handicap (Yasujima *et al.*, 1989).

Tumors

Various types of tumors may cause IS (Miyake *et al.*, 1986; Morimoto *et al.*, 1989). They involve either the cortex or the basal ganglia and include ependymomas (Ruggieri *et al.*, 1989), gliomas (Ruggieri *et al.*, 1989), gangliogliomas (Gabriel, 1983) and choroid plexus papillomas (Branch and Dyken, 1979), the latter often as a part of the Aicardi syndrome. These tumors are usually low grade and remain unchanged for many years or develop on cortical dysplasias; in our series, one such case was diagnosed 14 years after IS.

Vascular Malformation

As mentioned earlier, Sturge-Weber syndrome is only rarely associated with IS (Millichap and Bickford, 1962).

Calcifications

Cerebral calcifications associated with IS are usually due to tuberous sclerosis or to pre- or post-natal infection; in rare cases, they may be due to malformations, particularly hemimegalencephaly. However, isolated calcifications not clearly related to any of these disorders are rarely encountered.

Atrophy

Altogether, 47% (Curatolo *et al.*, 1982) to 49% (Singer *et al.*, 1982) of patients with IS exhibit diffuse cortical and/or subcortical atrophy. It remains difficult to determine strict criteria for brain atrophy. The investigation must be performed prior to steroid therapy, which is known to produce this type of image within a few days of treatment (Gastaut *et al.*, 1978). Although it is completely reversible, return to normal images may take several months (Ito *et al.*, 1983; Langenstein *et al.*, 1979). In addition, the size of the pericerebral space may vary considerably in normal infants (Fukuyama Y, 1979a), even when excluding the reversible phenomenon of external hydrocephalus (Kendall and Holland, 1981).

PROGNOSTIC VALUE OF NEURORADIOLOGICAL INVESTIGATIONS

The prognostic value of CT scan with respect to developmental outcome and seizure control in IS is variable. In two series, all the children with abnormal CT scan had cognitive delay, even when development had appeared normal prior to the onset of IS (Curatolo *et al.*, 1982; Singer *et al.*, 1982). However, in another series, there appeared to be no difference in cognitive outcome based on CT findings (Pedersen *et al.*, 1990). The remission rate was significantly higher in patients with normal CT in one series (Curatolo *et al.*, 1982). Singer *et al.* (1982) found no correlation between CT scan findings and either seizure control or occurrence of a second type of seizure. Thus etiology based on radiological findings is more likely than radiological findings *per se* to contribute to prognostic evaluation.

CONCLUSIONS

The data reviewed in this chapter help to determine the strategy for neurora-diological investigation, and provide some clues regarding the association between brain lesions and IS.

Indications for Neuroradiological Investigations

The neuroradiological investigation of IS should be performed in all cases and before steroid treatment is started, because the findings may help to decide which is the most appropriate drug to adminster and because shrinkage may appear early after the commencement of steroid therapy. The type of investi-gation – CT or MRI – largely depends on age. In the first year, CT scan is preferred as the initial examination because:

- it is easily obtained, widely available, has short exposure time (about 1 s) and high definition images:
- it correctly detects most major lesions that may be found in IS;
- it shows early calcifications which may be missed on MRI images; and
- it may guide the radiologist to choose optimum MRI sequences.

Thus, at onset, CT meets all the requirements for a first diagnostic classification and an immediate therapeutic decision.

Skull X-rays are no longer indicated except in cranial malformations. In Aicardi syndrome, cranial CT should be supplemented with bone X-ray studies to detect skeletal malformations, and in tuberous sclerosis sonography should be used to demonstrate associated cardiac and renal abnormalities.

When MRI is performed later in the evaluation of IS, its indication is generally more focused. This is to:

- Further define morphological abnormalities in patients with abnormal CT, such as the heterotopias in cases of Aicardi syndrome, the degree of structural disorganization of a hemimegalencephalic hemisphere with confirmation of the gross structural integrity of the contralateral hemisphere, or the associated cortical malformations in callosal agenesis.
- Pursue the possibility of cerebral anomalies as suggested by electroclinical signs, even though CT scan is normal. For example, cortical dysplasia may be suspected in patients whose spasms are preceded or followed by focal discharge.
- Determine whether myelination is normal, delayed or abnormal. Abnormal myelination may be observed in leukodystrophy, in focal destructive lesions and in malformations especially in the areas underlying cortical dysplasia.

Morphological studies are best performed using T1 or inversion recovery sequences, which should include views in the axial, coronal and sagittal planes. White matter maturation and lesions are best visualized on T2 sequences. To rule out tumor or infectious lesions, administration of the contrast medium DT-Gadolinium may be required.

Types and Topography of Abnormalities

The lesions associated with IS usually involve the cerebral hemispheres, and only very rarely the brainstem. Althouygh the cortex is typically involved, lesions can apparently be restricted to the white matter, particularly in leukomalacia, leukodystrophy and some cases of paraventricular porencephaly.

The extent of the lesions is quite variable, ranging from complete destruction of both hemispheres to the apparent lack of any lesion, even with MRI. When structural lesions are associated with IS, they are most often multifocal. When there is a single lesion, it more often involves the posterior half rather than the anterior half of the brain and mainly the occipital or temporal lobes, or the rolandic area. Extension to the frontal lobe due to wide or multifocal lesions seems frequently to be associated with intractability of the seizures: this is often the case in tuberous sclerosis and in sequelae following neonatal asphyxia after a full-term delivery.

11

Functional Imaging: SPECT

C. CHIRON, P. HWANG

Single photon emission computed tomography (SPECT) is a functional imaging method based on the study of the distribution of a radioactive tracer in the brain. SPECT measures an index of neuronal activity in different regions of the brain, the regional cerebral blood flow (rCBF), and therefore provides both functional and topographic data. SPECT is relatively easy to realize, moderately invasive, not particularly expensive and gives little irradiation. It can thus be used in pediatrics, even with infants.

Epilepsy is a disorder in which functional brain imaging is especially applicable, since it is sensitive enough to detect focal abnormalities in partial epilepsies – hypometabolism and hypoperfusion interictally, hypermetabolism and hyperperfusion ictally (Engel, 1984; Rowe *et al.*, 1989). Infantile epilepsy develops during the course of brain maturation and is therefore likely to change rapidly with age. Infantile spasms (IS) can be used as a model for the study of epilepsies in children, because of the polymorphism of its causes, of its clinical expression and of its outcome. SPECT imaging is particularly helpful in the study of these changes because of the ease with which it can be repeated during follow-up. But SPECT data are difficult to interpret because of the rapid development of the brain at this age, drug treatment and inter- and intra-individual variability.

The first rCBF studies were performed long after the acute stage of IS and steroid therapy, at the stage of sequelae, when rCBF defects are visually recognizable (Dulac *et al.*, 1987a). During the early phase of the disease, when functional variability and developmental changes are at their greatest, it is necessary to measure rCBFs so as to detect hypo- and/or hyperperfused areas. Knowledge of physiological changes in rCBF during infancy was therefore required. It has only recently become possible to address the onset of IS, once reference rCBF values had been established to which the data drawn from the IS group could be compared.

The following aspects will be addressed: SPECT methodology; physiological changes in rCBF during childhood; SPECT findings at different stages of IS; and pathophysiological hypotheses based on these data.

SPECT METHODOLOGY

Brain SPECT studies can be divided into two types. "Dynamic" studies refer to tomographic imaging performed with 133-xenon (^{133}Xe), which is a physiological blood flow indicator (Lassen, 1985). "Static" studies use tracers which behave somewhat like chemical microspheres; the images thus mimic a "snapshot" of CBF within 1 min of injection. ^{123}I-iodoamines (IMP, HIPDM) and ^{99Tc}-HMPAO are the tracers developed especially for static SPECT.

The static and dynamic methods have different advantages and disadvantages. Static SPECT uses a multipurpose SPECT system which is easy to manipulate and which is of relatively low cost. It gives images on cerebral sections usually 6–12 mm thick with a resolution of about 10 mm. Static SPECT is able to obtain ictal and postictal examinations because the isotope can be administered far from the imaging site. Its disadvantages include low sensitivity, uncertainties regarding the nonlinear relationship between count rate and true regional CBF, and therefore absolute quantification is difficult to obtain. Foci of hypoperfusion or hyperperfusion are usually recognized by comparing one side with the other and by referring to the images of normal subjects of the same age. Dynamic SPECT requires a more expensive and more complex SPECT system, which is only dedicated to the study of the brain. This system is sensitive enough to use a true blood flow indicator, as ^{133}Xe, whose cerebral transit time lasts only a few minutes, and therefore is able to provide absolute values of rCBF. However, because acquisition immediately follows injection of ^{133}Xe, it is difficult to perform ictal examinations. Dynamic SPECT gives images on 3–5 cerebral sections 20 mm thick with a resolution of 12 mm; CBF values can be calculated for every region of these images. The opportunity to measure rCBF values is of value in infants and young children because changes in rCBF are associated with the physiological maturation of the brain. The reference values now available enable one to interpret a patient's rCBF images and to locate accurately areas of decreased or increased flow. Dynamic SPECT studies are of particular interest in infantile epilepsy.

PHYSIOLOGICAL CHANGES IN rCBF DURING CHILDHOOD

All the functional brain markers studied in humans undergo modifications during childhood which are related to postnatal maturational processes: the number and density of synapses (Huttenlocher, 1979), cortical enzymatic activity (Farkas-Bargeton *et al.*, 1984), neuroreceptor density (McDonald and Johnson, 1990) and regional metabolism of glucose studied *in vivo* by positron emission tomography (PET; Chugani *et al.*, 1987). Modifications to cortical values are nonlinear but they exhibit four characteristics: (1) they are low at birth; (2) they increase rapidly during the first years of life to a maximum that is much higher than in adult life; (3) they decrease slowly during the second decade; (4) adult values remain quite stable. It has been hypothesized that the increase in these values is related to postnatal synaptic development (Chugani et al., 1987), whereas the following reduction is due to synaptic selection and stabilization (Changeux and Danchin, 1976; Purves and Lichtman, 1980).

SPECT studies in normal children show that rCBF follows the same pattern. A rapid increase in rCBF following birth has been reported with ^{123}I-IMP (Rubinstein et al., 1989) and [99Tc]HMPAO (Denays et al., 1992) and confirmed with [133]Xe (Raynaud et al., 1990). A more recent study involving the entire period of infancy and childhood, using ^{133}Xe has shown a peak in rCBF values at 6 years of age followed by a slow reduction to adult values (Chiron et al., 1992). This pattern of rCBF modifications related to age concerns the whole cortex, but there are topographic differences. Using a method in which each rCBF value is normalized to the global CBF, we were able to demonstrate that the increase appears earlier and more rapidly in the motor and posterior cortex than it does in the frontal cortex; that it appears from birth in the rolandic cortex, by the second and third month in the occipital and temporal cortex, and at the end of the first semester in the posterior associative occipito-temporal and parieto-occipital cortex. In contrast, the increase in rCBF in the frontal cortex is delayed, occurring at the end of the first and into the second year, and it is slower (Chiron et al., 1992). This development correlates with the maturation of cognitive functions supported by each of these areas: the sensorial, visual and auditory functions that are located in the posterior cortex mature mostly during the first year of life, whereas the frontal functions appear after the first year of life.

These regional findings are similar to those previously obtained in the study of regional metabolism with PET (Chugani et al., 1987). In addition, Chiron et al. (1992) have provided reference rCBF values with standard deviations (SD) according to age for each cortical region. It is the period from 0 to 2 years which has been documented the most, and it has become possible to study with sufficient reliability quantitative rCBF data obtained in infants with IS.

SPECT STUDIES IN IS

Overview

The most consistent findings in this generalized epilepsy are focal abnormalities. Although partly hypothetical, the following overview attempts to illustrate the various rCBF findings. At the onset of IS, patients exhibit hypoperfused areas that are epileptogenic foci related to cortical lesions mainly located in the posterior regions of the cortex. These areas remain hypoperfused during the evolution of the disease and are associated with sequelae that consist of focal epilepsy and/or selective cognitive deficits. Hyperperfused areas are also present from the onset of IS, even in the interictal period. These areas predominate in the frontal regions and could represent the spread of epileptic discharges originating in the posterior areas. They tend to decrease with steroid therapy, particularly those involving the frontal regions. Conversely, their persistence is correlated with an unfavorable outcome consisting of protracted generalized epilepsy, neurological deficits and severe mental retardation.

For methodological reasons, SPECT studies have not been able to follow the chronological development of IS, studies during the later stages having been performed before those during the earlier stages. We will first study the areas of hypoperfusion, then the areas of hyperperfusion.

Areas of Hypoperfusion

Demonstration of Hypoperfused Cortical Areas

Focal cortical abnormalities demonstrated by functional imaging were first reported in a study of 17 patients with IS who underwent ^{133}Xe SPECT investigation between 3 months and 6 years of age. Five of those patients were in the acute stage of the disease, whereas 12 had already passed through that stage (Dulac *et al.*, 1987a). Fourteen patients exhibited one or several areas of cortical hypoperfusion. Following this study areas of focal hypoperfusion were demonstrated in a series of 16 patients with tuberous sclerosis who were studied after IS, between 6 months and 16 years of age (Chiron *et al.*, 1990b). Fourteen of these subjects showed cortical areas of hypoperfusion, 13 of whom had multiple sites. Using [99Tc]HMPAO, Hwang *et al.* (in prep.) also found cortical abnormalities in 15 of 20 patients: they were focal in 7 cases and multifocal in 8, and they consisted of interictal hypoperfusion in 10 instances. In a series of 26 patients studied with ^{133}Xe, Chiron *et al.* (1993) were able to confirm these focal cortical perfusion abnormalities by quantification: 24 patients exhibited one or several areas of cortical hypoperfusion 9 months to 5 years (mean = 2 years) after the onset of IS (Fig. 11.1).

Areas of Hypoperfusion and Etiology of IS

Areas of hypoperfusion have therefore been demonstrated in studies involving IS with normal CT scan (Dulac *et al.*, 1987a), symptomatic IS due to tuberous sclerosis (Chiron *et al.*, 1990b), and both symptomatic (tuberous sclerosis, porencephaly, cortical malformations) and cryptogenic cases with normal MRI (Chiron *et al.*, 1993; Hwang *et al.*, in prep.). In symptomatic IS, lesions correspond to interictal hypoperfused areas. The areas that are overlooked by SPECT – about 25% in tuberous sclerosis – correspond either to tubers which are too small for the resolution of the system, or to tubers located in areas poorly studied by SPECT, for example the vertex (25% of cases) and the rolandic areas (50% of cases) (Chiron *et al.*, 1990b). In cryptogenic IS, hypoperfused areas have also been demonstrated in 14 of 17 patients studied by Dulac *et al.* (1987a), 5 of 8 patients studied by Hwang *et al.* (in prep.) and 6 of 8 patients studied by Chiron *et al.* (1993). Hypoperfused areas involving the cortical

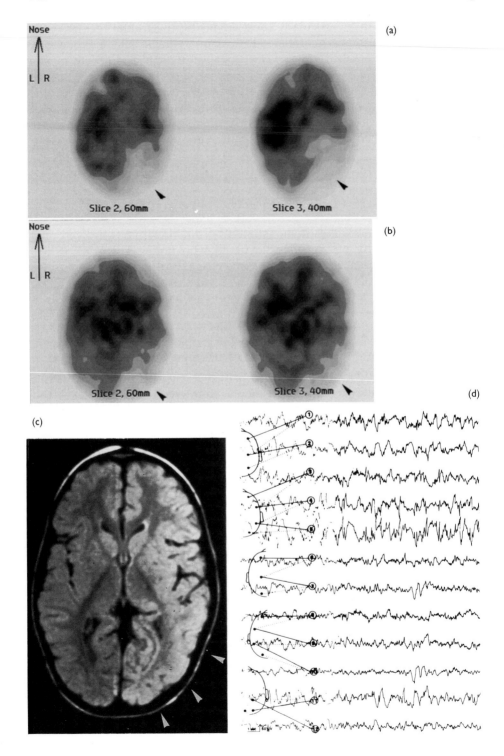

(a)

Nose

L | R

Slice 2, 60mm   Slice 3, 40mm

(b)

Nose

L | R

Slice 2, 60mm   Slice 3, 40mm

(c)

(d)

regions but without any apparent brain lesion have also been observed in symptomatic cases: in tuberous sclerosis, a quarter of hypoperfused areas did not correspond to any detectable lesion on MRI (Chiron *et al.*, 1990b).

Studies performed in both adult and child epilepsy have clearly demonstrated that functional imaging is more sensitive than structural methods of neuroimaging including CT and MRI. The percentage of cases with focal abnormalities disclosed by functional imaging without CT and MRI abnormalities ranges from 60 to 80% (Denays *et al.*, 1988; Chiron *et al.*, 1989a; Hwang *et al.*, 1990; Uvebrant *et al.*, 1991). Dulac *et al.* (1987b) suggested hypoperfused areas may be due to cortical lesions in IS, as in partial epilepsy. This assessment is supported in part by the neuropathological discovery of cortical dysgenesis following surgical resection of hypometabolic or hypoperfused areas (Chugani *et al.*, 1990; Adams *et al.*, 1992; Van Bogaert *et al.*, 1993; Otsubo *et al.*, 1993) (see Fig. 11.1).

Localization of Hypoperfused Areas

Areas of hypoperfusion that develop in the late stages of IS mainly involve the posterior cortex. In one study, focal or multifocal areas of hypoperfusion were posterior in 11 of 12 patients: it was occipito-temporal and/or parieto-occipital in 8, and temporal or parietal posterior in 3 (Dulac *et al.*, 1987a). In a quantitative ^{133}Xe study, 80% of the areas of hypoperfusion were posterior, for both symptomatic and cryptogenic cases (Chiron *et al.*, 1993) (Fig. 11.1). Hwang *et al.* (in prep.) also reported a predominance of occipital, temporal and parietal posterior areas of hypoperfusion. In all these series, the hypoperfused areas were unilateral in 50–70% of cases.

The Significance of Areas of Hypoperfusion

The significance of areas of hypoperfusion has been studied in relation to seizures, EEG foci, mental disorders and brain lesions.

Most of them seem to consist of epileptogenic foci. In partial epilepsies, the epileptogenic focus is hypoperfused interictally and hyperperfused during the ictal discharge (Rowe *et al.*, 1989). The topography of perfusion abnormalities

---

Figure 11.1 (a) ^{133}Xe SPECT imaging (levels OM + 60 mm and OM + 40 mm) in a 3-month-boy with infantile spasms. The scale from white to black correlates with low to high rCBF values. There is a clear hypoperfused area in the right temporo-parieto-occipital region. (b) ^{133}Xe SPECT imaging (levels OM + 60 mm and OM + 40 mm) in the same boy aged 4.5 years. The infantile spasms have been replaced by partial seizures (oculoclonia). The hypoperfused area is unchanged, involving the right temporo-parieto-occipital region. (c) MRI at 4.5 years shows a subtle abnormality in the right posterior associative region. The child underwent surgical focal exeresis at 5 years of age. Pathology revealed focal dysplasia. (d) EEG in the same boy at 4.5 years of age. There is a right temporo-occipital focus of spikes which corresponds to the rCBF defect (b) and the dysplasia (c).

was correlated with the semiology of seizures and with the interictal EEG foci in 50–70% of cases in various series (Denays *et al.*, 1988; Chiron *et al.*, 1989a; Uvebrant *et al.*, 1991; Adams *et al.*, 1992; Otsubo *et al.*, 1993); the correlation was higher for ictal discharges, ranging from 75 to 95% (Rowe *et al.*, 1989; Hwang *et al.*, 1990). Similar characteristics were present in IS. All those patients who later exhibited focal epilepsy had exhibited either interictal hypoperfusion or ictal hyperperfusion in the very area in which the discharges later took place: 2 patients (12%) in the study by Dulac *et al.* (1987a), 4 patients (25%) in the study by Hwang *et al.* (in prep.) and 12 patients (46%) in the study by Chiron *et al.* (1993). There was also a good correlation between perfusion abnormalities and persisting EEG foci, whether or not the focal seizures persisted: 9 of 12 (Dulac *et al.*, 1987a) and 21 of 24 (Chiron *et al.*, 1993) patients who had areas of hypoperfusion exhibited EEG abnormalities in the same area (Fig. 11.1). The correspondence was not as good as in the study by Hwang *et al.* (in prep.) or among the patients with tuberous sclerosis studied by Chiron *et al.* (1990b), in which only 47–58% of focal perfusion abnormalities were related to an EEG focus. However, Hwang *et al.* (in prep.) pointed out that a high proportion of EEG foci may have been overlooked in patients with hypsarrhythmia; in tuberous sclerosis, not all tubers are epileptogenic (Cusmai *et al.*, 1990a) and therefore hypoperfused areas do not always correspond to epileptic foci. The hypoperfused areas not sustained by a tuber are those that have the highest correspondence with EEG, since 75% of them correspond to a focus. It is therefore likely that in most cases hypoperfused cortical areas observed after IS underlie epileptogenic foci.

In addition, all series have shown that the best correlation involves posterior abnormalities. In one series, 100% of posterior hypoperfused areas corresponded to temporal and/or occipital EEG foci (Dulac *et al.*, 1987a). This percentage was 95% in a series with rCBF quantification (Chiron *et al.*, 1993) and 70% in the series of Hwang *et al.* (in prep). And among tuberous sclerosis patients, it was 63 and 87%, depending on whether or not there was a corresponding tuber (Chiron *et al.*, 1990b). Therefore, epileptogenic foci that persist after IS were mainly posterior in origin.

Hypoperfused areas sustain elective cognitive disorders. In adult focal epilepsy, the focal hypoperfused areas related to epileptogenic foci are associated with cognitive disorders corresponding to a dysfunction of this cortical area (Homan *et al.*, 1989). In children, the first demonstration of a correspondence between hypoperfusion and neuropsychological deficit involved IS (Chiron *et al.*, 1987); since then, case reports with or without epilepsy have shown the same correspondence (Jambaqué and Dulac, 1989; Lou *et al.*, 1990). In the first study that dealt with cryptogenic IS (Chiron *et al.*, 1987), persistent neuropsychological deficits consisted of dysphasias, agnosias or dyspraxic disorders; the patients had hypoperfused areas that involved corresponding cortical areas – temporal in dysphasic patients, parieto-occipito-temporal in dyspraxic patients. More recently, in three patients with visuomotor incoordination, rCBF as measured by ^{133}Xe has demonstrated the persistence of a hypoperfused area in the temporo-occipital cortex, a region that is known to contribute to visuospatial function (Jambaqué *et al.*, 1993). It is also important to note that the neurospsychological sequelae of IS mainly involve functions sustained by the posterior cortex.

Hypoperfused areas are present from the very beginning of IS. From the first qualitative study with ^{133}Xe, it was suspected that these abnormalities were present at the onset of IS, since in seven of the eight patients who exhibited a hypoperfused area, its topography was that of the predominant abnormalities disclosed by the first EEG recording (Dulac *et al.*, 1987a). The same applied to four of the five patients with elective neuropsychological troubles, whereas the four patients without persistent hypoperfusion had not exhibited any EEG focus at onset (Chiron *et al.*, 1989b).

A more recent quantitative study confirms this hypothesis: 18 of 20 patients who underwent SPECT investigation at the onset of IS exhibited at least one hypoperfused area (Chiron *et al.*, 1993). These rCBF defects have the same characteristics as those discovered at later stages: they are observed in both symptomatic and cryptogenic cases, they mainly involve the posterior cortex (80%), and in 75% of patients they correspond to an EEG focus in the same area, a focus disclosed by intravenous administration of diazepam. As shown on some hypometabolized areas using PET (Chugani *et al.*, 1990), these hypoperfused areas remain unchanged throughout the evolution of IS; they are observed in the same proportion and in the same areas up to 3 years after onset. They are indeed epileptogenic, since five of seven patients with a long follow-up developed focal epilepsy precisely in the same areas (Fig. 11.1).

The hypoperfused areas are likely to correspond to a cortical lesion. PET and SPECT studies in surgical cases showed that part of the hypometabolism and hypoperfusion in the epileptogenic focus most often corresponded to a cortical lesion which could be overlooked on CT or MRI (Engel *et al.*, 1982; Stefan *et al.*, 1990). In patients with tuberous sclerosis who were qualitatively studied with ^{133}Xe, 85% of the hypoperfused areas were sustained by a tuber (Chiron *et al.*, 1990b). In Hwang and co-workers' (in prep.) series, two patients underwent surgery, and they both had focal cortical dysplasia; MRI was normal but SPECT showed hypoperfusion of this area. Chugani *et al.* (1990) were the first to show that hypometabolic areas in IS could result from focal dysplasia.

Therefore, rCBF–SPECT studies suggest that some hypoperfused areas discovered throughout the evolution of IS are due to epileptogenic foci resulting from cortical lesions that precede the onset of the disease.

Areas of Hyperperfusion

Hyperperfused areas have not been noted interictally in IS up until now, but small foci of increased rCBF are difficult to recognize on SPECT images and rCBF quantification is needed to detect them. The following data are based on preliminary results only (Chiron *et al.*, 1993).

Hyperperfused Areas in IS

All 20 patients who underwent ^{133}Xe investigation in the acute phase of IS exhibited at least one area of cortical hyperperfusion. It was not a mild phenomenon, in that a mean of 3.5 foci of hyperperfusion were observed per patient and the increase of perfusion involved nearly 10% of the cortical areas compared with 6% for the decrease in perfusion mentioned previously. rCBF studies in partial epilepsies in both adults and children have shown that hyperfusion results from an ictal discharge in the epileptogenic focus (Rowe *et al.*, 1989; Hwang *et al.*, 1990). Although these 20 IS patients were interictally investigated – that is, without any concomitant spasms or partial discharge recorded on simultaneous EEG – they all had at that point an intense spiking activity, and 13 had a typical hypsarrhythmic pattern. Hyparrhythmia has been considered a special type of nonconvulsive status epilepticus, because it comprises diffuse and continuous slow spikes and waves (Beaumanoir, 1973). The multiple foci of hyperfusion are likely to express the continuous and diffuse paroxysmal cortical activity of hypsarrhythmia.

The hyperactivity is independent of whether or not there is any brain lesion (apparent on MRI) and of the number of lesions. Multiple areas of hyperperfusion are indeed observed in both cryptogenic and symptomatic West syndrome, and in tuberous sclerosis with multiple tubers as well as in porencephaly with a single lesion (Chiron *et al.*, 1993).

The topography of the areas of hyperperfusion is consistent. In contrast with the hypoperfused areas, they are mostly bilateral (85% of cases) and mainly involve the anterior cortex: 78% of them are frontal, with about the same percentage in cryptogenic (80%) and symptomatic (73%) cases (Chiron *et al.*, 1993; Fig. 11.2).

Evolution with Steroid Therapy

High-dose steroids, as usually administered in IS, seem to decrease global cortical perfusion (Futagi *et al.*, 1988). We obtained similar findings, with a decreased global perfusion from 2.5 SD to 1.25 SD at the end of steroid treatment (Chiron *et al.*, 1993). In three control patients who were not epileptic but received the same steroid therapy for cerebello-opsomyoclonic syndrome, the perfusion decreased by 2 SD after 1 month of steroid treatment. The decrease in cortical perfusion is therefore a nonspecific effect of steroids. This action could underlie some of the adverse effects of steroids on the CNS, such as decreased EEG activity and the radiological aspect of pseudo cortico-subcortical atrophy, which are known to reverse after cessation of treatment (Satoh *et al.*, 1982).

Regionally, this decrease in perfusion produces on the one hand a discrete increase in the number and size of hypoperfused areas, some of which may be disclosed by steroid treatment, and on the other a discrete reduction in the number and extent of hyperperfused areas. This is compatible with a global effect and suggests that there is no specific effect on particular regions of the cortex. But the frontal regions showed remarkable behaviour: after steroid treatment, the number of frontal hyperperfused foci decreased from 76 to 63%. It is interesting to note that this reduction concerned in the main those patients who ceased having spasms (from 76 to 55%), whereas there was no change for those whose spasms persisted (from 76 to 71%).

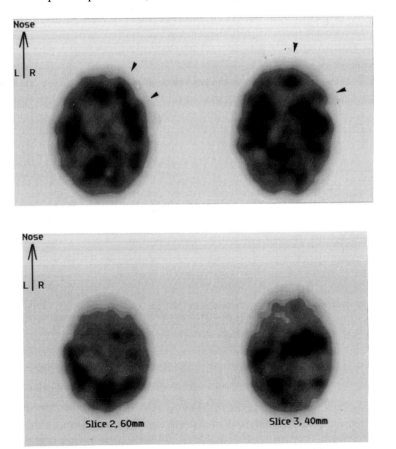

Figure 11.2 (a) ^{133}Xe SPECT imaging (levels OM + 60 mm and OM + 40 mm) in a 6-month-girl with infantile spasms. The scale from white to black correlates with low to high rCBF values. There are numerous foci of hyperperfusion, mainly located in the frontal lobes. (b) ^{133}Xe SPECT imaging at the same levels in a normal 6-month-old girl. The low frontal rCBF is physiological at this age and completely different from the high activity observed in (a) in this area.

The frontal lobe would seem, therefore, to support multiple foci of hyperperfusion at the onset of IS. Corticotherapy reduces this hyperperfusion, but in patients for whom this effect is insufficient, spasms tend to persist. This frontal hyperperfusion would seem, therefore, to play an essential role in the long-term prognosis of IS.

SPECT Studies and Prognosis of IS

Prognostic Value of the Number of Lesions

The epileptic and mental prognosis of IS is partly related to the number and extent of cortical lesions. In tuberous sclerosis, there is a negative relationship between the number of tubers and IQ, behaviour and severity of epilepsy (Jambaqué *et al.*, 1991). The same relationship applies to the number of hypoperfused areas observed at the later stage of IS. Among 16 tuberous sclerosis cases with IS investigated qualitatively with [133]Xe (Chiron *et al.*, 1990b), 12 evolved favorably with cessation of epilepsy and 3 had normal SPECT, whereas 6 exhibited areas of hypoperfusion that were restricted to the tubers. On the other hand, the four whose severe secondary generalized epilepsy persisted had at least four wide areas of hypoperfusion which clearly exceeded the size of the corresponding tubers and which involved cortical areas devoid of tubers in two patients. In addition to severe epilepsy, these patients suffered from global mental retardation, whereas the other 12 had either normal ($n = 6$) or mildly delayed ($n = 6$) mental development.

Conversely, the absence of any lesion correlated with favourable outcome, without epileptic or mental sequelae, can be used to define idiopathic West Syndrome (Dulac *et al.*, 1993a; Vigevano *et al.*, 1993). The six patients reported with a normal rCBF either were no longer epileptic (Hwang *et al.*, in prep.) or exhibited normal neuropsychological status (Chiron *et al.*, 1987). Such a favorable outcome can be predicted based on a normal rCBF pattern at the onset of WS (Chiron *et al.*, 1993).

Prognostic Value of the Topography of Lesions

Evolution of epilepsy. Frontal abnormalities are associated with a poor prognosis of IS. Spasms are more resistant in patients with frontal lesions than in those with posterior lesions only (Cusmai *et al.*, 1988). The majority of patients with bilateral frontal lesions continue to experience severe symptomatic generalized epilepsy of the Lennox-Gastaut type or secondary generalized epilepsy after the spasms (Jambaqué *et al.*, 1991; Koo *et al.*, 1993.) The predominant EEG abnormalities that persist in those intractable epilepsies are located in the frontal areas: slow spike waves predominate in the frontal lobes in LGS, and secondary bisynchrony mainly results from frontal involvement (Gastaut and Zifkin, 1988).

In patients with tuberous sclerosis who underwent ^{133}Xe investigation, 75% of those with persistent generalized epilepsy exhibited extensive areas of bilateral frontal hypoperfusion and bisynchrony; in contrast, among the 12 patients who had a favorable outcome, only one exhibited bilateral frontal hypoperfusion and 3 unilateral frontal hypoperfusion, and none of the 12 exhibited bisynchrony. In addition, 2 of 4 patients with severe epilepsy had hypoperfusion without tubers, compared with 2 of 12 in the favorable group. In a qualitative ^{133}Xe study including the latter 16 patients together with tuberous sclerosis patients who had not exhibited IS, we were able to show that such areas of hypoperfusion without tubers correspond to epileptic foci, which mainly involve the temporal region (60%); these temporal hypoperfused areas mainly concern patients with intractable epilepsy (Chiron *et al.*, 1990b). These abnormalities are likely to be secondary, since the temporal cortex is known to be particularly vulnerable and epileptogenic.

It appears that frontal lesions put patients at high risk of further epilepsy which is intractable because of secondary generalization due to bisynchronism, and which is likely to produce secondary temporal lesions. The latter would be epileptogenic themselves and would help to worsen the epilepsy and prolong it.

Mental evolution. The mental evolution of IS also seems to be worsened by frontal abnormalities, either because of the persistence of severe epilepsy which is always associated with severe mental retardation, or because of the frontal involvement of the initial lesions (Jambaque *et al.*, 1991). These authors suggest that the involvement of the frontal lobe may contribute to the development of autism.

In a qualitative ^{133}Xe study involving 13 cryptogenic patients who were studied neuropsychologically, severe mental retardation only persisted in those five patients with frontal hypoperfusion (Chiron *et al.*, 1987). In contrast with those patients who only had posterior areas of hypoperfusion, they suffered from global, not elective cognitive disorders. They also had particular behavioral problems, four of them being autistic. This relationship between frontal hypoperfusion and autism has recently been confirmed in a quantitative study (Jambaqué *et al.*, 1993): the three autistic patients in this series were the only ones to have frontal hypoperfusion. However, frontal hypoperfusion was not their only feature, since in both studies there were also posterior, temporal or parieto-occipito-temporal involvement. This double localization supports the hypothesis of a double involvement in autism which consists of sensorial and verbal dysfunction sustained by the posterior part of the brain on the one hand, and a perceptivo-frontal disorganization sustained by the prefrontal cortex and posterior-anterior connections on the other. Indeed, in autism without epilepsy, abnormalities of the relationship between posterior parietal and frontal cortex have been reported although no area of hypometabolism could be disclosed (Rumsey *et al.*, 1985; De Volder *et al.*, 1987). In patients with IS, the regions supposed to produce seizures sustain hypoperfusion and their special topography produces autism (Chiron et al., 1987). The epilepsy could therefore be considered as a topographic marker that visualizes the areas of cortical dysfunction in autistic patients.

HYPOTHESIS CONCERNING IS

These rCBF findings need to be confirmed in a larger series and particularly in longer term follow-up studies, but it is presently possible to elaborate a coherent physiopathological hypothesis of IS. The anomalies disclosed by SPECT in cortex complement the PET findings that clarify subcortical functioning and cortico–subcortical relations at a given moment in the evolution of IS (Chugani et al., 1992).

The onset of IS results from the combination of two pathological phenomena, a posterior cortical lesion and frontal hyperactivity. The posterior lesion could be the *primum movens*: this lesion precedes the spasms, and is located in a region that reaches functional maturity in the second trimester of life, the very age of onset of IS. Thus this lesion becomes epileptogenic at that age because of physiological maturation and it produces discharges. Since the immature brain is less able than the adult brain to suppress the generalization, these discharges tend to diffuse and to enhance the development of bilateral foci (Haas et al., 1990). Since the inhibitory systems are underdeveloped and myelinization of the corpus callosum is not complete, the discharges follow both the homolateral and contralateral fibers, resulting in intra- and inter-hemispheric diffusion without any synchronism (Moshé, 1987). Therefore, the multiple foci of hyperactivity result in an apparently anarchic generalized activity of spikes and slow waves. As a result of this diffuse dysfunction, the cortex loses the ability to exert its normal inhibitory role upon subcortical structures and lets them produce clusters of brief tonic phenomena, the spasms. If the level of cortical activity remains high, particularly on the frontal lobes, spasms persist. The myelination of transcallosal fibers that starts at the age of 2 years and continues until the end of the first decade, helps to synchronize frontal foci and induce secondary generalized epilepsy in the original sense of the term. This epilepsy, usually intractable, hinders mental development and can produce secondary lesions in the temporal regions. The temporal cortex is indeed highly epileptogenic and the discharges at this level produce axonal sprouting and reactive synaptogenesis (Sutula et al., 1989); these synapses constitute epileptic foci that maintain the epilepsy and worsen its consequences.

Infantile spasms therefore constitute a particular model of focal epilepsy that, as a consequence of physiological processes of cortical maturation and of the asynchronism of antero-posterior development, results during the second trimester of life in a generalized epilepsy consisting of spasms and hypsarrhythmia. In idiopathic cases, the phenomenon of generalization occurs, although there is no focal lesion; it could be purely functional, due to the particular genetic or biochemical background of some patients. This model of infantile epilepsy is different from that of adults; in the mature brain, the pathophysiology includes reactive synaptogenesis that maintains the epileptic processes (Represa *et al.*, 1989), whereas in IS the epilepsy prevents the normal regression of redundant neurophysiological pathways.

12

Functional Imaging: PET

H.T. CHUGANI

The development of high-resolution tomographic imaging of the brain in the past 10 years has had a significant impact on the diagnosis and management of West syndrome. The use of anatomical neuroimaging with computed tomography (CT) and magnetic resonance imaging (MRI) to detect structural abnormalities in patients with West syndrome is described in Chapter 10. However, many of the microscopic cytoarchitectural abnormalities alluded to and described in some detail in Chapter 9 are not detected by CT and MRI. Functional neuroimaging with single photon emission computed tomography (SPECT) may detect perfusion abnormalities associated with some of the more widespread microscopic disturbances or cortical lamination defects seen in West syndrome (described in Chapter 11). High-resolution functional neuroimaging with positron emission tomography (PET) can detect even small areas of focal cortical dysplasia, and also has provided some insight into the neuroanatomical circuitry involved in the generation and propagation of the epileptic spasms in West syndrome. The important role of PET in the preoperative evaluation and surgical treatment of medically refractory spasms is discussed in Chapter 23.

BASIC CONCEPTS OF PET METHODOLOGY

PET is a noninvasive imaging method which can be used to measure local chemical functions in various body organs. This technique employs a camera consisting of multiple pairs of oppositely situated detectors which are used to record the paired high-energy (511 KeV) photons travelling in opposite directions as a result of positron decay (Hoffman and Phelps, 1986). Tracer kinetic models which mathematically describe physiological or biochemical reaction sequences of compounds labeled with positron-emitting isotopes permit a characterization of the kinetics and the mathematical expression for calculating actual rates of the biological process being studied (Huang and Phelps, 1986). Because of the short half-life (minutes to hours) of the isotopes commonly used in PET, it is essential that the cyclotron used to generate these isotopes be

156

situated either on-site or within 1–2 h driving distance from the PET scanning facility. The clinical and research applications of PET methodology have been steadily increasing, and at present over 300 substrates and drugs labeled with positron-emitters are available for the study of various biological functions *in vivo* (Fowler and Wolfe, 1986). In the brain, PET has been applied in the study of local glucose and oxygen utilization, blood flow, protein synthesis, and neurotransmitter uptake and binding (Phelps and Mazziotta, 1985). With most current PET scanners (e.g. CTI 831 positron tomograph, Knoxville, TN), it is possible to obtain relatively high-resolution images (15 images, spatial resolution of 4.2 mm in plane of section, 6.3 mm slice thickness) (Hoffman *et al.*, 1987). However, a more recently developed PET scanner (CTI-713, Knoxville, TN) provides 15 slices at 3.4 mm spacing, with intrinsic resolution of 3.5 mm (transaxial) by 4.4 mm (axial) (Cutler *et al.*, 1992).

Dosimetry

The major PET tracer applied in the study of epileptic spasms is 2-deoxy-2[^{18}F]fluoro-D-glucose (FDG), which provides a measure of local cerebral glucose utilization. With the usual injected dose (0.143 mCi/kg) of this tracer, the whole body radiation dose to the child is only about 300 mrad (0.3 cGy). Peak dose is to the bladder and is about 2 rad (2 cGy). The dose to the brain is 500 mrad (0.5 cGy), and compares favorably to the dose in CT scanning, which is on the order of 1–3 rad (1–3 cGy) (Chugani, 1992).

FOCAL CORTICAL ABNORMALITIES

Studies using PET in children with West syndrome and normal CT and MRI scans have shown that a number of patients previously diagnosed with "cryptogenic" spasms have focal cortical regions of decreased glucose utilization on *interictal* PET (Fig. 12.1a) (Chugani *et al.*, 1990, 1992). When PET is performed in the ictal state, or if frequent interictal spiking occurs during the tracer uptake period (first 30 min after tracer administration) of the PET study, increased glucose utilization may be seen instead (Fig. 12.1b). Focal ictal and/or interictal EEG abnormalities correspond to the PET focus in virtually all of these cases. In infants with hypsarrythmia, these focal EEG abnormalities may either precede or follow the presence of hypsarrythmia in the evolution of the infants' EEGs. Longitudinal studies of PET in the same infants indicate the persistent and stable nature of these focal metabolic abnormalities (Fig. 12.2).

When the PET study is performed too early in the course of West syndrome, however, focal hypometabolism may be difficult to detect due to the fact that glucose metabolism of immature cerebral cortex is typically low in the first year of life (Chugani and Phelps, 1986; Chugani *et al.*, 1987). We have encountered several infants with intractable spasms and normal MRI whose initial PET scans (performed prior to 15 months of age) were nonfocal despite the presence of interictal and/or ictal focal features on the EEG. In each case, when the PET study was repeated 6–12 months later, a metabolic focus corresponding to EEG localization became apparent (Fig. 12.3). Based on this experience, we recommend that infants with West syndrome, intractable seizures and lateralizing features on EEG or clinical examination, and who fail to show focal abnormality on PET, should have the PET study repeated after age 15 months when cerebral glucose metabolism shows its normal maturational increase (Chugani *et al.*, 1987).

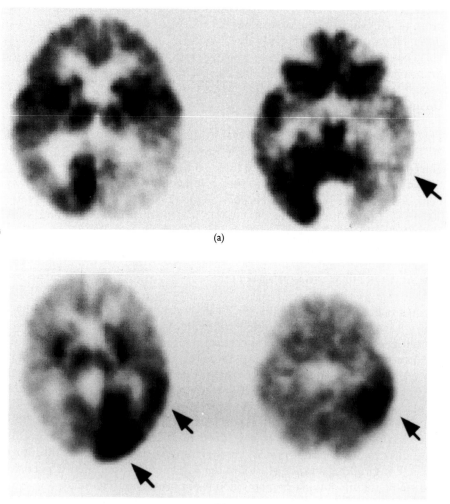

(a)

(b)

Figure 12.1   (a) Interictal PET scan of a 9-month-old baby with infantile spasms showing decreased glucose metabolism in the parieto-occipito-temporal distribution. The MRI scan was normal. (b) Increased glucose utilization seen in the left parieto-occipito-temporal region of a 5-month-old baby with spasms whose PET scan was performed in the ictal state. The MRI scan showed left occipito-temporal pachygyria.

Whereas our initial report of PET-defined focal cortical abnormalities indicated a parieto-occipito-temporal topography (Chugani *et al.*, 1990), further experience shows that any cortical area can be involved (Chugani *et al.*, 1993). In some cases, an entire hemisphere can be hypometabolic on PET and documented to be epileptogenic. In addition, although our earlier report included only females, it is now clear that males as well as females can harbor these metabolically defined lesions associated with epileptic spasms. When PET is the sole neuroimaging modality to identify the epileptogenic area, neuropathological examination of the brain tissue shows a high incidence of malformative and dysplastic lesions affecting the cortex and underlying white matter (Vinters *et al.*, 1992).

SUBCORTICAL ACTIVATION PATTERNS

A number of features distinguish the spasms of West syndrome from most other epileptic disorders. These include the age-specificity, the typically poor

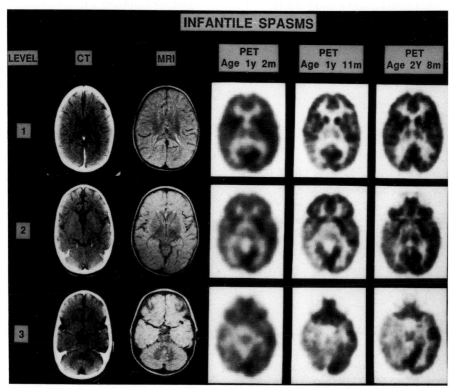

Figure 12.2 Computed tomography (CT), MRI and PET scans of a child with intractable infantile spasms. PET was performed three times between 1 year 2 months and 2 years 8 months, and revealed a persistent decrease in glucose metabolism in the right occipito-temporal region.

response to conventional anticonvulsants, and the relatively symmetric myoclonus-like semiology of the spasms. The latter feature suggests that subcortical brain areas may be important to the neuronal network involved in the pathophysiology of spasms. Indeed, there is considerable evidence based on clinical, physiological and pharmacological studies to suggest that the brainstem, particularly structures near sleep-regulating centers in the pons, may be essential components of this neuronal circuitry.

Studies analyzing sleep patterns in infants with West syndrome have documented decreased rapid eye movements (REM) sleep and less total sleep time when compared with normal infants (Fukuyama *et al.*, 1979b; Hrachovy *et al.*, 1981). Only infants whose spasms and hypsarrythmic pattern on EEG improved with ACTH or prednisone showed a reversal of the REM sleep abnormality. These observations suggest that anatomical substrates in close proximity to centers that regulate sleep cycles in the pons may be involved in the generation or propagation of spasms. Coleman (1971) induced infantile spasms in patients with Down syndrome by administering the serotonin precursor 5-hydroxytryptophan, and Silverstein and Johnston found lower cerebrospinal fluid concentrations of the serotonin metabolite 5-hydoxyindole acetic acid (5-HIAA) in infants with spasms compared with age-matched controls (Silverstein and Johnston, 1984). These findings suggest a state of supersensitivity of serotonin receptors in infants with spasms resulting in

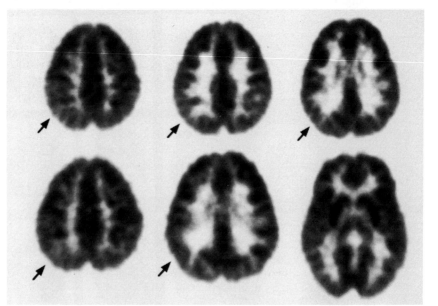

Figure 12.3 Two PET studies from the same child with intractable infantile spasms. At age 15 months (top three images), there was a suggestion of decreased glucose utilization in the right parieto-occipito-temporal distribution (arrows), but the study was interpreted as normal. At age 21 months (bottom three images), the hypometabolic area (arrows) was slightly more prominent and corresponded to the EEG focus.

diminished presynaptic serotonin turnover and release from serotonin-containing neurons which are concentrated in the raphe region of the pons (Silverstein and Johnson, 1984). It should be noted that there is also a well-established relationship between abnormal serotonin metabolism and myoclonic disorders, which epileptic spasms have been said to resemble clearly (Klawans *et al.*, 1973; Chadwick *et al.*, 1975; Nausieda *et al.*, 1982) (for a review, see Chapter 1).

With PET technology, the participation of brainstem structures in the neuronal network of spasms was directly demonstrated (Chugani *et al.*, 1984). Although it is often difficult to distinguish between the pons and other brainstem regions with the current spatial resolution of PET, glucose metabolism in the brainstem region was clearly increased in 21 of 44 infants with West syndrome (Chugani *et al.*, 1992). This study also demonstrated activation of the lenticular nuclei, seen with even higher frequency (32 of the 44 infants) than brainstem activation. The pattern of lenticular nuclei activation on PET was quite characteristic, consisting of symmetrically increased glucose utilization even when focal hypo or hypermetabolism was present in the cortex (Fig. 12.4).

It is not clear why a subcortical activation pattern is not *always* present on the PET scans of infants with West syndrome. Detailed analyses of age and sex of infant, EEG pattern at various times (including during the tracer uptake period of PET), and exposure to various pharmacological agents, however, failed to uncover any factor that could predict the presence or absence of subcortical activation on PET (Chugani *et al.*, 1992). It is possible that the pattern of lenticular nuclei and brainstem activation corresponds to a pathophysiological state that predisposes to infantile spasms. Further studies using PET in infants prior to treatment of the spasms may provide further insight into clinical and electrographic correlations of subcortical metabolic pattern seen in West syndrome.

NEURONAL NETWORK IN EPILEPTIC SPASMS

As alluded to above, it is widely believed that the brainstem is an essential component of the neuronal network involved in the generation and propagation of epileptic spasms. In fact, some investigators believe the brainstem to be the *primary* site responsible for the generation of spasms (Hrachovy *et al.*, 1981; Hrachovy and Frost, 1989b). Studies on the neuropathological findings in West syndrome, however, have not suggested a *primary* role for the brainstem. By far the majority of anatomical abnormalities detected in patients with West syndrome have been in the cerebral cortex (Meencke and Gerhard, 1985; Jellinger, 1987; Palm *et al.*, 1986). There is only one report indicating a number of pontine abnormalities in patients who had earlier manifested infantile spasms. (Morimatsu *et al.*, 1972).

The emerging concept is that the spasms of West syndrome are age-specific seizure manifestations of a wide variety of structural or metabolic *cortical* abnormalities (Dulac *et al.*, 1987b), which initiate abnormal cortical–subcortical interactions. This cortical "triggering" mechanism is supported by several reports documenting that epileptic spasms can be provoked by, or associated with, a partial seizure (Dulac *et al.*, 1987b, Yamamoto *et al.*, 1988; Carrazano *et al.*, 1990; Donat and Wright, 1991a). Furthermore, spasms typically do not occur in the neonatal period even in the presence of a structural cortical abnormality. Rather, the timing of spasms seems to coincide with the onset of cortical maturation or "encephalization" as seen on PET studies of the ontogeny of cerebral glucose utilization, i.e. 3–4 months in posterior cortical regions and 6–10 months in frontal cortex (Chugani and Phelps, 1986; Chugani *et al.*, 1987). If the brainstem were to play a primary role in generating epileptic spasms, one would expect spasms to occur in the neonatal period when

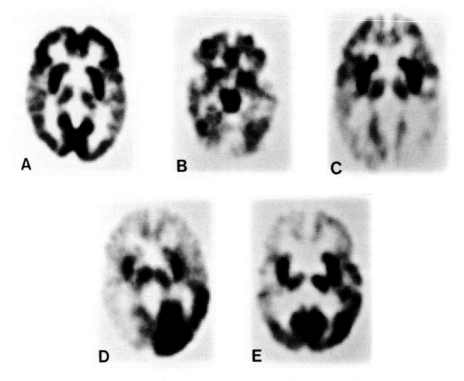

Figure 12.4 PET images of five patients with infantile spasms illustrating increased glucose utilization patterns in lenticular nuclei and/or brainstem regardless of associated abnormalities in cerebral cortex. (A) Lenticular nuclei hypermetabolism and bilateral temporal cortex hypometabolism; (B) brainstem hypermetabolism; (C) lenticular nuclei hypermetabolism and left occipito-temporal cortex hypometabolism; (D) lenticular nuclei hypermetabolism and left occipito-temporal cortex hypermetabolism; (E) lenticular nuclei hypermetabolism associated with right frontal, temporal and lateral occipital and left frontal cortex hypometabolism.

brainstem function is relatively mature (Chugani and Phelps, 1986; Chugani *et al.*, 1987). The notion that epileptic spasms result from abnormal cortical–subcortical interactions is neither novel nor unique. In fact, such an interaction is essential for seizure generation in some animal models of epilepsy (Gale, 1985; Browning 1985).

Any model describing the neuronal network for the origin and propagation of epileptic spasms, however, must also accommodate the finding of lenticular nuclei activation seen on PET studies (Chugani *et al.*, 1992). Figure 12.5 summarizes our attempt to provide such a model. A key feature in this model is that the cortical abnormality exerts a noxious influence over the brainstem, from where discharges spread rostrally to lenticular nuclei and caudally to spinal cord, accounting for the *relative* symmetry of the spasms (Chugani *et al.*, 1992). The primary cortical abnormality can be either focal or diffuse. At a critical stage of maturation, the abnormal cortical substrate initiates abnormal functional interactions with brainstem raphe nuclei. These nuclei house a large number of serotonin-synthesizing neurons which project widely throughout the brain (Nieuwenhuys, 1985).

One serotonergic pathway, the raphe–striatal pathway, has strong connections in humans between raphe neurons and putamen bilaterally, and its involvement in spasms may account for the lenticular nuclei and brainstem metabolic activation seen on PET studies. Increased activity of this projection would be consistent with the finding of decreased 5-HIAA in the cerebrospinal fluid of infants with West syndrome (Silverstein and Johnston, 1984). The fact that the raphe–striatal projection may be tonically modulated by corticosteroids (Defiore and Turner, 1983; Schwartzberg and Nakane, 1983; Sarrieau *et al.*, 1988) provides a convenient mechanism of action of steroid therapy in suppressing infantile spasms.

Ascending cortical projections from the raphe area could possibly be involved in producing the pattern of hypsarrythmia seen on the EEG in West syndrome. Since the region around the raphe nuclei is believed to be involved in sleep organization, dysfunction in this area may account for the sleep disturbances in infants with West syndrome (Fukuyama *et al.*, 1979b; Hrachovy *et al.*, 1981) and the fact that infantile spasms often occur soon after arousal from sleep (Kellaway *et al.*, 1979). In contrast, descending spinal pathways from raphe or from the closely associated reticular formation, and the ascending raphe–striatal projections, may be more involved with the relatively symmetric motor manifestations of the spasms.

Knowledge of the neuronal circuitry associated with spasms in West syndrome may offer new therapeutic approaches through pharmacological manipulation. However, the serotonin projection system is complex, with the existence of multiple receptors which bind to this neurotransmitter in the central nervous system. It is now recognized that there are at least six types of serotonin receptors in the brain (Peroutka, 1988), of which 5-HT$_{1D}$ receptors are the predominant type in the terminals of the raphe-striatal projections (Herrick-Davies *et al.*, 1989; Waeber *et al.*, 1988, 1989).

The development of specific antagonists to 5-HT$_{1D}$ receptors may offer a rational novel approach to the suppression of epileptic spasms. In fact, broad-spectrum serotonin receptor antagonists have already been attempted, but have failed to demonstrate clinical efficacy possibly because of low binding affinity to the 5-HT$_{1D}$ receptor (Hrachovy *et al.*, 1988a, 1989).

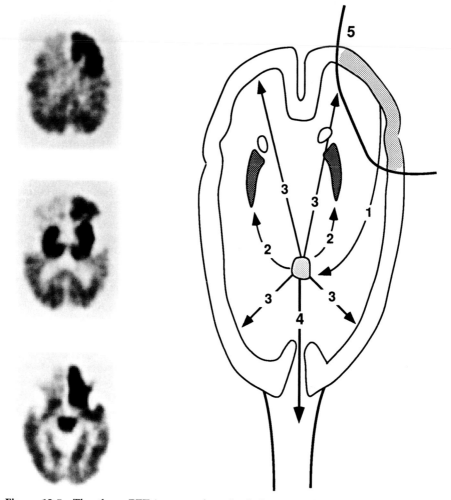

Figure 12.5 The three PET images of cerebral glucose utilization on the left of the figure illustrate hypermetabolism of the left fronto-temporal cortex, bilateral symmetric hypermetabolism of the lenticular nuclei and the brainstem in a patient with intractable infantile spasms. On the right of the figure is a schematic diagram describing the proposed neuronal circuitry involved in the pathogenesis of infantile spasms: (1) noxious influence of abnormal cortical region on brainstem (raphe area); (2) raphe–striatal pathway, serotonergic (5HT$_{1D}$), under tonic control by corticosteroids; (3) generation of hypsarrythmic pattern; (4) spinal cord propagation (direct or indirect) and lenticular nuclei involvement result in clinical infantile spasms; (5) surgical resection of primary cortical abnormality abolishes activation of circuitry.

Finally, the cortical origin of epileptic spasms proposed in the neuronal network summarized in Fig. 12.5 is both entirely consistent with, and supported by, accumulating evidence that surgical resection of a focal structural or metabolic cortical abnormality abolishes both the spasms and hypsarrythmic EEG pattern (Chugani *et al.*, 1990, 1993; Branch and Dyken, 1979; Palm *et al.*, 1988; Mimaki *et al.*, 1983; Ruggieri *et al.*, 1989; Uthman *et al.*, 1991), presumably as a result of ablation of the cortical generator depicted in the model shown in Fig. 12.5. Surgical management of West syndrome is discussed in further detail in Chapter 23.

13

Introduction to Etiology

B. DALLA BERNARDINA, O. DULAC

No list of the identified causes of infantile spasms (IS) could ever be exhaustive, given the increasing number of single case reports related to various specific brain diseases. Indeed, it has been said that IS are an age-related but non-specific reaction of the brain to any kind of brain damage. However, most of these single patient case reports, although well studied from the etiological point of view, are poorly documented from the electroclinical point of view, with regard to the ictal and interictal characteristics. As stressed in Chapter 6, although patients with Angelman syndrome (Bower and Jeavons, 1967) or biotinidase deficiency (Colamaria *et al.*, 1989) are considered on occasion to exhibit IS, the electroclinical pattern is usually different from that of IS, since the type of seizure consists of massive myoclonus, not epileptic spasms. This distinction has therapeutic implications. Therefore, it is likely that the list of potential etiologies of IS is somewhat overestimated.

CAUSES OF INFANTILE SPASMS

Etiologies of IS are usually classified into symptomatic cases due to pre-, peri- and postnatal causes, and cryptogenic cases. Perinatal causes account for 15% of cases, the 25% incidence rate classically suggested clearly being overesti-mated, as shown by modern neuroimaging (Aicardi, 1986a). The frequency of postnatal causes has been widely overestimated due to the erroneous interpre-tation of so-called post-immunization IS that are now known to be cryptogenic in most cases.

Cerebral malformations account for 30–34% of neuropathological cases (Jellinger, 1987). They occur in isolation or as part of various neurocutaneous syndromes – tuberous sclerosis, neurofibromatosis or sebaceous naevus (Martin-Blasquez *et al.*, 1988). They include midline defects such as holopro-sencephaly (Jellinger, 1970), callosal agenesis both due to (Yamamoto *et al.*, 1985) and not due to Aicardi syndrome (Diebler and Dulac, 1987) – septal agenesis (Kuriyama *et al.*, 1988), hypothalamic hamartoma (Gomibuchi *et al.*, 1990), schizencephaly (Yakovlev and Wadsworth, 1946), hydranencephaly

166

(Neville, 1972), four-layered micropolygyria (Jellinger, 1970; Meencke and Gerhard, 1985), Rett syndrome (Hagberg, 1993), subcortical laminar heterotopia (Moutard *et al.*, 1994) and congenital bilateral perisylvian syndrome (Kuzniecky *et al.*, 1991b). Dysplastic disorders range from lissencephaly, particularly of the Miller-Dieker type with 17p13 chromosomal deletion (Bordarier *et al.*,1986), to more focal dysplasia (Chugani *et al.*, 1990) or hemimegalencephaly (Robain *et al.*, 1989), and microdysgenesis. Microdysgenesis has been suggested as a cause of infantile spasms (Meencke and Gerhard, 1985; Palm, 1986) and of mental retardation in nonepileptic patients (Martin Palida, 1975; Huttenlocher, 1974; see Chapter 9). It is not clear, however, whether the latter abnormalities have a pathogenic role, since they may be observed in normal controls (Lyon and Gastaut, 1985). Vascular malformations are rarely involved (Cusmai *et al.*, 1988), occasionally as part of Sturge-Weber syndrome (Millichap *et al.*, 1962).

Congenital infectious diseases comprise diffuse lesions produced by toxoplasmosis (Christensen and Melchior, 1960), cytomegalovirus (Watanabe *et al.*, 1973), rubella (Riikonen, 1984a) and syphilis (Finkelstein, 1938).

Perinatal brain damage accounts for 36–40% of neuropathological cases (Jellinger, 1987). Although this cause is estimated to account for 18% (Baird and Borofsky, 1957) to 80% (Watanabe *et al.*, 1973) of cases, it is most likely to be overestimated, being about 15% when only patients with marked abnormalities of birth followed by persistent neurological disorders are considered (Aicardi and Chevrie, 1978). They comprise porencephaly (Alvarez *et al.*, 1987; Cusmai *et al.*, 1988; Palm *et al.*, 1988), multicystic encephalomalacia (Harris and Pampiglione, 1962; Jellinger, 1970; Meencke and Gerhard, 1985), ulegyria (Bignami *et al.*, 1964) leukomalacia (Jellinger, 1970; Meencke and Gerhard, 1985), scars and gliosis of the cerebral hemispheres, basal ganglia, white matter and cerebellum, while brainstem lesions are rare (Tominaga *et al.*, 1986). Small-for-date infants have been said to be three times more likely to develop IS than true prematures (Crichton, 1968), as a result of uterine hemorrhage or toxemia. Neonatal hypoglycemia was reported as a major cause in one series (Riikonen and Donner, 1979).

Postnatal insults mainly comprise anoxic–ischemic, infectious and traumatic disorders, particularly subdural hematoma (Millichap *et al.*, 1962a) and formerly Reye syndrome (Garcia de Alba *et al.*, 1989). Anoxia–ischemia results from near drowning (Ganji *et al.*, 1987; Hrachovy *et al.*, 1987), near miss sudden death syndrome (Aubourg *et al.*, 1985) or surgery for cardiac malformation.

Various metabolic diseases account for 10% (Meencke and Gerhard, 1985) to 17% (Jellinger, 1987) of IS cases. They include Van Boggaert-Bertrand's spongy dystrophy (Meencke and Gerhard, 1985; Poser and Low, 1960), Krabbe's disease (Andrews *et al.*, 1971; Williams *et al.*, 1979), neonatal adrenoleukodystrophy (Aubourg *et al.*, 1986), Leigh's disease (Diebler and Dulac, 1987; Kamoshita *et al.*, 1970), orthochromatic leukodystrophy (Bignami, 1966), pyridoxine deficiencies (French *et al.*, 1965), and various aminoacidopathies including nonketotic hyperglycinemia (Dalla Bernardina *et al.*, 1979), pyruvate carboxylase deficiency (Rutlege et al., 1986), hyperornithinemia, hyperammonemia and homocitrullinemia (Shih et al., 1969), and phenylketonuria that used to be commonly associated with hypsarrhythmia prior to routine neonatal screening (Jellinger, 1987; Poley and Dumermuth, 1968). The potential involvement of histidinemia (Duffner and Cohen, 1975) has not been confirmed.

Various types of tumors may cause IS (Miyake et al., 1986; Morimoto et al., 1989). They involve either the cortex or the basal ganglia and include ependymomas (Ruggieri et al., 1989), gliomas (Ruggieri et al., 1989), gangliogliomas (Gabriel, 1983) and choroid plexus papillomas (Branch and Dyken, 1979), the latter often as part of Aicardi syndrome.

Neonatal bacterial meningitis, brain abscess (Lombroso, 1983a) and herpetic encephalitis (Ohtaki et al., 1987) may also result in IS (Diebler and Dulac, 1987). For various postnatal viral diseases, including cytomegalovirus (Midulla et al., 1976) and Epstein-Barr virus (Bialek et al., 1990), it is more difficult to assess a causal relationship without firm evidence that the virus has produced any brain damage. The same applies to pertussis immunization that was formerly claimed to be a major cause of IS (Melchior, 1977). Recent epidemiological studies have failed to support these assertions based on a lack of modification of age of onset of IS following changes in the immunization calendar: vaccination therefore seems to trigger the onset of IS in infants in whom the disease is destined to develop (Bellman et al., 1983). One report of three cases described lesions similar to those of subacute spongiform encephalopathy, thus suggesting the involvement of a slow virus (Toga and Gambarelli, 1982), but this finding has to be confirmed. Acute inflammatory lesions may not be causally related to IS, but may represent intercurrent or superimposed lethal disorders due to ACTH-related immunosuppression (Jellinger, 1987).

FROM THE ELECTROCLINICAL PATTERN TO ETIOLOGY

This classification into pre-, peri- and postnatal causes is of limited use in clinical practice, unlike the cryptogenic group that can itself be split into two subgroups (see Chapter 20). Indeed, prenatal causes include malformative, metabolic, clastic and even mixed causes (due for instance to the combination of porencephaly and heterotopias). As shown in Chapter 6 and in the following chapters of this section, the electroclinical pattern and the evolution vary according to these different causes. The same applies to peri- and postnatal causes that may both be either clastic or metabolic. Indeed, from a clinical point of view, it is more beneficial to distinguish four groups: clastic, degenerative (metabolic), malformative and cryptogenic/idiopathic.

Regarding the diagnostic work-up, some conditions can easily be recognized from their onset because they are characterized by very specific features (e.g. hypopigmented cutaneous areas in tuberous sclerosis, chorioretinal lacunae of Aicardi syndrome). In most instances, however, the diagnostic approach requires the combination of a whole range of congruent clinical and EEG characteristics, each of which in isolation would fail to establish the diagnosis. Tables 13.1 to 13.3 list the clinical EEG ictal and interictal items that should be taken into consideration. By studying these tables, one is able to identify some of the specific patterns of the clastic, degenerative, malformative and cryptogenic/idiopathic categories of IS.

1. *Clastic IS*. The history comprises acute neurological distress early in life, and the first seizures are often delayed, occurring in the second semester of life or even later. Neurological examination often discloses focal abnormalities and nonepileptic jerks. The EEG shows abnormal background activity, multifocal spikes, focal and generalized tonic seizures. Abnormal interictal EEG activity and focal seizures combined with epileptic spasms are more likely to occur if brain lesions are due to a prenatal cause and are combined with brain malformation (e.g. in cytomegalovirus fetopathy).
2. *Degenerative disease*. Neurological signs increase progressively, and the patients may exhibit erratic myoclonus. The EEG shows progressive disorganization of the background activity, suppression bursts, focal seizures and massive myoclonus. Neuroradiology reveals progressive atrophy.
3. *Malformations*. The patient is hypotonic and may show specific cutaneous stigmata, but there is usually no focal motor deficit. Epileptic spasms occur early in life, often preceded by partial seizures. The EEG shows asymmetrical or unilateral hypsarrhythmia, eventually combined with abnormal background activity, asynchrony and the disappearance of interictal activity between consecutive spasms. The interictal pattern may be specific to a

Table 13.1 Neurological and neuroradiological findings

Etiology	Clastic	Degenerative	Malformative	Cryptogenic/idiopathic
Age of onset of neurological signs	Early	Early	Variable	Late or none
Moderate to severe hypotonia	+	+	+++	−
Focal deficit	++	+++[a]	+/−	−
Progressive impairment	+	++++	−	−
Microcephaly				
congenital	+/−	−	+	−
acquired	++	++	−	−
Specific clinical signs	−	+/−	++	−
Subcontinuous erratic myoclonus	+/−	+++	+/−	−
Abnormal startles	++	+++	+	−
Audiogenic startles	+/−	+++	−	−
Neuroradiology	+++	+/−	++	−

[a]Only following severe seizures.

given malformation, independent of the occurrence of spasms. Epileptic spasms may occur without hypsarrhythmia, and clusters of pseudoperiodic epileptic spasms may be intermingled with a focal seizure.

4. *Cryptogenic idiopathic IS*. There is no unusual history and the development is normal until the first epileptic spasms. Neurological and neuroradiological investigations are negative. The asymmetrical ictal or interictal EEG features, including after benzodiazepine use, indicate cryptogenic IS (Dulac *et al.*, 1986a). Idiopathic cases exhibit only independent spasms.

More specific clinical or EEG aspects may be encountered in given etiologies, as shown in the following chapters.

COURSE ACCORDING TO ETIOLOGY

Four different patterns can be distinguished:

1. *Protracted epileptic spasms*. Malformations involving most of the cerebral cortex (e.g. lissencephaly or Aicardi syndrome) and major destruction (e.g. hydranencephaly) are characterized by intractability and the persistence of clusters of spasms many years after the first seizures occurred.

Table 13.2 Interictal EEG findings

	Clastic	Degenerative	Malformative	Cryptogenic/idiopathic
Hypsarrhythmia as first manifestation	−	−	+/−	+++
Background abnormalities	++	++	+/−	−
Mixed slow waves, fast spikes, focal/multifocal	++	++	+/−	−
Unilateral asymmetric hypsarrhythmia	+/−	−	++	−
Asynchronous hypsarrhythmia	+/−	+/−	++	−
"Sleep" hypsarrhythmia	−	−	++	−
Unusually ample and fast/age activities	+/−[a]	−	++	−
Typical hypsarrhythmia	+/−	−	−	+++[b]
Ictal "vanishing" hypsarrhythmia	+/−	−	+++	+/−[b]
Suppression–burst	+	++	+	−

[a] Cytomegalovirus; [b] see Chapter 1.

Table 13.3   Ictal features

	Clastic	Degenerative	Malformative	Cryptogenic/idiopathic
Spasms as first symptom	−	−	+/−	+++
Partial seizures	++	+++	+++	−
Partial evolving into spasms	+/−	+/−	+++	−
Unilateral/focal spasm	+/−	−	++	−
"Subclinical" spasms	+/−[a]	−	+++	−
Spasms without hypsarrhythmia	+/−[a]	+/−	+++	−
Tonic spasms	+++	+	+/−	−
Massive myoclonic jerks	++	+++	+	−
Other seizures	+	+	+/−	−
Bilateral symmetrical spasms	+/−	+/−	+	+++

[a]Cytomegalovirus.

2. *Multifocal epilepsy.* Multiple epileptogenic cortical lesions, such as tuberous sclerosis or term delivery ischemia, evolve into multifocal or secondarily generalized epilepsies, which are difficult to treat.
3. *Focal epilepsy.* Cases with single epileptogenic foci such as proencephaly, cortical dysplasia, or tuberous sclerosis with single epileptogenic cortical tubers may evolve into, or be preceded by partial seizures.
4. *Lennox-Gastaut syndrome.* The combination of several types of generalized seizures including tonic seizures and atypical absences together with frequent episodes of status epilepticus, and a slow spike and wave pattern, may characterize the outcome of West syndrome, particularly in cryptogenic cases. Differentiation from secondary generalized epilepsy may be difficult, since the latter also frequently follows IS.
5. *Seizure-free patients.* Cessation of seizures may include patients with complete recovery (idiopathic IS) and patients with various degrees of cognitive deficiencies (cryptogenic and symptomatic IS).

14

Genetic Basis

J. FEINGOLD, O. DULAC

Infantile spasms (IS) result from various causes, most of which are associated with brain lesions, and are an age-related syndrome. In most instances, they occur in the first year of life, combined with typical or modified hysarrhythmia, and the combination is called West syndrome. However, a sizable number of patients with genetically determined encephalopathy producing spasms as one major component of the clinical pattern do not exhibit hypsarrhythmia. Therefore, for the study of genetic predisposition, it is preferable to deal with the age-related seizure type, IS, rather than with the more restrictive syndromic concept.

In a study of 77 probands with IS, the incidence of IS observed in their relatives was 7.4 ± 0.52% for first-degree relatives, 0.28 ± 0.28% for second-degree relatives and 0% for third-degree relatives (Fleiszar *et al.*, 1977). The authors suspected a polygenic mode of transmission together with environmental factors. However, since the genetic background varies according to etiology, the genetic predisposition to IS is a mixture of a variety of genetic predispositions, and it may serve as a model for the study of multifactorial genetic predispositions in epilepsy. Indeed, some of the lesions that produce IS are genetically determined, as in tuberous sclerosis. However, its occurrence is also age-related. The age-relationship is reminiscent of several idiopathic and genetically determined epilepsy syndromes, such as absence epilepsy and febrile convulsions. Linkage to a precise chromosomal region is likely for some epilepsy syndromes, for example benign familial neonatal convulsions (Leppert *et al.*, 1989) and juvenile myoclonic epilepsy (Delgado-Escueta *et al.*, 1989). Therefore, the study of the genetic bases of IS needs to consider both the genetically determined diseases that produce IS, and familial antecedents of epilepsy and febrile convulsions.

GENETICALLY DETERMINED DISEASES THAT PRODUCE IS

Monogenic transmission

Many diseases that are either usually or only occasionally associated with IS are genetically determined, involving all modes of inheritance of single genes. IS has occasionally been reported in diseases with autosomic recessive transmission, including various types of leukodystrophy (Andrews *et al.*, 1971; Bignami *et al.*, 1966; Poser and Low, 1960). Leigh's disease (Kamoshita *et al.*, 1970), pyridoxine dependency (French *et al.*, 1965) and various aminoacidopathies such as phenylketonuria (Poley and Dumermuth, 1968). IS has also been reported in diseases with autosomic dominant transmission, including various neurocutaneous syndromes, particularly linear sebaceous syndrome (Martin Blasquez *et al.*, 1988) and neurofibromatosis (Huson *et al.*, 1988), and in rare sex-linked dominant diseases such as incontinentia pigmenti (Simonsson, 1972).

In some genetically determined diseases that frequently produce IS, familial recurrence of IS appears to be quite rare. For example, tuberous sclerosis is often associated with IS, and although several family members may have tuberous sclerosis and epilepsy, it is rare for the combination of tuberous sclerosis and IS to occur in the same family. We are aware of only four families having such a combination, in three of which the affected siblings were twins (Pavone *et al.*, 1980; Pinsard, personal communication; Wilson and Carter, 1978), suggesting that tuberous sclerosis alone may be insufficient for determining the familial recurrence of IS.

Some genetically determined syndromes produce IS as a major component. This is the case in the dominantly inherited CHARGE syndrome, which includes microphthalmy, coloboma, cardiac malformation, mental retardation and deafness together with IS (Curatolo *et al.*, 1983; Pagon *et al.*, 1981), and in several families with X-linked recessive encephalopathy and IS (Menkes *et al.*, 1964; Feinberg and Leahy, 1977; Rugtveit, 1986); in one of the latter there was also partial agenesis of the corpus callosum (Menkes *et al.*, 1964).

Finnish authors have reported a series of familial cases of encephalopathy comprising progressive mental deterioration, limb edema, optic atrophy and hypsarrhythmia. They have called this disease the PEHO syndrome: Progressive encephalopathy with Edema, Hypsarrhythmia and Optic atrophy (Salonen *et al.*, 1991; Somer and Sainio, 1993). In addition, there were specific dysmorphic features that allowed recognition of these patients. Pregnancy and perinatal course were unremarkable. During the first few weeks after birth, patients usually appeared normal, although some had edema of the hands and feet, and others hypotonia. The onset of neurological symptoms ranged from 2 weeks to 4 months with loss of visual contact or with twitching of the extremities that evolved to IS with hypsarrhythmia at 6 months of age. The IS were poorly controlled with ACTH. Pyramidal signs and axial hypotonia appeared in all infants, and the patients neither learned to site or crawl.

Dysmorphism included a long and a low narrow face, epicanthus, midfacial hypoplasia, a small chin and a high and narrow palate with striking gingival hyperplasia. Optic atrophy and microcephaly typically occurred later, and by 2–3 years of age the disease seemed to stabilize with clonic or tonic–clonic and absence seizures. Various biochemical and histological studies have failed to disclose the etiology, and karyotypes have been normal. From the pedigrees it appears that autosomal recessive inheritance is involved.

We have identified four families in which siblings seemed to share a similar neurological disorder, consisting of early onset of spasms together with, or preceded by, either erratic myoclonus or alternating focal clonic or tonic–clonic seizures (Dulac *et al.*, 1993b). Following infancy, erratic myoclonus and spasms persisted in all the patients. Progressive microcephaly from the middle of the first year of life was the second major feature of this syndrome, which may be due to an inborn error of metabolism. Whether this syndrome consists of a single disease or of several genetically determined encephalopathies is not clear at present.

Chromosomal Translocation

Some chromosomal translocations may produce complex malformations associated with IS. Examples include the Miller-Dieker syndrome (Dobyns *et al.*, 1984; see also Chapters 10 and 15), Down syndrome (Pollack *et al.*, 1978), and other chromosomal disorders (Hattori *et al.*, 1985; see also Chapter 20).

Unknown Mode of Inheritance

In some diseases involving siblings with IS, the mode of transmission is difficult to determine. This is the case in syndromes in which IS is associated with congenital microcephaly, psychomotor retardation and nephrotic syndrome (Roos *et al.*, 1987), IS associated with broad thumbs (Tsao and Ellingson, 1990), agenesis of corpus callosum, spastic quadriplegia and microcephaly associated with IS (Cao *et al.*, 1977), and in some rare cryptogenic cases (Cotte-Ritaud and Delafin, 1965).

Frequency and Etiology of IS Recurring in Siblings According to Etiology

Very few data are available: In one study (Dulac *et al.*, 1993b), 4/223 probands had a sibling with IS, compared with 0/223 control epileptic patients without IS and 0/223 nonepileptic control patients. Familial cases of IS in this series included twin pregnancy in one case, tuberous sclerosis and twin pregnancy in another, undetermined congenital encephalopathy in a third case, and it was cryptogenic in a fourth.

A retrospective series of all familial cases of IS over 15 years disclosed 11 families. Two were sets of premature monozygotic twins, a third was a twin pregnancy with tuberous sclerosis, two had cryptogenic West syndrome, two had recurrent maternal toxemia, and four had a progressive encephalopathy different from the PEHO syndrome (Dulac *et al.*, 1993b).

FAMILIAL ANTECEDENTS OF EPILEPSY AND FEBRILE CONVULSIONS

The familial incidence of epilepsy in patients with IS is low. It ranges from 3% (Trjaborg and Plum, 1960) to 6% (Watanabe *et al.*, 1973). When the combined familial history of epilepsy and febrile convulsions (FC) is considered, the incidence rises to 7–17% (Lacy and Lenry, 1976).

In one study (Dulac *et al.*, 1993b), the antecedents of epilepsy or occasional seizures including FC in first-degree relatives of 223 patients with IS were compared with those of two age-matched control groups of 223 patients each – one group with epilepsy other than IS, and one without epilepsy. The group of patients with spasms had an increased familial incidence of spasms, but not of FC, compared with both control groups. The familial incidence of epilepsy was intermediate between the epileptic and the nonepileptic control groups. The control group with epilepsy had an increased familial incidence of epilepsy and FC compared with both the study and the nonepileptic control groups.

Regarding the type of epilepsy in the families of patients with spasms, one-third of the probands with familial antecedents of epilepsy had tuberous sclerosis (Dulac *et al.*, 1993b). Thus, excluding cases in which spasms are the expression of an identifiable epileptogenic disease transmitted as a Mendelian trait, the familial incidence of epilepsy in the parents dropped to twice the incidence in the general population, and in siblings it was similar to that of the control group without epilepsy.

However, in various subgroups of children with spasms, a stronger link with epilepsy and FC may be observed. Matsumoto *et al.* (1981b) found a positive history of epilepsy in 40% of their "cryptogenic" cases, compared with 9.5% in the "perinatal" group. This was also the case for the idiopathic West syndrome group in the study of Vigevano *et al.* (1993), in which 29% of the combined idiopathic and cryptogenic cases and 4.7% of the symptomatic cases had a familial history of FC; 19.3% and 12.5%, respectively, also had a familial history of epilepsy. However, in the latter series, tuberous sclerosis was included, thus increasing the proportion of familial antecedents in the symptomatic group, reaching 43.7% for tuberous sclerosis. In addition, Vigevano *et al.* (1993) found that 5/31 combined idiopathic and cryptogenic cases had FC in first-degree relatives. In this series, 27 patients experienced complete recovery and met the characteristics of idiopathic epilepsy (Commission, 1989); 5 exhibited a photo-convulsive response and 2 others a spike focus several years after recovery. However, since idiopathic cases involve less than 10% of all cases of West syndrome, only a study which is selective by including this group could disclose the link. Based on present data, this is the only group in which a genetic predisposition to epilepsy may play a role. In contrast, we found no difference in the familial incidence of epilepsy and FC in a series of 30 patients with idiopathic West syndrome compared with a series of 15 cryptogenic cases (unpublished data). Further clarification of this point would require an epidemiological study of IS stratified by etiology, specifically focusing on idiopathic cases, and including a sufficient number of patients.

Contradictory results were obtained when studying the HLA system: one study found no relation (Howitz and Platz, 1978), whereas another found that there was a significant increase in the frequency of DRw52 in patients with spasms compared with controls. The authors suggested that immunological mechanisms could thus be involved in the pathophysiology of spasms (Hrachovy et al., 1988b).

NONGENETIC FAMILIAL RECURRENCE

Presently identified maternal factors consist of twin pregnancy and recurring maternal toxemia. Sets of twins with West syndrome have been reported (Pavone et al., 1980; Senga et al., 1986). Twin pregnancy is known to predispose to leukomalacia, and the latter to West syndrome (Cusmai et al., 1993). It is therefore difficult to determine in cases of West syndrome due to twin pregnancy whether a similar genetic background or leukomalacia played the more important role. In two families from our own series (Dulac et al., 1993b), recurrent maternal toxemia was associated with spasms. Such a condition had not been reported previously.

GENETIC COUNSELLING

For those families with a member suffering from epileptic spasms including West syndromes, genetic counselling requires a precise etiologic diagnosis of the underlying diseases whenever possible – for example, whether it results from an inborn error of metabolism or a neurocutaneous syndrome. In the latter case, the expression of the disease may be variable and involve other kinds of epilepsy in addition to West syndrome. According to the mode of transmission, the findings in the parents should determine whether the disease is likely to result from a mutation. When the precise etiology cannot be determined, some clinical features suggest a specific encephalopathy with recessive autosomic transmission: edema, optic atrophy of facial dysmorphia (retrognathism, hypertrophy of the gums) suggesting the PEHO syndrome, or erratic myoclonus as in the cases reported above. In the absence of these findings, the risk of recurrence is probably under 1%, similar to the order of magnitude of IS itself.

CONCLUSIONS

Although the incidence of infantile spasms is higher in the siblings and parents of patients with spasms than in the general population, this seems to be largely the result of various kinds of familial encephalopathies that are both genetically determined and which often cause epileptic spasms by themselves. This is the case with tuberous sclerosis, agyria and progressive encephalopathy from various causes. The higher incidence of epilepsy in the parents and siblings of children with spasms also seems to result from the same mechanism.

On the other hand, it is difficult to determine from the present data whether there is any specific genetic predisposition to infantile spasms which is independent of the genetic predisposition to various epileptogenic encephalopathies, and which is shared by other epileptic syndromes, particularly the idiopathic ones. For FC, it seems clear that the familial incidence of IS is in the same range as that for the general population, and lower than that for children suffering from other kinds of epilepsy. The higher familial incidence of other kinds of epilepsy and of FC in idiopathic West syndrome needs to be confirmed in wider and more focused studies because of the suggestion that the latter may, at least in part, be genetically determined.

15

Dysplasias

F. VIGEVANO, L. FUSCO, S. RICCI, T. GRANATA, F. VIANI

INTRODUCTION

The term dysplasia has more than one meaning. It is sometimes considered to be a synonym of "malformation", referring to any tissue that is imperfectly developed in embryonic or fetal life (Sarnat, 1992). According to Spranger *et al.* (1982), dysplasia should only be used to refer to "an abnormal organization of cells into tissue(s) and its morphological result(s)".

Here we use the term dysplasia in its wider sense. Cerebral dysplasias may be diffuse (as in lissencephaly), involve one hemisphere alone (as in hemimegalencephaly), or be localized to part of a hemisphere (as in focal dysplasia). Their etiology varies; broadly speaking, we can distinguish between "intrinsic", genetically programmed factors, and "extrinsic" factors, induced by a chemical, infectious, vascular or mechanical influence. Whatever the cause, the ultimate result is that the structure and cytoarchitecture of the affected cerebral tissues suffer marked changes, which severely compromise their function.

Cerebral dysplasia may occur as an isolated disorder or in association with malformations of other organs, as in genetic syndromes with multisystemic involvement, or in association with cutaneous anomalies, as in neurocutaneous syndromes.

From a clinical point of view, dysplasias may be responsible for motor deficits, mental retardation and seizures. Epilepsy secondary to dysplasia poses a difficult clinical problem because of its early onset and its notable resistance to treatment. Here we deal with the general characteristics of epilepsy secondary to cerebral dysplasia, centering our attention on the spasms that are such a frequent feature.

This and other chapters in this book deal also with some of the malformation syndromes, for which it has been possible to identify more or less constantly recurring clinical and electroencephalographic patterns.

EPILEPSY SECONDARY TO DYSPLASIA

In a recent review, Cowan and Hudson (1991) report that the frequency of prenatal etiologic factors in infantile spasms ranges from 15 to 56%. Besides cerebral malformations, this category includes neurocutaneous syndromes, intrauterine infections, chromosomal abnormalities, metabolic diseases, and sequelae of prenatal cerebral ischemia. More specifically, the frequency of cerebral dysplasias ranges from 2 to 21%. These figures illustrate the importance of malformation as an etiologic factor.

For general, epilepsy secondary to cerebral malformations has the following presenting characteristics:

- partial seizures and spasms occurring as isolated or closely linked events;
- an interictal EEG determined by the type of malformation;
- frequent resistance to treatment.

Even though published reports mention adult onset cases, epilepsy resulting from cerebral dysplasia most commonly appears in the early neonatal period. In Aicardi syndrome, for example, the seizures invariably begin within the first 3 months of life (Chevrie and Aicardi, 1986b). In our recent review of 14 cases of hemimegalencephaly (Vigevano *et al.*, 1991b), 13 patients had epilepsy; in 8 cases, the seizures began in the first week of life.

The onset can be difficult to identify exactly, because of the subtle appearance of the symptomatology. The first indication may be nothing more than a lateral deviation of the eyes or chewing movements, only recognized as ictal events much later on. An early onset of disease may indicate a poor prognosis. All our patients with hemimegalencephaly who were resistant to drug treatment began having seizures in the neonatal period.

Epilepsy due to dysplasia is manifested by two types of seizures: partial seizures in addition to spasms. The partial seizures are predominantly motor events, with the most common manifestations being psychomotor arrest, lateral eye deviation with ocular jerks, automatisms such as sucking and chewing, and unilateral or bilateral limb myoclonus. Impaired consciousness, cyanosis and diffuse tonic contractions are rarely seen in the early months of life.

Most of these seizures have a duration of minutes. Long-term EEG monitoring usually indicates that many seizures are largely, and some seizures completely, subclinical. These patients tend to have numerous seizures with a stereotypical pattern of clinical expression and EEG counterpart (Fig. 15.1). Status epilepticus, or prolonged partial seizures, are rare. These events occur in patients with focal dysplasia or hemispheric lesions, for example those with Sturge-Weber syndrome, in whom epilepsy begins at the age of about 1 year, with partial status precipitated by fever.

The other type of seizures often observed are spasms. Spasms have one clinical and EEG characteristic common to other etiologies: a muscular contraction lasting about 1 sec, corresponding on the EEG to diffuse slow-wave

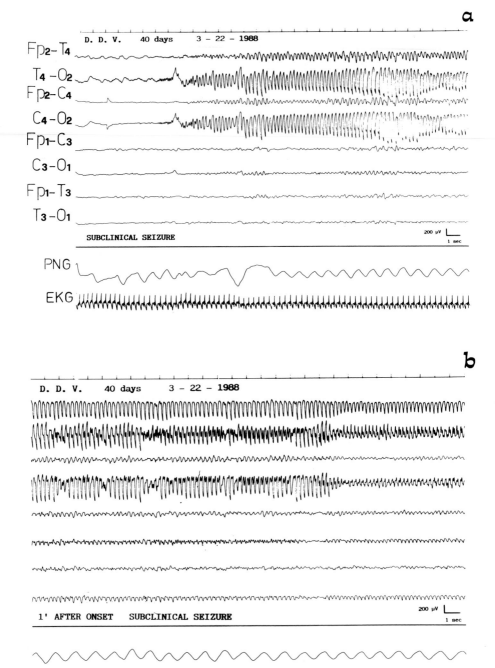

Figure 15.1 Right hemimegalencephaly in a 40-day-old infant. Continued pp. 181–2.

c

D. D. V.   40 days   3 – 22 – 1988

2' AFTER ONSET   LEFT EYES DEVIATION WITH OCULAR JERKS

200 µV
1 sec

d

D. D. V.   40 days   3 – 22 – 1988

3' AFTER ONSET   EATING AUTOMATISMS

200 µV
1 sec

Figure 15.1   *continued*   A sequence of six EEGs (a–f) shows a partial seizure beginning in the right parieto-occipital area and spreading to the temporal area; for the first 2 min the seizure is subclinical, then ocular jerks and eating automatisms occur.

e

D. D. V.   40 days   3 – 22 – 1988

5' AFTER ONSET   END OF THE SEIZURE   200 μV
                                                            1 sec

f

D. D. V.   40 days   3 – 22 – 1988

20" LATER   200 μV
                                                            1 sec

Figure 15.1 *continued.* (f) The first seizure is followed within seconds by another identical seizure.

activity (Fusco and Vigevano, 1993). However, spasms also have distinctive features of their own. Above all, they may have a very early onset. Figure 15.2 shows a spasm recorded in a newborn infant on day 13 of life.

The muscular contractions can consist of flexion, extension or mixed flexion–extension of the limbs. These movements are nearly always asymmetric or even unilateral, and can be accompanied by focal manifestations. In other words, the spasm reflects the type of malformation: hemispheric lesions lead to a more marked muscular contraction, sometimes affecting the contralateral side of the body only; bihemispheric lesions give rise to asymmetric spasms; and agenesis of the corpus callosum produces spasms that either involve both sides of the body in an asynchronous manner or which predominate alternately from one side to the other (Fig. 15.3).

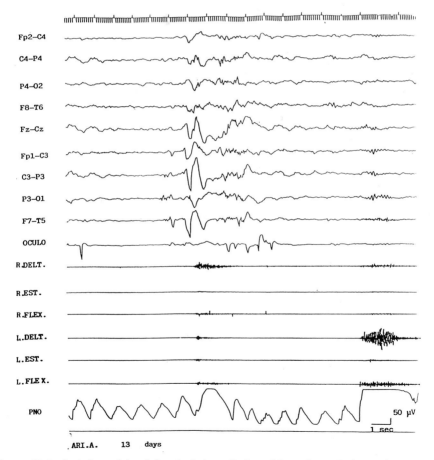

Figure 15.2 Left frontal focal dysplasia in a 13-day-old newborn. Polygraphic recording of an asymmetric spasm predominantly affecting the right side of the body; the ictal EEG shows a very high-amplitude slow wave, more evident over the left hemisphere.

True spasms are sometimes followed by a tonic contraction that lasts a few seconds and has as its EEG correlate a low-amplitude recruiting rhythm. Like the spasm itself, the EEG correlate of a spasm reflects the underlying malformation. The diffuse slow-wave activity, often associated with a fast low-amplitude rhythm, generally has an asymmetric representation or appears only on one hemisphere, as happens in focal dysplasia and hemimegalencephaly. In Aicardi syndrome and in most cases of agenesis of the corpus callosum, the EEG shows series of spasms originating over each hemisphere at different times, without contralateral spread, and also spasms with an ictal EEG discharge, asynchronous on the two hemispheres.

One distinctive feature of epileptic attacks arising from dysplasia is the unusual admixture that one observes between partial seizures and spasms. These two seizure types may appear as isolated events, but more often appear to be closely interlinked. One observes diverse combinations. During a series of spasms, one spasm may be followed immediately by a partial seizure (Fig.

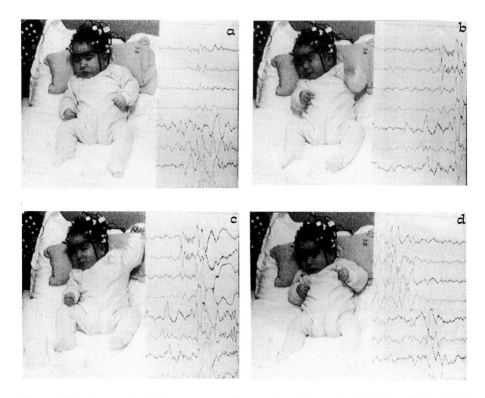

Figure 15.3 Agenesis of the corpus callosum in a 3-month-old infant. Video/EEG recording of a spasm. The eight channels (from top to bottom) correspond to the following derivations: Right Fp2-T4, T4-02, Fp2-C4, C4-02; Left Fp1-C3, C3-01, Fp1-T3, T3-01. During this asymmetric spasm, the child raises the left arm and extends the right arm downwards. In (a)–(d), note the asynchronous interictal EEG anomalies.

15.4). In some cases, it seems as though the partial seizures are always triggered by a spasm; in others, the spasms follow a partial seizure. At times, the spasms were already present, as in Fig. 15.4. When this happens, the partial seizure appears never to have interrupted the series of spasms. Occasional reports

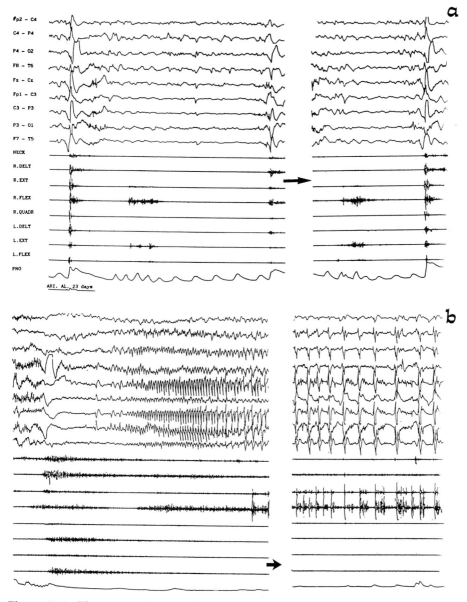

Figure 15.4 The same patient as in Fig. 15.2 at 23 days old. (a) A series of spasms; (b) a spasm triggers a left motor partial seizure; (c) a few seconds after the end of the partial seizure, spasms reappear.

c

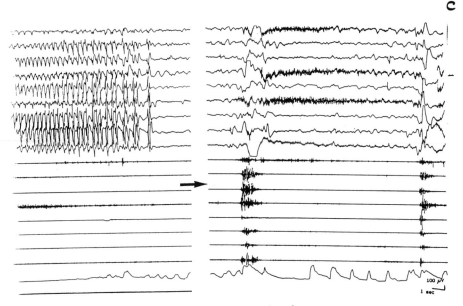

Figure 15.4 *continued*

mention persisting spasms and partial seizures that coexist (Donat and Wright, 1991). More frequently, one observes partial seizures followed by spasms; that is, the reverse phenomena – the partial seizures apparently trigger the spasms. The phenomenon needs to be looked for very carefully. The partial seizures may be subclinical with only the spasms clinically evident (Fig. 15.5). Hence it is important to perform long-term monitoring in patients with spasms, so that the EEG characteristics can be defined with utmost precision.

This unusual relation between partial seizures and spasms is of great interest. Whereas a partial seizure is an electrical phenomenon originating at the cortical level, little is known about the site of origin of spasms. Some authors attribute infantile spasms to subcortical structures (Martin, 1964; Hrachovy and Frost, 1989b). Their close association with partial seizures, as described above, could confirm this hypothesis.

Interictal EEG recordings provide important information on cerebral dysplasia. Diffuse and focal forms of neuronal migration disorders give rise to unusually fast EEG activity.

Various authors (Dulac *et al.*, 1983a; Gastaut *et al.*, 1987) have described the EEG characteristics of lissencephaly, emphasizing the typical presence of diffuse high-amplitude fast activity. This pattern is already recognizable in the early months of life, because the frequencies are unduly fast for such an age. Similar findings may be seen in band heterotopia (Moutard *et al.*, 1994). Abnormally fast activity is seen in focal and hemispheric neuronal migration disorders; in focal dysplasia, it may be localized to one area of the brain (Fig. 15.6b), in hemimegalencephaly to a whole hemisphere (Fig. 15.7; see Paladin *et* al., 1989). Complete agenesis of the corpus callosum results in an EEG pattern of asymmetric, asynchronous background activity over the two hemispheres (Fariello *et al.*, 1977).

The interictal abnormalities consist of spike and spike-wave discharges and theta waves. Initially, these represent the site of the lesion, but later they tend to invade other regions of the brain. The abnormalities are already obvious within days of birth, and become progressively more numerous. In the first months of life, sleep recordings show that these abnormalities tend to cluster together in bursts, which alternate with periods of EEG depression. This unusual pattern, often termed "suppression–burst", can have a focal (Fig. 15.6a), hemispheric or bilateral localization. It recurs constantly in the first months of life in patients with hemimegalencephaly, and the term "unilateral hypsarrhythmia" or "hemihypsarrhythmia" has been coined to describe it (Fig. 15.8). In Aicardi syndrome and generally in agenesis of the corpus callosum, the suppression–burst pattern may be present as a bihemispheric asynchronous abnormality (Fig. 15.9).

Clinically, cerebral dysplasia may generate a form of epilepsy that has a

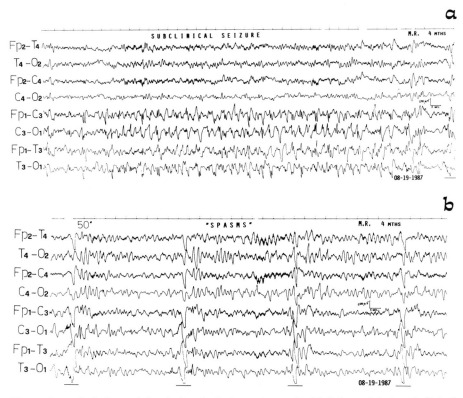

Figure 15.5 Left frontal focal dysplasia in a 4-month-old infant. (a) A subclinical seizure recorded in the left anterior region; (b) a few seconds later, a series of spasms begins.

particularly poor evolution. The clinical picture so far described is typical of the first months of life. Although treatment may lead to seizure control, the seizures more often persist. Treatment-resistant patients continue to have seizures, particularly focal seizures. In some cases, spasms may also persist

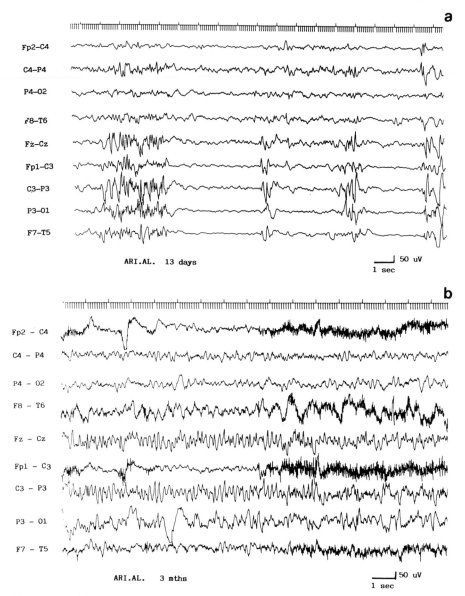

Figure 15.6 The same patient as in Fig. 15.2 and 15.4. (a) An interictal EEG recorded at 13 days during sleep shows a focal suppression–burst pattern localized over the left anterior region; (b) a recording at 3 months of age, during wakefulness shows, in the same area, prominent fast activity.

throughout infancy and adolescence. Patients with focal and hemispheric lesions, in whom the rest of the cerebral parenchyma appears healthy, may benefit from neurosurgical treatment (King *et al.*, 1985; Vigevano *et al.*, 1989b).

SPECIAL SYNDROMES

The characteristic features of some malformations have led to the identification of a number of electroclinically distinct syndromes. The prototype of these disorders is Aicardi syndrome, a disorder characterized by infantile spasms, peculiar fundoscopic lesions described as "chorioretinal lacunae", and agensis of the corpus callosum. This association has been observed only in girls.

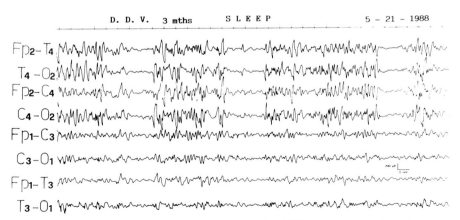

Figure 15.7 Right hemimegalencephaly in a 6-month-old infant. An EEG recorded during sleep shows very high-amplitude fast activity over the right hemisphere. Sleep spindles over the right hemisphere also have a higher amplitude.

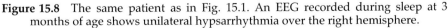

Figure 15.8 The same patient as in Fig. 15.1. An EEG recorded during sleep at 3 months of age shows unilateral hypsarrhythmia over the right hemisphere.

Aicardi syndrome is almost invariably associated with an early onset of spasms and partial seizures that precede the occurrence of spasms in the first 3 months of life. In general, we find partial seizures and spasms occurring concurrently or as isolated events, asymmetric or unilateral spasms, and interictal and ictal "split brain" EEG due to agenesis of the corpus callosum (Bour *et al.*, 1986).

In the lissencephaly syndromes, the most prominent clinical features are severe mental retardation, diffuse hypotonia, microcephaly and seizures. The EEG is almost invariably diagnostic, because it is dominated by "major fast dysrhythmia" – in other words, abnormally fast, very high-voltage activity. The epilepsy consists mainly of spasms, and myoclonic and atonic seizures; partial seizures are very rare, and erratic myoclonus may occur. One does not generally observe hypsarrhythmia, only bilateral paroxysmal abnormalities intermingled with fast activity.

Most patients with hemimegalencephaly have hemiparesis, hemianopsia, mental retardation, cranial asymmetry and seizures. Epilepsy starts in the first days of life with partial seizures, followed in 50% of cases by infantile spasms. The spasms are always asymmetric or unilateral. The EEG over the malformed hemisphere shows increasing paroxysmal abnormalities, and unilateral hypsarrhythmia during sleep. In later months, continuous spikes and spike-and-

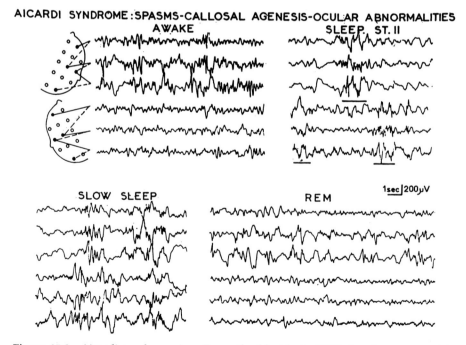

Figure 15.9 Aicardi syndrome in a 5-month-old girl. An EEG showing asymmetric, asynchronous background activity and irritative anomalies, most evident during sleep.

wave complexes occur in waking and during sleep. These anomalies tend progressively to involve the contralateral hemisphere and produce an asymmetric suppression – burst pattern. Also in hemimegalencephaly, the fast activity typical of neuronal migration disorders is recognizable over the malformed hemisphere.

The foregoing examples illustrate certain recognizable clinical and EEG features that recur almost constantly in these malformation disorders and which are of help in formulating a diagnosis. Other syndrome-specific electroclinical pictures, among them that of tuberous sclerosis, are discussed in other chapters of this book. In conclusion it is important to recognize the general characteristics of epilepsy associated with cerebral dysplasia because they help to identify the etiology, choose the treatment and formulate the prognosis.

16

Tuberous Sclerosis

P. CURATOLO

Tuberous sclerosis (TS) is a congenital hamartomatosis with variable expression in multiple organs, transmitted by autosomal dominant inheritance. Based on population studies, its prevalence is reported to be 1:7000. Tuberous sclerosis shows genetic heterogeneity with linkage to 9q34 and recently to 16p13.

Pathologically, TS is a disorder of cellular migration, proliferation and differentiation. Cortical tubers constitute the hallmark of the disease and are pathognomonic of cerebral TS. There is variability in the range and extent of the neurological problems; symptoms caused by cortical tubers may include partial or generalized seizures, mental retardation, hemiplegia and abnormal behavior. Seizures are the most common neurological symptom of TS, occurring in 92% of a large clinical series (Gomez, 1988).

INFANTILE SPASMS AND TUBEROUS SCLEROSIS

The high incidence of infantile spasms (IS) in TS has long been emphasized. In fact, IS has been reported to be the presenting symptom in up to 69% of patients with TS (Pampiglione and Pugh, 1975; Hunt, 1983). Conversely, TS has been found in 7–25% of infants with symptomatic IS (Pampiglione and Moynahan, 1976; Matsumoto *et al.*, 1981b). We found the incidence of TS to be 11% in a series of 164 infants affected by IS who underwent computerized tomography (Curatolo *et al.*, 1987). These data suggest the existence of an important association between TS and IS and that TS should be suspected in children with IS (Chevrie and Aicardi, 1977). However, in recent years, important advances in the understanding of seizures associated with TS have indicated that infants with TS exhibit some characteristic clinical and EEG features, distinguishing these infants from those with classical West syndrome including hypsarrhythmia, and suggesting a malformative etiology. In this chapter, an attempt is made to delineate the main clinical and EEG characteristics and the natural history of IS associated with TS.

CLINICAL FEATURES AT ONSET

Epilepsy in TS often begins in the first year of life and in most cases in the very first few months of life. At this time, the most common seizure types are partial motor and IS. Although the number of TS patients evaluated by video/EEG examination is small, video/EEG monitoring has shown that a sizable proportion of IS are preceded by partial seizures (Stephenson, 1988). Furthermore, in the same child partial seizures may precede, coexist or evolve into IS, and partial seizures together with IS may occur. One of the most commonly observed patterns in early onset IS associated with TS is the presence of apparently bilateral and symmetrical flexor tonic contraction of the limbs lasting for a few seconds preceded by eye deviation. A vast number of subtle partial seizures, such as unilateral tonic or clonic phenomena, mainly localized to the face or limbs, can be missed by the parents until the third or fourth month of life, when IS occur (Dulac *et al.*, 1984). Isolated attacks develop within weeks into a typical cluster, most commonly on awakening.

The three main types of spasms (flexor, extensor, mixed) may occur in infants with TS (Roger *et al.*, 1984). The type of spasms depends upon whether it is the flexor or extensor muscles which are most affected and the extent of the contraction.

Typical IS associated with TS are rare. Lateralizing features such as tonic eye deviation, nystagmus, head turning, unilateral grimacing and inequality of movements of the limbs may be observed. The tonic or atonic components displayed in IS are often asymmetrical. In some cases, the spasms may be unilateral, often with an adversive component (Dulac *et al.*, 1984).

Almost all cases of IS associated with TS have their onset between the end of the second and the eleventh months of life; the appearance of IS before the age of 3 months is uncommon and the greatest incidence is between 4 and 5 months (Dulac *et al.*, 1984). Rare cases begin in the second year of life or later in the first decade. Familial cases of IS reported in children with TS are the expression of the autosomal dominant transmission of the disease. At the age of occurrence of the spasms, TS can be recognized by the presence of cutaneous hypopigmented macules. Associated neurological abnormalities include hemiparesis and subtle asymmetric motor deficits. The incidence of abnormal mental and motor development prior to the onset of IS is lower than in other groups of symptomatic IS, such as brain malformations. However, at this age, it may be difficult to identify a mild degree of cognitive delay.

INTERICTAL EEG FINDINGS

Focal or multifocal epileptiform abnormalities may be found when EEG is performed between the neonatal period and the development of IS. Infants with IS due to TS exhibit a particular awake interictal EEG characterized by a multifocal asynchronous pattern of spike discharges and irregular slow activity of 2–3 Hz (Westmoreland, 1988; Curatolo, 1991). Reducing the amplification and increasing the number of electrodes make it easier to recognize focal abnormalities. Although the EEG foci can be located in any region of the brain, the most common location for IS is the posterior temporal and occipital regions (Cusmai *et al.*, 1990a; see Figs 16.1 and 16.2). Drowsiness increases slow-wave activity (Fig. 16.3). During NREM sleep, an increase in the amount of epileptiform activity is observed, multifocal and focal abnormalities tend to generalize, and bursts of more synchronous polyspikes and waves separated by sudden voltage attenuation become evident resembling hypsarrhythmia (Dulac *et al.*, 1984; see Figs 16.4 and 16.5). Spindle activity may (Fig. 16.5) or may not be recorded (Fig. 16.4) in these patients due to the amount of epileptiform abnormalities. In REM sleep, by comparison, the epileptiform activity is decreased, the generalized discharges are usually suppressed, and there is a definite tendency for the EEG foci to become spatially very restricted (Fig. 16.6). High time resolution topographic analysis of EEG has shown that a multifocal pattern may arise from a single dominant focus, related to a prominent neuroimaging abnormality in the temporo-occipital region detected by magnetic resonance imaging (Fig. 16.7) or by positron emission tomography (Fig. 16.8; Curatolo and Cusmai, 1987a; Seri *et al.*, 1991).

Severe sleep problems are frequent after the onset of IS and are mainly due to sleep-related epileptic events. All night polysomnographic recordings in children suffering from IS have shown an increased number and duration of awakenings after sleep onset, and a marked reduction in total sleep time and in REM sleep time (Fig. 16.9).

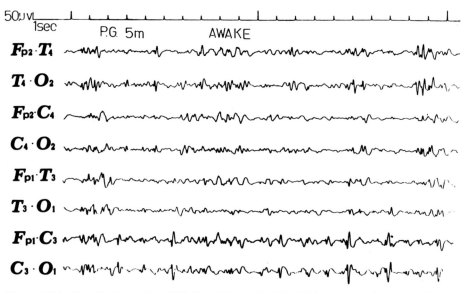

Figure 16.1   Interictal awake EEG in a 5-month-old child. Independent multifocal spikes can be identified, mainly in the left occipital region.

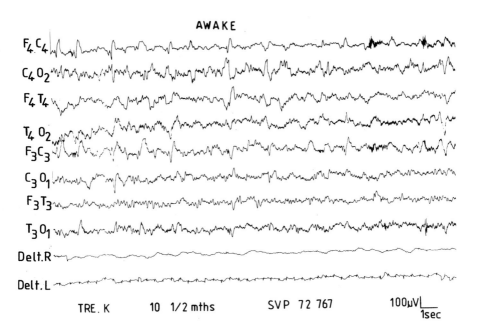

Figure 16.2 Spasms since the age of 8 months. There is no hypsarrhythmic pattern. Note the right central spike wave focus in the awake recording.

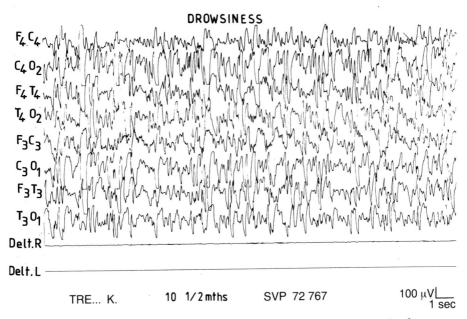

Figure 16.3 Same patient and recording as in Fig. 16.2. The increase in slow-wave activity during drowsiness produces a tracing that resembles hypsarrhythmia.

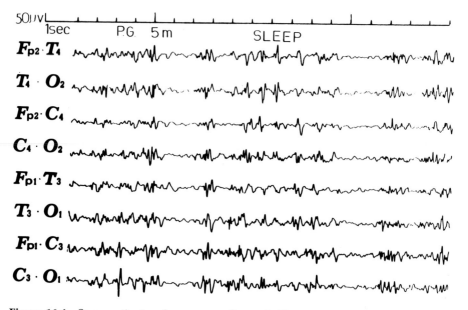

Figure 16.4   Same patient and same recording as in Fig. 16.1. During NREM sleep, the EEG abnormalities generalize. Note the lack of spindles.

These interictal EEG abnormalities are reproducible in terms of topography and tend to persist in serial records.

ICTAL EEG FINDINGS

Video/EEG and polygraphic recordings of the spasms, as well as 24 h EEG monitoring, have shown that a cluster of spasms is a single seizure consisting of a series of spasms often associated with several other clinical manifestations. Each seizure consists of a combination of both focal and bilateral manifestations, for example a hemiclonic or motor adversive phenomenon followed by a cluster of spasms; the involvement of the limbs is bilateral, but often asymmetrical (Dulac *et al.*, 1984; Plouin *et al.*, 1989). Ictal EEG starts with a focal discharge of spikes and polyspikes, often originating from the temporal, rolandic or occipital regions, followed by a generalized irregular slow wave transient and an abrupt flattening of background activity in all regions. In other instances, the first spasm coincides with the disappearance of interictal activity throughout the cluster. Although there is no evidence of focal discharge during the cluster, the whole cluster is likely to be a single seizure, since the interictal activity only recurs at the end of it.

SLEEP Ⅱ

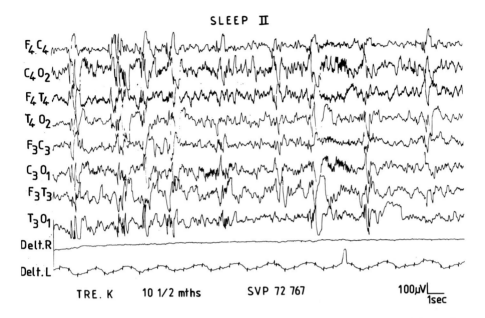

F₄C₄

C₄O₂

F₄T₄

T₄O₂

F₃C₃

C₃O₁

F₃T₃

T₃O₁

Delt.R

Delt.L

TRE. K   10 1/2 mths   SVP 72 767   100μV ⌐ 1sec

Figure 16.5 Same patient and same recording as in Fig. 16.2. During NREM sleep, the EEG abnormalities generalize. Note the presence of spindles.

REM

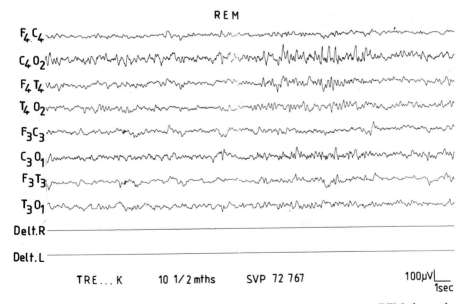

F₄C₄

C₄O₂

F₄T₄

T₄O₂

F₃C₃

C₃O₁

F₃T₃

T₃O₁

Delt.R

Delt.L

TRE... K   10 1/2 mths   SVP 72 767   100μV ⌐ 1sec

Figure 16.6 Same patient and same recording as in Fig. 16.2. During REM sleep, the generalization disappears and the focus is restricted to the right central area.

EVOLUTION OF CLINICAL AND EEG FEATURES

The vast majority of children with TS who had IS at onset eventually develop either partial motor or complex partial seizures, or apparently generalized tonic, atonic or tonic–clonic seizures. However, a video/EEG study has shown that almost all the epileptic seizures associated with the TS can be described as partial (partial motor, complex partial or having some form of secondary generalization) (Stephenson, 1988).

In the EEG of older patients with TS, the pseudotype pattern of hypsarrhythmia tends to disappear and the tracings tend to exhibit focal spikes or slowing, with transitional stages from unifocal to bifocal and multifocal discharges. However, the occipital and posterior temporal spikes prevailing at the onset tend to persist in morphology and location in serial EEG records, and after 2 years of age additional foci with a frontal localization become progressively evident. During sleep, the EEG is characterized by multifocal abnormalities associated with bursts of bilateral and more synchronous slow spike waves,

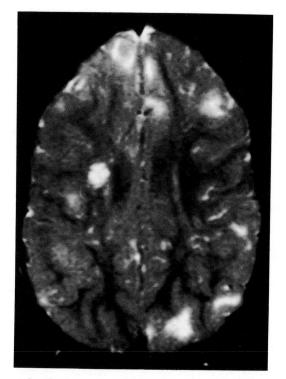

Figure 16.7 T2-weighted images on MRI. Multifocal hyperintensities may be seen in both hemispheres, mainly in the left parieto-occipital region.

with a pattern similar to that seen in Lennox-Gastaut syndrome. At this stage, the recognition of focal origin of these apparently generalized abnormalities on standard EEG is difficult, but high time resolution topographic analysis of EEG and dipole localization methods may detect the presence of a secondary bilateral synchrony (SBS), often originating in the frontal regions and corresponding to prominent tubers detected by MRI (Seri *et al.*, 1991).

PATHOPHYSIOLOGICAL ASPECTS

Although the pathophysiological mechanisms responsible for the coexistence of IS and partial motor seizures are still uncertain, IS associated with TS may be of a focal nature, suggesting a secondary generalization from partial seizures (Blume and Pillay, 1985). The age of onset of seizures and the age when epileptiform activity becomes apparent on the EEG depend upon the location of cortical tubers detected by MRI, and may coincide with functional maturation of the cortex, with an earlier expression for the temporo-occipital regions than for the frontal ones. Therefore, it is not paradoxical that cortical lesions

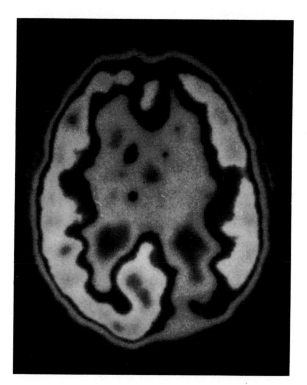

Figure 16.8   PET reveals a hypometabolic region in the left occipital area.

which are associated with IS at a certain age are not epileptogenic later in life and that, in the same child, complex partial seizures originating from a more anterior cortical tuber may not begin for a number of years.

Although a topographic correspondence between EEG foci and the largest tubers detected by MRI has been reported (Curatolo and Cusmai, 1988; Cusmai *et al.*, 1990a; Tamaki *et al.*, 1990), MRI is as yet unable to detect all the cortical tubers that can be identified pathologically (Nixon *et al.*, 1989). Positron emission tomography or single photon emission computed tomography may reveal hypometabolic or hypoperfused regions not predicted by MRI, demonstrating that the disturbance of cerebral function may be more extensive than indicated by morphological imaging alone (Szélies *et al.*, 1983; Chiron *et al.*, 1990b).

MENTAL OUTCOME

Neuropsychological and cognitive dysfunction, as well as behavioral disorders, are common in TS and are related to findings on morphological and functional imaging (Curatolo and Cusmai, 1987b). Infants with transient IS and isolated cortical tubers located in the parietal and rolandic regions may have normal intelligence. In contrast, children with persistent IS preceded or followed by partial seizures and with multiple bilateral tubers often develop drug-resistant epilepsies and severe mental retardation (Curatolo *et al,*, 1991; Jambaqué *et al.*, 1991).

Transient cognitive dysfunction and behavioral changes in association with the onset of IS are common. However, subjects with a stable mental retardation and behavioral regression tend to show a consistent pattern of multiple strategically localized cortical tubers.

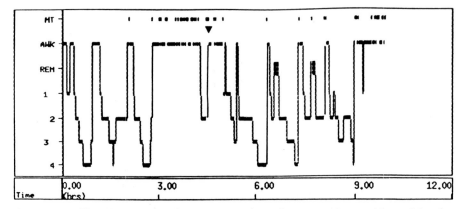

Figure 16.9 Hypnogram showing extreme sleep fragmentation, evidenced by frequent sleep stage shiftings and an increased number of awakenings (AWK) during sleep.

A very high incidence of autism has been found in children with TS and IS (Hunt, 1983). Autism appears to be more common in infants with parieto-temporal and frontal tubers, and it has been suggested that an early dysfunction in the associative areas due to the location of cortical tubers may be responsible for the autistic features (Curatolo and Cusmai, 1987b; Jambaqué *et al.*, 1991). Limbic epilepsy due to TS may in other cases produce autism (Deonna *et al.*, 1993).

TREATMENT

Antiepileptic drug treatment should be used rationally in children with TS, in that the choice of drugs should be adopted according to the electroclinical pattern. ACTH and steroids do not seem to be the drugs of choice when IS have been preceded by other seizure types. In such cases, antiepileptic drugs active against partial seizures may prove to be of greater benefit than steroid treatment, and carbamazepine and vigabatrin alone or in combination may become the drugs of choice (Chiron *et al.*, 1990a). Although nearly half of patients with spasms develop drug-resistant partial seizures, their overall condition is improved. Great variability has been reported in response to therapy, and recovery from the spasms or appearance of other types of seizures may depend more on the characteristics of cortical tubers than on the pharmacotherapeutic strategy (Curatolo, 1994).

Selected drug-resistant patients with persisting partial epilepsy and a well-recognized unifocal abnormality can be considered for surgical resection (Bebin *et al.*, 1990). Surgical treatment may also occasionally be useful despite the presence of multifocal EEG and neuroimaging abnormalities. Complete removal of large single cortical hamartomas corresponding to the most active epileptogenic foci can result in either cessation of seizures or better control (Dalla Barnardina *et al.*, 1993). However, the delayed epileptogenicity of the most anterior tubers must be borne in mind when surgery is discussed for infantile epilepsy in a very young child. Combined studies by means of topographic mapping of EEG, high field MRI and PET may provide more accurate localization of epileptogenic zones and result in better selection of candidates for focal cortical resection. When intractable drop attacks constitute a major seizure type, corpus callosotomy should be considered.

CONCLUSION

Most infants with IS and TS exhibit clinical and EEG characteristics that are different from typical West syndrome. Total events at onset are mainly characterized by partial motor seizures and infantile spasms. IS are often asymmetrical and preceded by lateralizing features. Visual recording techniques have led to significant progress in the classification of seizures associated with TS, demonstrating that they have a focal or multifocal origin in the vast majority of cases. In most cases, an awake interictal EEG shows focal or independent multifocal spike and slow-wave activity at onset and later a pseudo-hypsarrhythmic pattern. The age of onset of seizures and the age of occurrence of EEG foci depend on the localization of cortical tubers with an earlier expression of the parieto-occipital than of the frontal regions. Early recognition of these distinctive features appears worthwhile for therapeutic and prognostic implications. Although vigabatrin has led to a breakthrough, focal seizures may persist. Studies using combined topographic mapping of EEG, MRI and PET may provide new strategies for selecting candidates suitable for surgery.

17

Other Neurocutaneous Syndromes

C. BILLARD, J. MOTTE, L. VALLEE

The definition of neurocutaneous syndrome is quite broad and usually includes congenital diseases which have both cutaneous and neurological manifestations. Among the numerous causes of infantile spasms (IS), various neurocutaneous syndromes (NCS) have been described. A sizable literature describes the frequency of clinical and EEG patterns and the etiology of IS in tuberous sclerosis (see Chapter 15). In contrast, there are few reports of the other neurocutaneous syndromes. According to personal experience and a review of the literature, two groups can be distinguished with a different frequency, profile and course of the disease. The first group, which is the most common, consists of neurofibromatosis type-1 (NF1) associated with infantile spasms. The frequency with which cases are reported would seem to eliminate coincidence. In the second group, very few cases have been reported and they are distributed among the various rare neurocutaneous syndromes.

NEUROFIBROMATOSIS TYPE-1

In contrast to the bad outcome of West syndrome in other NCS (Riikonen, 1982; Hrachovy *et al.*, 1984), cases of West syndrome with neurofibromatosis type-1 (NF1), as defined by the National Institutes Consensus (1982), have a good outcome (Dulac *et al.*, 1983b; Huson *et al.*, 1988; Larregue *et al.*, 1977; Pou Serrdel and Salez-Vasquez, 1971; Pou Serradel, 1984). Our experience of 15 such cases supports this impression (Motte *et al.*, 1993).

Most cases have a family history of NF1 without familial epilepsy. Virtually all patients with IS exhibit epileptic seizures in the first year of life, and only very few have partial seizures before spasms, the majority of them having spasms as the first epileptic manifestation. The spasms occur in infants with previously normal psychomotor development, except for very rare cases of patients with partial seizures at onset of the disease.

The behavioral regression – sometimes very mild – is usually concomitant with the onset of spasms or can occur later. Some children may remain free of behavioral regression throughout the evolution of their disease.

Spasms may be quite frequent in infants with NF1 and IS. In the majority of children, they are symmetrical, with no focal features on examination of history or on EEG/video recording. It is very unusual for the spasms to be associated with lateral head-turning. Ictal EEG recording showed that clusters of spasms consisted of independent spasms in all cases in our series except one patient who later developed complex partial seizures (Motte *et al.*, 1993). The interictal EEGs showed typical hypsarrhythmia in all our patients. Few infants have mild focal slow waves when awake or brought on by sleep or by intravenous administration of diazepam.

A computed tomography scan does not reveal any central manifestation of neurofibromatosis. It is entirely normal in the majority of cases. Magnetic resonance imaging has shown no abnormalities in a few cases.

It is our experience that corticosteroids achieve an immediate and dramatic response, whatever the time lapse from onset of spasms. Duration of steroid treatment (1–3 months) does not seem to produce any difference in the evolution of the epilepsy. Prospective data for determining whether or not the treatment should be prolonged are required. In one patient, after 2 weeks of ineffective ACTH, nitrazepam was added and successfully controlled the spasms. In another patient, spasms disappeared without treatment. The children in our series remained seizure-free after withdrawal of steroids. They had classical anticonvulsant drug treatment for 1–10 years. No fits were observed after withdrawal of all drugs after a mean follow-up of 7 years (range 2–19 years). Only one child with mental retardation before onset of spasms continued to have complex partial seizures for 3 years, but eventually became seizure-free and medication was successfully withdrawn. Another child had partial epilepsy which remained intractable for 5 years.

The intellectual outcome is also usually good. Two-thirds of the children in our series aged over 6 years have normal intelligence and normal educational achievement. We observed one child who had a severe intellectual deficit: his MRI was abnormal and his mother also had an intellectual deficit. In such cases, the intellectual impairment is probably related to the NF1 rather than to the infantile spasms. Long-term EEG recordings usually remain normal. In a few cases, they show transient focal paroxysmal abnormalities between 1 and 3 years of age. Permanent focal discharges are seen in those few children who remain epileptic.

Despite the small number of patients in our series and the limited data that are available, some general statements may be made:

1. The frequency of IS in NF1 is clearly greater than the frequency of IS in the general population (Riikonen and Donner, 1979). In the only prospective epidemiological study of NF1, there were two patients with IS among the 135 cases selected (Huson *et al.*, 1988). In contrast, in the general population, the frequency of IS is estimated to be between 1:2000 and 1:4000 (Cowan and Hudson, 1991) (see Chapter 2). On the other hand, the frequency of NF1 in series of consecutive IS is extraordinarily high: Eeg-Olofsson and Sidenvall

(1992) found two cases in an epidemiological study of 66 cases of IS, Nolte *et al.* (1988) found one among 54 consecutive cases, Ferraz *et al.* (1986) found one in a series of 66 cases of IS, and Matsumoto *et al.* (1981b) found two in another series of 200 cases of IS.

2. Our experience of IS in NF1 is similar to that of Huson *et al.* (1988). In general, among such patients there is:
   - normal psychomotor development before the onset of spasms;
   - symmetrical spasms without associated partial seizures;
   - typical hypsarrhythmia and a good response to corticosteroid therapy;
   - no relapse after long-term follow-up and after withdrawal of all drugs;
   - good intellectual outcome, which is clearly better than in other symptomatic cases of IS.

   Therefore, IS associated with NF1 fulfills the characteristics of West syndrome (see Chapter 1).
3. Our data suggest that IS in NF1 is very different from that described by Dalla Bernardina *et al.* (1984) for IS due to cerebral malformations. In fact, IS in NF1 meets most clinical, EEG and outcome characteristics of idiopathic West syndrome (see Chapter 21), including response to treatment. The characteristics of IS associated with NF1 suggest that the spasms are not related to cerebral malformations. We doubt that this is a coincidence and speculate that the spasms in NF1 have a similar mechanism to those of idiopathic West syndrome. It is possible that there is a genetic or biochemical relationship between NF1 and West syndrome.

OTHER NEUROCUTANEOUS SYNDROMES

In this group, the outcome is usually unfavorable due to intractable epilepsy and severe cognitive dysfunction. Tuberous sclerosis (discussed in Chapter 16), Sturge-Weber syndrome, naevus linearis sebaceous, incontinentia pigmenti, Sjögren-Larsson syndrome and Ito's hypomelanosis involve these features. Brain malformations are usually demonstrated by means of neuroradiological investigations (Levin *et al.*, 1984; Avrahami *et al.*, 1985; Ardinger and Bell, 1986; Diebler and Dulac, 1987; Barkovich, 1990) or neuropathological studies (De Recondo and Haguenau, 1972; Hauw *et al.*, 1977; Choi and Kudo, 1981; Ross *et al.*, 1982; Meencke and Gerhard, 1985; Jellinger, 1987).

Sturge-Weber Syndrome

Children with Sturge-Weber syndrome (SWS) often exhibit severe epilepsy several weeks or months after birth. Although IS have been observed in some children (Millichap *et al.*, 1962; Fukuyama and Tsuchiya, 1979), their occurrence is much less frequent than the acute onset of focal or generalized severe and prolonged seizures. The characteristics of the spasms have not been fully described but they are intractable, usually associated with hemiparesis, and followed by epilepsy and mental retardation. In Fukuyama and Tsuchiya's (1979) study, spasms began at 4.6 months; 3 months later, left-sided status epilepticus associated with hemiparesis occurred. Although the spasms were symmetrical, interictal spike activity was more pronounced in one hemisphere.

Sjögren-Larsson Syndrome

Infantile spasms were observed by us in one case of typical Sjögren-Larsson syndrome with the classic diagnostic criteria (cutaneous ichthyosis with desquamation in strips, retinal degeneration, spastic quadriplegia with profound mental retardation and microcephaly). In this case, spasms began at 4 months. The patient's clinical records noted that they were symmetrical but a video-recording was not performed; EEG showed bilateral spikes, polyspikes and sharp waves with focal paroxysmal activity appearing after intravenous diazepam. There was cortical atrophy on CT scan.

The outcome was very poor, with refractory epilepsy despite various drugs, no progress of any sort and finally death. Autopsy was not performed. However, focal EEG discharges, cortical atrophy and poor outcome suggested that IS were due to a brain lesion.

Ito's Hypomelanosis

Infantile spasms were observed in association with Ito's hypomelanosis in two cases followed by the authors and in several others from the literature. The typical cutaneous symptomatology was always associated with mental retardation and neurological signs (e.g. hemiplegia, quadriplegia, microcephaly), suggesting cerebral lesions.

Symmetrical and asymmetrical spasms appeared early (before 3 months). All therapy was ineffective and partial or secondary generalized seizures completed the poor outcome. Although incompletely described, the epilepsy is usually intractable and linked to severe encephalopathy (Larregue *et al.*, 1977). Simonsson's (1972) case is the only one in which spasms began after 6 months and were controlled by treatment.

Some arguments confirm the existence of cerebral lesions. Lissencephaly, with typical EEG characteristics and MRI aspects, was seen in one case followed by us. In Ross and co-worker's (1982) study, severe abnormalities of neuronal migration were seen on neuropathological study, with gray matter heteropias, suggesting that there was a common mechanism in the pathology of the development of the skin and the brain. In the case documented by Larregue *et al.* (1977), the outcome was poor and the coexistence of severe encephalopathy also suggested brain malformation.

Naevus Linearis Sebaceous Syndrome

Two cases followed by the authors and 12 other cases of IS with naevus linearis sebaceous syndrome have been described (Moynahan and Wolff, 1967; Herbst and Cohen, 1971; Lovejoy and Boyle, 1973; Leyh and Loewel, 1973; Larregue *et al.*, 1977; Kurokawa *et al.*, 1981; Vigevano *et al.*, 1984; and Nuno *et al.*, 1990).

In addition to the typical camel-colored cutaneous stains, severe encephalopathy was always present. In the cases studied by ourselves, spasms began early and were asymmetrical, associated in one case with multifocal epileptiform discharges and in the other with unilateral hypsarrhythmia. Partial seizures were always observed and the outcome was always poor. There have been reports of cases with early onset of spasms, frequent hypsarrhythmia, sometimes unilateral (Leyh and Loewel, 1973; Kurokawa *et al.*, 1981). Apart from one case in which MRI was normal but quadriplegia suggested a radiologically nondetectable cerebral lesion, most reports clearly confirm cerebral lesions. Vigevano *et al.* (1984) reported a case in which the CT scan showed hemimegalencephaly. In another case, the low density of the left parieto-temporal region indicated extensive lateralized cerebral lesions (Kurokawa *et al.*, 1981).

Woolly hair naevus and nevoid basal cell carcinoma syndrome (Larrègue *et al.*, 1977; Murphy and Tenser, 1982) are also associated with various kinds of epileptic seizures and epileptic spasms, but these diseases are classified as hamartomas rather than neurocutaneous syndromes.

CONCLUSIONS

Infantile spasms are rarely associated with neurocutaneous syndromes apart from tuberous sclerosis and more rarely NF1 neurofibromatosis (Matsumoto *et al.*, 1981b; Riikonen and Donner, 1979). In the other rare neurocutaneous syndromes, the frequency of IS is low and they are usually associated with brain lesions (neurological signs, MRI lesions, brain malformation on neuropathology), as described in Meencke and Gerhard (1985) and Jellinger's (1987) review of morphological aspects. The clinical and EEG profiles of spasms, the poor outcome of epilepsy and the mental evolution indicate that in these cases infantile spasms are probably an early expression of severe focal or multifocal symptomatic epilepsy, and that apart for NF1 they rarely meet the diagnostic criteria of West syndrome.

18

Perinatal Insult

R. CUSMAI

In the past, a prominent role in the etiology of infantile spasms (IS) was attributed to anoxic–ischemic insults. Chevrie and Aicardi (1977), studying the etiological factors of convulsive disorders occurring in the first year of life, found a higher incidence of abnormalities during pregnancy and delivery in children with IS than in patients with febrile or other occasional seizures. In a neuropathological study of IS, Jellinger (1987) found that perinatal brain damage accounted for 36–40% of the cases. Indeed, the reported incidence of perinatal brain damage in IS varies from 18 to 80% (Lacy and Penry, 1976). Aicardi (1986a, pp. 17–38) emphasized that these percentages are hard to assess because a difficult birth or an abnormal event occurring in the perinatal period does not necessarily imply a causal relationship. In Aicardi and Chevrie's (1978) series, if one considers severe abnormalities at birth followed by persistent neurological deficits, the percentage of IS caused by perinatal insults drops to 15%.

Perinatal insults, most of which have been reported to produce IS, include diffuse lesions due to hypoxic–ischemic encephalopathy and focal lesions, such as porencephaly (Alvarez *et al.*, 1987; Palm *et al.*, 1988; Cusmai *et al.*, 1988), caused by cerebrovascular disorders. Volpe (1987) classified the major neuro-pathological forms of hypoxic–ischemic encephalopathy as selective neuronal necrosis, status marmoratus, parasagittal cerebral injury, periventricular leuk-omalacia, focal and multifocal ischemic brain necrosis including porencephaly, and multicystic encephalomalacia.

PATHOPHYSIOLOGICAL MECHANISMS OF PERINATAL ASPHYXIA

The most common cause of perinatal ischemic disease is asphyxia. Several pathophysiological mechanisms may explain perinatal cerebral lesions of circulatory origin, such as a reduction or dysregulation of cerebral blood flow and sudden obstruction of the cerebral vessels (for a review, see Volpe, 1987). Acute fetal hypovolemia may be a consequence of hemorrhage as in placenta previa at the end of pregnancy, or of materno-fetal infections. Abruptio placenta, eclampsia, mechanical dystocia and complicated breech delivery may all cause acute fetal anoxia. Other disorders known to be responsible for cerebral injury are increased fetal blood viscosity and chronic placental insufficiency associated with maternal diabetes and toxemia. These disorders of fetal circulation may lead to cerebral damage by compromising arterial autoregulatory mechanisms. Arterial territories differ between premature and term infants, and cerebral lesions tend to occur in different regions of the brain at different ages. In the brain of the premature infant, the watershed areas are periventricular, mainly in the posterior part of the hemispheres. Metabolic activity in this region is intense and makes the periventricular region more susceptible to injury. Therefore, in compromised premature infants, periventricular leukomalacia is a common pathological finding, whereas epileptogenic cortical lesions are mild. In term infants, the watershed areas are localized in the regions between the anterior and middle cerebral arteries, and between the middle and posterior arteries. Thus cerebral lesions in term neonates mainly involve the cortex, and they are more common in the frontal and parieto-occipital regions. For these reasons, the clinical features of hypoxic–ischemic encephalopathy vary with gestational age and with the nature of the insult.

NEURORADIOLOGICAL FINDINGS

Computer tomography (CT) and magnetic resonance imaging (MRI) are useful in diagnosing different forms of perinatal insults (for a review, see Diebler and Dulac 1987, 1990; see also Chapter 10). CT findings of periventricular leukomalacia in premature infants are ventriculomegaly with an irregular outline of lateral ventricles due to reduced periventricular white matter, mainly at the trigones. MRI shows the same abnormalities, with a periventricular white matter hyperintense signal on T2-weighted sequences. In term infants, MRI is able to detect some conditions only described in the past by neuropathologists, such as status marmoratus and ulegyria. In status marmoratus, MRI shows clumps of myelinated fibers, which appear as areas of high signal intensity in the basal ganglia in T1-weighted sequences. In ulegyria, MRI identifies the characteristic gyral pattern of necrosis of the deepest part of the sulci, and the underlying tissue loss and gliosis.

In reviewing the CT and MRI scans in a series of 32 children presenting with symptomatic IS due to perinatal insult, we found diffuse as well as focal brain lesions (Cusmai *et al.*, 1993). Unilateral porencephalic lesions were present in 15 patients, but their topography and extent varied. Eight children had circumscribed cysts involving the rolandic or parieto-occipital regions (Fig. 18.1). Seven patients had large lesions involving the frontal lobe, which were associated with unilateral hemispheric atrophy in four cases (Fig. 18.2). Periventricular leukomalacia was noted in 12 patients, all of whom were premature

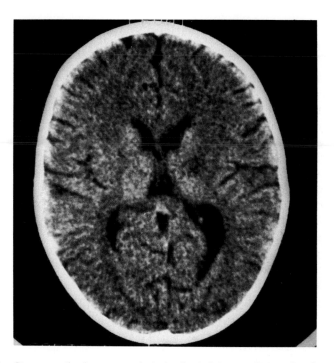

Figure 18.1   Circumscribed porencephaly in the left internal capsule of a patient with right hemiplegia and West syndrome who recovered completely from epilepsy and developed no seizures after steroids.

infants (Fig. 18.3), and 5 of them had diffuse bilateral atrophy with status marmoratus in one patient and bilateral ulegyria in another (Fig. 18.4).

CLINICAL FEATURES

In the neonatal period, full-term infants have seizures after a hypoxic–ischemic event more frequently than do premature infants, and CT scan shows brain swelling. Following this acute event, the patient's condition improves for several weeks before the first spasms appear, although CT scan shows atrophy and ventricular dilatation. Some EEG features suggest a high risk of IS: a markedly depressed tracing followed by multifocal spikes or sharp waves in the full-term neonate (Watanabe *et al.*, 1987a), and numerous positive rolandic spikes lasting several weeks in the prematurely delivered neonate (Radvanyi-Bouvet *et al.*, 1987).

   The clinical and prognostic features of IS following perinatal insult have been studied extensively (Matsumoto *et al.*, 1981b; Watanabe *et al.*, 1982). This group is heterogeneous with respect to radiological and clinical presentations. In the literature, age of onset of infantile spasms in the perinatal group is reported to

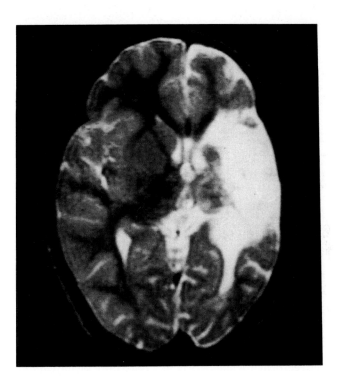

Figure 18.2 Large left porencephaly with hemiatrophy in a patient who suffered intractable focal epilepsy following infantile spasms.

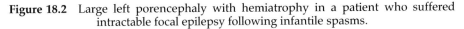

be slightly later in relation to other symptomatic causes of IS. Meencke and Gerhard (1985) reported that the mean age of onset of spasms following perinatal insult was 8 months, and in the study by Velez *et al.* (1990) the spasms appeared at 7 months. In our series, however, spasms appeared between 4 and 9 months of age (mean 5.5 months).

Spasms related to perinatal insults may be symmetric or more frequently asymmetric. Video/EEG recordings may define the exact semiology. Spasms appear in clusters, often preceded by partial seizures. Partial seizures preceding spasms are suggestive of focal brain damage. In diffuse brain lesions, spasms are asymmetrical or show focal signs such as eye or head deviation. Ictal EEGs may show focal seizures followed by a cluster of spasms, or a cluster of spasms with asymmetric recruiting rhythms or with asymmetric decremental activity (Cusmai *et al.*, 1993; Fig. 18.5). Interictal EEGs at the onset of spasms show diffuse or multifocal abnormalities with the characteristics of symmetrical or asymmetrical hypsarrhythmia (Fig. 18.6). Thus IS in patients with perinatal brain damage, particularly prematurely born patients, usually meet the characteristics of West syndrome (see Chapter 1). Neurological deficits are

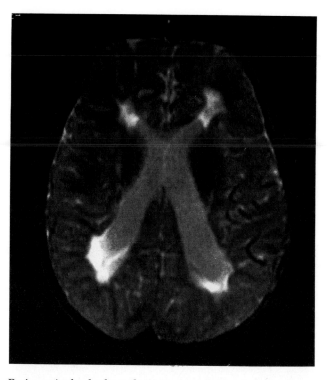

Figure 18.3 Periventricular leukomalacia in a premature infant who recovered from West syndrome and who suffered no seizures after steroid treatment.

often present in the first months of life or at birth. These typically include hemiplegia, diplegia or tetraplagia, dystonic movements, strabismus and various degrees of developmental delay.

Several investigators have studied the long-term outcome of children with IS, with respect to epilepsy and mental retardation (Riikonen, 1982; Jeavons *et al.*, 1990). Seizure relapse in the perinatal group occurred in 55.2% of patients after ACTH therapy (Matsumoto *et al.*, 1981b). A good prognosis for seizure control after steroid therapy was reported by Velez *et al.* (1990). These studies did not consider the neuroradiological features in relation to outcome of epilepsy.

In our series of 32 patients, 25% developed chronic epilepsy after IS. In correlating the CT and MRI scans of these patients with outcome of epilepsy, we divided the children into two groups (Table 18.1): those with unilateral porencephalic lesions (15/32) and those with diffuse cerebral lesions (17/32). In the group of 15 patients with porencephaly, we observed that the outcome of epilepsy was favorable in those patients with circumscribed lesions (Fig. 18.1). The patients who presented with seizure relapse had large porencephalic cysts involving the frontal lobe with cerebral hemiatrophy (Fig. 18.2). In the group with diffuse lesions, 12 were premature with periventricular leukomalacia (Fig.

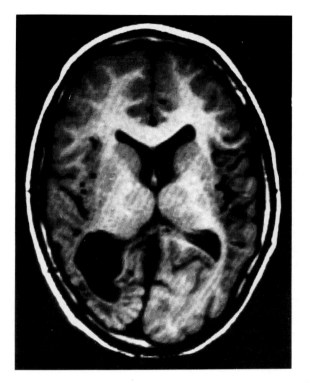

Figure 18.4 Right occipital and left rolandic ulegyria in an infant who, following term delivery, exhibited neonatal asphyxia followed by infantile spasms. The spasms remained intractable until callosotomy. Following surgery, the seizures occurred only occasionally for the next 5 years of follow-up (see Chapter 23).

18.3), and 5 were term infants with diffuse cerebral atrophy. In the subgroup of children with periventricular leukomalacia, most were seizure-free after steroid treatment. In the subgroup of children with diffuse cerebral atrophy, 3 of 5 had presented with epilepsy at follow-up (Fig. 18.4).

Very few data are available with regard to long-term outcome. Palm *et al.* (1987) reported an improvement in resistant cases of IS with porencephaly following the uncapping surgical procedure (see Chapter 23).

SUMMARY

Hypoxic–ischemic brain damage is an important neurological problem in the perinatal period. Neurological morbidity in patients with hypoxic–ischemic encephalopathy is high. Neurological sequelae include nonprogressive syndromes with mental retardation, seizures and motor deficits. CT and MRI may disclose focal as well as diffuse cerebral lesions, and may show various degrees of damage corresponding to different stages of evolution of cerebral hemorrhagic and ischemic lesions. MRI may show some brain morphological aspects due

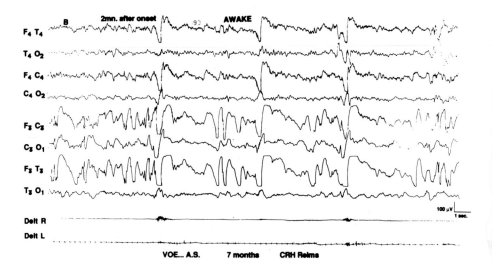

Figure 18.5 A girl with right congenital hemiplegia due to porencephaly. Spasms from 6 months of age. Note that there is persisting focal delta activity on the left hemisphere between consecutive spasms recorded on deltoid EMGs, and that there is no recurrence of hypsarrhythmia between consecutive spasms. Rapid response to steroids. No epilepsy 5 years later.

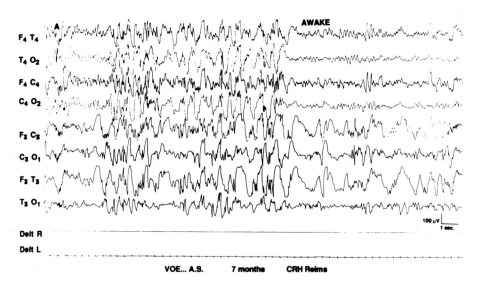

Figure 18.6 Same patient as in Fig. 18.5. Note the left slow-wave focus combined with the hypsarrhythmic pattern.

Table 18.1 Correlation of neuroradiological findings with outcome of epilepsy

	Porencephaly		Diffuse hemisphere lesions	
Outcome of epilepsy	Circumscribed ($n = 8$)	Large ($n = 7$)	Premature ($n = 12$)	Term delivery ($n = 5$)
Favorable	8	3	11	2
Unfavorable	0	4	1	3

to hypoxic–ischemic encephalopathy, such as ulegyria diagnosed in the past only by neuropathologists. MRI spectroscopy and positron emission tomography have improved the knowledge of the metabolic features of brain damage.

Perinatal brain damage may lead to various types of epilepsy with different age of onset and with different clinical features. Infantile spasms – usually West syndrome in this condition – is the most typical age-dependent epileptic disorder. The incidence of West syndrome has varied widely in a number of studies, from 15 to 80% of patients with IS in Lacy and Penry (1976) depending upon the clinical and EEG inclusion criteria. The decrease in incidence of perinatal anoxic–ischemic encephalopathy associated with IS is probably due to improvements in obstetric care and to the ability of recent neuroradiological investigations to distinguish prenatal lesions with incidental delivery complications from severe perinatal insults. In our series, taking into account only those patients with severe perinatal complications, we found the percentages of patients with IS following perinatal insults to be comparable with those reported by Aicardi and Chevrie (1978). The outcome of epilepsy is probably related to the extent, severity and topography of brain lesions. In premature infants with periventricular leukomalacia, the neurological deficits are more severe than epileptic disorders because of the predominantly white matter involvement. West syndrome may occur in these patients whose response to steroids is prompt and the outcome of epilepsy favorable. It is remarkable that leukomalacia often predominates in the posterior areas of the brain, those which are most usually involved in the development of West syndrome, probably as a consequence of maturational chronology (see Chapters 11 and 12).

In patients presenting with diffuse cortical atrophy and in some patients with porencephalic lesions, cortical involvement is responsible for the most severe epileptic outcome.

19

Infectious Disorders Associated with West Syndrome

R. RIIKONEN

The known causes of infantile spasms are multiple and it is often stated that infantile spasms are but a response of the immature brain to multiple types of insults. One or more of the congenital central nervous system infections have been cited in 16 reports (Christensen and Melchior, 1960; Feldman and Schwartz, 1968; Jellinger, 1970; Watanabe et al., 1973; Lacy and Penry, 1976; Midulla et al., 1976; Oates and Harvey, 1976; Riikonen, 1978; Riikonen and Donner, 1979; Kurokawa et al., 1980; Matsumoto et al., 1981; Lombroso, 1983a; Dyken et al., 1985; Meencke, 1985; Jellinger, 1987; Prats et al., 1991): congenital cytomegalovirus (CMV, $n = 4$ reports), congenital toxoplasmosis ($n = 5$), congenital rubella ($n = 2$) and congenital syphilis ($n = 2$). One or more meningitides or encephalitides have been cited as etiologic factors in 13 reports (Millichap et al., 1962; Jellinger, 1970; Lacy and Penry, 1976; Riikonen and Donner, 1979; Kurokawa et al., 1980; Matsumoto et al., 1981; Lombroso, 1983a; Fois et al., 1984; Dyken et al., 1985; Meencke, 1985; Jellinger, 1987; Glaze et al., 1988; Prats et al., 1991). The most frequent were measles encephalitis ($n = 4$), varicella ($n = 2$), pertussis ($n = 2$), tuberculosis ($n = 3$) and meningococcal meningitis ($n = 21$). Infections were considered to be the etiology of infantile spasms in 3–11% of patients in large series: 27/757 patients of 3.5% (Kurokawa et al., 1980) 6/200 patients of 3% (Matsumoto et al., 1981), 22/214 patients or 10% (Riikonen, 1982), 18/165 patients or 11% (Lombroso, 1983a) and 11/191 patients or 5.7% (Fois et al., 1984). In their epidemiological studies of infections and infantile spasms, Hughes and Long (1986) raised the possibility that infectious diseases play a more significant role in infantile spasms than had previously been thought. The successful treatment of some cases of infantile spasms with immunoglobulins (Echenne et al., 1987; Ariizumi et al., 1987) indicates that immunological events may play a role in the pathogenesis of infantile spasms in some patients.

Although infections are often mentioned as etiological factors of infantile spasms, surprisingly little information is available on the diagnostic work-up, course and outcome of these children. At the Children's Hospital, University of Helsinki, all cases with infantile spasms were studied carefully with regard to infections and followed for many years (Riikonen, 1978, 1982; Riikonen and Donner, 1979). This series involved 29 patients: congenital CMV ($n = 5$), congenital or acquired CMV ($n = 1$), acquired CMV ($n = 5$), congenital rubella ($n = 2$), herpes simplex virus ($n = 5$), enterovirus ($n = 1$), adenovirus ($n = 1$), viral encephalitis with unknown agent ($n = 3$), meningococcus ($n = 4$), pneumococcus ($n = 1$) and pertussis ($n = 1$).

TYPES OF INFECTIONS

Cytomegalovirus

In 1968, Feldman and Schwarz reported a possible association between CMV infection and infantile spasms. Subsequently, Midulla *et al.* (1976) described three children with infantile spasms who had concomitant CMV viruria and suggested that spasms are sometimes the result of acquired, primary infection. Although seizures may accompany congenital CMV infection, an association between infantile spasms and CMV virus remains difficult to assess because at the age when infantile spasms usually begin, up to 36% of normal children excrete CMV in their urine (Granström *et al.*, 1977). Furthermore, there is evidence that acquired CMV infections generally cause no acute clinical symptoms and are without sequelae (Granström *et al.*, 1977; Stagno, 1990; Alford *et al.*, 1990).

In Finland, Riikonen retrospectively reviewed data on 205 children with infantile spasms (Riikonen, 1978). In 11 children (5%), spasms were attributed to CMV infection. At least five of the infants had congenital CMV, and three of them exhibited intracranial calcifications. Infection in the remaining infants appeared to be acquired postnatally. CMV viruria was recorded in 9 of the 11 infants. Although all but one of the infants exhibited intellectual impairment, the symptoms were less severe in those infants thought to have acquired CMV infection. Remarkably, in two infants, severe (in one case fatal) disseminated CMV infection developed during corticotrophin therapy. Furthermore, two children with CMV infection – one congenital and the other acquired – still showed signs of chronic central nervous system (CNS) infection many years later. In both cases, the CSF IgG and IgG albumin ratios were increased. Using the sensitive ELISA method, intrathecal CMV antibody production was demonstrated in one case. The same patient also showed signs of chronic infection at autopsy.

The detection of CMV-specific IgG or IgM antibodies in the cerebrospinal fluid (CSF) may also indicate ongoing CNS infection. The nucleic acid hybridization technique may ultimately prove valuable as a rapid diagnostic method for detecting CMV virus, or for determining whether or not CMV latently infects the CNS (Bale, 1984; Chou, 1990).

Congenital Rubella

Rubella infection as an etiological factor in infantile spasms has been reported by Oates and Harvey (1976) and Riikonen and Donner (1979). The diagnosis should be considered in any infant with evidence of intrauterine growth retardation and other stigmata consistent with congenital infection, regardless of maternal history. Congenital infection can be confirmed by laboratory tests (Preblud and Alford, 1990). First, in children with encephalitis, the virus may persist in the CSF for several years. Second, the CSF may also be examined for the presence of rubella-specific IgM. In general, detectable IgM antibody is a reliable indicator of congenital infection because IgM is fetally derived. Third, the persistence of IgG antibody at the age of 6–12 months, especially in high titers, is presumptive evidence of intrauterine infection with rubella virus. Sera should be drawn at 3 and 5–6 months, with a repeat specimen at 12 months if necessary.

Congenital Toxoplasmosis

Toxoplasmosis has in only a few cases been mentioned as an etiological factor in infantile spasms (Christensen and Melchior, 1960; Dumermuth, 1961; Riikonen and Donner, 1979; Kurokawa et al., 1980; Meencke, 1985). The most widely used serological tests for the diagnosis of toxoplasmosis are the Sabin-Feldman dye test, the complement fixation (CF) test, the indirect hemagglutination test, the IFA test, the double-sandwich IgM-ELISA and the IgM-immunosorbent agglutination assay (Vesikari et al., 1980). Recently, measurement of the avidity of IgG antibodies against *Toxoplasma gondii* has proved valuable in the diagnosis of toxoplasma infection (Hedman et al., 1989). The ELISA technology has been adapted for serodiagnosis of toxoplasmosis and appears likely to replace much of the present methodology. Persistent CSF pleocytosis, an elevated protein content and the persistence of IgM antibodies for toxoplasma may also suggest continued active infection. Such persistence of IgM antibodies has also been reported in congenital rubella (Vesikari et al., 1980).

Herpes Simplex Virus

To the best of our knowledge, no reports have been published of infantile spasms after herpes encephalitis. The diagnosis of herpes simplex virus (HSV) infection is often delayed. Cytosine arabinoside was given to three of five patients in the Finnish series, but it did not prevent a severe brain lesion and onset of infantile spasms, which appeared very soon after the onset of encephalitis.

The clinical diagnosis of HSV infection is difficult in neonates in particular, because of the frequent absence of skin vesicles as an initial component of the disease. Serial demonstrations of increased CSF cell counts and protein concentrations, negative bacterial cultures of CSF and negative antigen studies of CSF acid in the diagnosis of HSV infection of the CNS (Kohl, 1988; Whitley, 1990). The use of α-interferon has long been the most rapid method for diagnosing HSV. Every effort should be made to confirm infection by viral isolation (skin lesions, CSF, stool, urine, throat, nasopharynx and conjuctivae). A definite diagnosis is only made by the detection of HSV in brain biopsies or, more recently, by the demonstration of HSV-DNA in CSF using the polymerase chain reaction technique (Aurelius *et al.*, 1991). Serological diagnosis of HSV infection is not of great clinical value because therapeutic decisions must be made before the results of serological studies are known. Electroencephalography, computed tomography (CT) and magnetic resonance imaging (MRI) are all useful for detecting CNS abnormalities (Koskiniemi and Ketonen, 1981; Sainio *et al.*, 1983; Mikati *et al.*, 1990). Because immunoglobulin production in the CNS may continue for years after the primary infection (Koskiniemi *et al.*, 1984; Vandvik *et al.*, 1985; Riikonen and Meurman, 1989), estimation of the IgG index may provide important clues as to past HSV infection at the age when infantile spasms appear.

Because toxoplasmosis and herpes infections can now be successfully treated, early diagnosis is important. Toxoplasmosis and rubella as causes of infantile spasms can be prevented if maternal screening, prenatal diagnosis of toxoplasmosis (Remington and Desmonts, 1990) and vaccination against rubella are carried out.

Enterovirus and Adenovirus

Enterovirus and adenovirus infections in the Finnish series had a similar clinical picture to that of HSV encephalitis. Acyclovir was commenced in two patients before the viral infection was definitely diagnosed – $ECHO_{22}$ in one patient and adenovirus in the other. Both patients also showed progressive degenerative lesions on their brain CT.

Other Viral Etiology

Three patients in the Finnish series showed encephalitis with gastrointestinal symptoms, but the search for viral agents failed to disclose a specific agent.

Bacterial Meningitis

Like other severe insults to the brain, meningitis can result in infantile spasms. Bacterial meningitis has often been considered a cause of infantile spasms; for example, in 21/757 patients in the series of Kurokawa *et al.* (1980).

EVALUATION FOR INFECTION

Table 19.1 summarizes the diagnostic work-up of infection in children with infantile spasms at presentation.

Head circumference can be taken as a measure of brain growth, and the brain injury can be timed from a point at which head growth ceases (Riikonen and Donner, 1979). Impairment of vision, sensorineuronal hearing loss and congenital heart malformations are often seen in congenitally infected children. Every child with infantile spasms should be examined by fundoscopy. Retinal changes can lead to the suspicion of infectious etiology (rubella, CMV and toxoplasma).

EEG is a sensitive test for the diagnosis of neonatal HSV encephalitis. It is superior to radiological procedures in detecting cerebral involvement. The paroxysms consist typically of sharp or triangular waves at pseudoperiodic intervals of 0.5–1.5 s (Sainio et al., 1983; Mikati et al., 1990). Skull X-ray, CT or MRI are able to show calcifications typical for toxoplasmosis and CMV. CT and MRI may show progressive atrophic lesions in the temporal region typical of HSV encephalitis (Koskiniemi and Ketonen, 1981). They are also able to show brain malformations. However, a diagnosis of brain malformation does not exclude a viral etiology. A neuroradiological suggestion of lissencephaly of the brain has been reported in association with CMV but without neuropathological demonstration of the four-layered malformation (see Ch. 9) (Hayward et al., 1991). In addition, in our series, lissencephaly was associated with herpes infection in one patient. Aicardi syndrome has many clinical similarities with congenital infections (Willis and Rosman, 1980), in particular toxoplasmosis, but the outcome may be quite different. Furthermore, serial serum titers of rubella, toxoplasmosis and HSV can lead to the diagnosis of congenital infections. Because one-third of infants are infected with CMV by the age of onset of infantile spasms, the measurement of serum antibodies or virus isolation in urine does not lead to a diagnosis. CMV antibodies should, however, be measured before starting steroid therapy, because in cases of infection (pneumonitis, encephalitis) a rise in antibodies confirms the diagnosis of CMV infection, which can be fulminant during therapy.

Table 19.1 Etiology of infantile spasms: diagnostic work-up of infections at presentation

1. History and physical examination
   – growth of the head (microcephaly, hydrocephaly)
   – examination of eyes, hearing, heart
2. EEG
3. Skull X-ray, CT or MRI
4. Serum titers of rubella, toxoplasma, cytomegalovirus and herpes
5. CSF: cell count, glucose, protein, bacterial culture, IgG index, virus antibody index (CSF/serum levels of virus-specific IgG: CSF/serum levels of albumin)
6. CSF: rubella IgM, toxoplasma IgM, virus isolation when specific infections are suspected.

CSF examination is able to detect chronic CNS infections by leukocytosis, high protein and/or a high IgG index. In our experience, a high IgG index led to the diagnosis of herpes infection 2–3 weeks later in one patient. In this case, HSV isolation and fluorescent antigen were negative. The rise in CF titers occurred only later. EEG was nondiagnostic. If there is any suspicion of chronic CMV infection, a high viral antibody index may lead to diagnosis even years later (Riikonen and Donner, 1979). Rubella and toxoplasma IgM should be studied and virus isolation attempted when specific infections are suspected.

SEIZURES AND EVOLUTION OF EEG FEATURES

The following is based on a Finnish study of 29 children with infectious etiology for the spasms (Riikonen, 1978, 1982; Riikonen and Donner, 1979).

Seizures

The children with congenital CMV infection ($n = 5$) and congenital rubella infection ($n = 2$) had very early signs of CNS irritation: long-lasting tremors despite normal blood sugar and calcium, or generalized convulsions. The mean age of onset of infantile spasms in the whole group was 7.2 (range 2–16) months. All but three patients (90%) continued to experience seizures after a mean follow-up of 7 (range 0.4–13) years. The mean interval between viral encephalitis and onset of infantile spasms was short, only 2.2 (range 0.5–3.5) m04ths.

EEG

EEG abnormalities preceded hypsarrhythmia in 10/11 patients where EEG was carried out before the onset of infantile spasms. The first EEG showed findings characteristic of herpes encephalitis in 4/5 patients. No other characteristic EEG patterns were seen in other patients. At the end of follow-up, EEG was normal in only three patients (10%). In five patients, the EEG showed a pattern of generalized slow spike-wave complexes (1.5–2.5 complexes per second) of the Lennox-Gastaut syndrome type.

The children with infectious etiology continued to have seizures and had an abnormal EEG more often than children with other etiology, 32% of whom were seizure-free and 21% of whom had a normal EEG at follow-up (Riikonen, 1982).

NEUROPATHOLOGICAL FINDINGS

The number of reported autopsies of children with infantile spasms associated with infections is small. In his review of the neuropathological findings of 264 patients with a history of infantile spasms, Jellinger (1987) noted five series in which one or more children had an infection (see Table 19.2). The neuropathological findings were as follows: immature ganglion cells and delayed stratification of cortex in one patient (Christensen and Melchior, 1960), and a diminished number of Purkinje cells in another, subependymal cystic necroses and calcifications suggesting the sequelae of toxoplasmosis (Dumermuth, 1961); microdysgenesis in suspected connatal toxoplasmosis and chronic meningitis (Meencke, 1985); severe vascular or hypoxic brain damage due to early infections (Jellinger, 1970); spongy lesions of the neuropil similar to those in transmissible spongiform subacute encephalopathies caused by slow viruses (three patients) (Dumermuth, 1961). The causal relationship between infantile spasms and acute meningitis or meningoencephalitis has, however, been questioned (Lacy and Penry, 1976; Jellinger, 1987).

These autopsies did not yield any new data on the genesis of infantile spasms. It may be that very large (cortical) lesions of the brain of any etiology can cause infantile spasms at a certain stage of brain maturation. However, inflammatory changes in the brainstem were found in one patient reported by Kellaway (1959) and in the patients of Morimatsu et al. (1977). These abnormalities were thought to be operative in the pathogenesis of infantile spasms (Kellaway et al., 1983). Unfortunately, the brainstem has not been studied specifically in most autopsies. However, in careful neuropathological examinations by Christensen and Melchior (1960), the brainstem was normal in all six autopsies.

TREATMENT AND COURSE

In the Finnish series, ACTH therapy was not given to 8/29 children with infectious etiology because of severe mental retardation. In the remaining 21 children, the response was good (total cessation of spasms and disappearance of hypsarrhythmia) in 8 patients (38%) and poor in the remaining 13 patients (62%). A better response to ACTH (60%) was seen in the series of infantile spasms from Finland (Riikonen, 1982). Severe disseminated CMV infection developed in two patients during therapy. The response was poor in the two patients with congenital CMV infections treated with ACTH, and in all five children with preceding HSV infection.

It would appear advisable, then, to avoid ACTH therapy in children with congenital or symptomatic acquired CMV infection. Children with a proven history of congenital infection (virus isolated in the urine before the age of 2–3 weeks) and children strongly suspected of having a congenital infection because of their clinical symptoms (microencephaly, retardation, brain calcifications, chorioretinitis, virus isolation) should be treated with more conventional anticonvulsants and not with ACTH. Furthermore, children with meningoencephalitis, pneumonitis or other clinical manifestations of a possible CMV infection should be immediately evaluated for CMV infection. If antibody titers rise to or exceed four-fold, CMV infection must be suspected

Table 19.2 Autopsy series of infantile spasms and infections

	Diagnosis	No. of patients	Neuropathology
Christensen and Melchior (1960)	Encephalitidis seq.	2	*Case 1*: immature ganglion cells and delayed stratification of cortex *Case 2*: diminished number of Purkinje cells in the granular layer of cerebellum
Dumermuth (1961)	Toxoplasmosis	1	Subependymal cystic necroses and calcifications
Jellinger (1970)	Postmeningitic encephalopathy	1	Ulegyria, thalamic, cerebellar and cortical atrophy
Riikonen and Donner (1979)	CMV and toxoplasmosis	1	Multifocal necroses in brain, CMV inclusion bodies in brain, kidney, lungs
	Toxoplasmosis	1	Large meningeal and intracerebral calcifications
Toga and Gambarelli (1982)	Encephalopathy	3	Spongy lesions of the neuropil[a]
Meencke (1985)	Toxoplasmosis	1	Cortical microdysgenesis
	Chronic meningitis	1	Cortical microdysgenesis, meningitis, scar within hippocampus, gliosis within brainstem dendate nucleus

[a]Ultrastructurally similar to those in transmissible spongiform subacute encephalopathies caused by slow virus.

and ACTH therapy should not be given or it should be discontinued. It is recommended that CMV antibody titers for comparison of later titers should be determined in all patients before starting a course of ACTH. The demonstration of CMV-induced early antigen in cell culture permits the rapid detection of CMV in urine, blood, bronchoalveolar fluid or CSF (Chou, 1990).

It has been shown that good results with immunoglobulin therapy are seen in some patients with intrathecal IgG or IgM synthesis or in postencephalitic patients (Sandstedt et al., 1984). It may be that patients with herpes virus infections (CMV and herpex simplex virus) benefit more from immunoglobulin therapy than from corticosteroid treatment, which may potentially be hazardous because of its immunosuppressive properties (Haynes, 1990; Abraham and Manho, 1977) and because herpesviruses tend to persist in the host. Toxoplasma gondii can also be reactivated by steroid therapy. It is also known that in transplantant recipients in which corticosteroids have remained a part of the immunosuppressive regime, Toxoplasma gondii can cause meningoencephalitis or progressive brain lesions (Ho and Dummer, 1990).

In the study of Glaze et al. (1988), all three children with infantile spasms following meningitis had very severe developmental and intellectual impairment (Glaze et al., 1988). In our study, all but 3 of the 29 children (2 with acquired CMV infection and 1 with encephalitis with unknown etiology) became mentally retarded after follow-up. These children had a less favorable outcome compared with the 214 children in the earlier reported Finnish series in which 78% were mentally retarded (Riikonen, 1982). Cerebral palsy was also frequent (20/29 children or 69%). Many children with severe mental retardation also had a severe visual and hearing impairment and autistic-like behavior.

CAUSAL RELATIONSHIP BETWEEN INFANTILE SPASMS AND INFECTIONS

In the Finnish series, most of the children had an uneventful history and normal mental development prior to meningitis or encephalitis but cognitive status deteriorated and spasms developed soon thereafter. The causal relationship between infantile spasms and infections in these children seems evident. Our series also supports the conclusion that infantile spasms may be associated with CMV infection, but only a small proportion (5% or less) of cases would appear to be the result of acquired or symptomatic congenital CMV infection. Whether preceding nonspecific or subclinical infections act as triggering events for infantile spasms as suggested by Hughes and Long (1986) remains to be seen.

CONCLUSIONS

1. Infectious diseases may play a more significant role in infantile spasms than previously thought. New virological methods have made a more accurate

diagnosis possible. A careful etiological evaluation, including a search for infections, should be undertaken for every child with spasms of unknown cause.

2. Brain malformations may also be caused by viruses.
3. It is advisable not to give steroid therapy to children with congenital or postnatal symptomatic CMV infections because steroids have immunosuppressive properties that may make the infections fulminant. This may also be true for other herpes viruses. It remains to be seen if postencephalitic patients in particular benefit from immunoglobulin therapy for infantile spasms.
4. The outcome of children with infectious etiology seems to be particularly poor. This makes the prevention and specific diagnosis of infections especially important. The infections caused by CMV, HSV, toxoplasma, syphilis, pertussis, tuberculosis, meningococcus and pneumococcus are now treatable. Vaccinations against rubella, measles, pertussis and tuberculosis – and hopefully against CMV and other infectious agents in the future – will help to reduce the number of infections.

20

Miscellaneous Causes

O. DULAC

It has been said that infantile spasms (IS) are but an age-related and nonspecific response of the brain to various types of insult (Kellaway, 1959). Indeed, a great variety of brain lesions may produce IS. Although the great majority of cases are due to diseases discussed in specific chapters of this book, a sizable number of less common causes remain to be addressed. They can be classified into a few etiologic groups: chromosomal aberrations, complex malformative syndromes, inborn errors of metabolism, tumors and postnatal disorders.

CHROMOSOMAL ABERRATIONS

A number of chromosomal aberrations may produce major brain malformations that cause IS; for example, 17p deletion producing agyria–pachygyria (see Chapter 15), trisomy 13 producing holoprosencephaly (see Chapter 15), and a number of chromosomal abnormalities producing callosal agenesis (see below). On the other hand, chromosomal aberration may produce IS, although there is no neuroradiological evidence of brain malformation, e.g. t(6;14)(q27;q13.3) (Hattori et al., 1985). The same applies to cases supposed to result from chromosomal deletion, i.e. some cases of Rett syndrome (Hagberg, 1993). In all these cases, there is developmental delay prior to the occurrence of the first spasms.

The incidence of epilepsy is slightly higher in *Down syndrome* (DS) than in the general population. About 2.5–3% of cases exhibit epilepsy, and two to three times as many exhibit occasional seizures (Pueschel et al., 1991; Staftstrom et al., 1991) related to ischemia or intracranial infection, whereas febrile convulsions are rare. Epileptic spasms (ES) are the most frequent types of seizures that occur in infancy, accounting for over half the seizures beginning before 2 years and the majority of those occurring in the first year of life. In a study of 32 patients with DS and epilepsy, 10 patients exhibited ES, with most of the others suffering from myoclonic, tonic and/or generalized tonic–clonic seizures; only 19% had focal seizures (Guerrini et al., 1989). Reflex seizures are frequent (Guerrini et al., 1990).

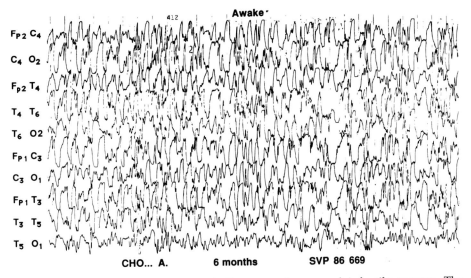

Figure 20.1 A 6-month-old boy with Down syndrome and infantile spasms. The awake tracing shows typical hypsarrhythmia.

The combination of ES with DS was first reported in 1963 by Coriat. In this series, 1% of DS patients were affected. Psychomotor delay precedes the first seizures that occur at a mean age of 6 months (range 5–8 months), and consists of symmetrical spasms and no other type of seizure is combined with the spasms (unpublished personal series). In the latter series, the EEG showed a typical hypsarrhythmic pattern in five cases (Fig. 20.1), which disappeared in one of the three cases administered diazepam intravenously. Spasms were recorded in three cases in which hypsarrhythmia reappeared between consecutive spasms of a cluster (Fig. 20.2). No major psychomotor deterioration was noted, although the patients became agitated.

Following steroid treatment, outcome is favorable in most instances: 8/10 cases in one series (Guerrini *et al.*, 1989), 4/5 in another (unpublished personal series). The spasms disappear at a mean age of 4 months, hypsarrhythmia at 5 months, with recovery of the previous psychomotor condition.

MALFORMATIONS

Callosal agenesis is a neuropathological finding common to a number of more or less specific brain malformations. Although the combination of IS and callosal agenesis is characteristic of Aicardi syndrome (see Chapters 9 and 15), it may be observed in other conditions, including cases similar to Aicardi syndrome from the clinical, EEG and neuropathological points of view, but occurring in boys (Curatolo *et al.*, 1980; Billette de Villemeur *et al.*, 1992), a variety of chromosomal aberrations (for a review, see Diebler and Dulac, 1987), a rare condition with

Spasm

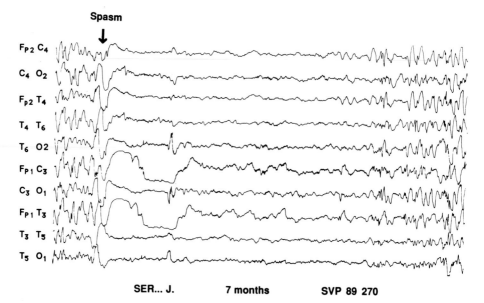

SER... J.   7 months   SVP 89 270

Figure 20.2   A 7-month-old girl with Down syndrome. The ictal tracing shows high-amplitude slow waves. The hypsarrhythmic tracing recurs before the following spasm of the cluster, as in idiopathic West syndrome.

sex-linked inheritance (Menkes *et al.*, 1964) and in rare cases of agyria (Josephy, 1944).

Seizures are particularly frequent in callosal agenesis. In one series, over 50% of the patients exhibited seizures, and 17/96 had IS, 10 of whom did not have Aicardi syndrome (Diebler and Dulac, 1987). The clinical and EEG character-istics of these patients were very variable, though not one patient had typical or modified hypsarrhythmia. The seizures remained intractable and all the patients either died or remained severely retarded.

A single case of IS with *hamartoma of the tuber cinereum* has been reported, although over 24 cases with epilepsy are on record (Garcia Alvarez, 1992).

Hydranencephaly: One detailed clinical study reported flexor and asymmetri-cal spasms with the head and eyes moved to the right, lasting 1–2 s and repeated in clusters at approximately 5 s intervals for up to 5 min, from the age of 4 months (Neville, 1972). The EEG showed a complete absence of phasic activity over the entire head, even during the spasms which on the poly-EMG, showed both flexor and extensor involvement.

ANGIOMAS

A single case of multiple neonatal hemangiomas complicated at the age of 4 months with infantile spasms has been reported (McShane *et al.*, 1990). The EEG tracing was defined as hypsarrhythmic and CT scan showed a right temporoparietal calcified lesion which enhanced with intravenous contrast. After steroid treatment, follow-up at 24 months was favorable.

INBORN ERRORS OF METABOLISM

In one case of *Pyruvate carboxylase deficiency*, Rutledge *et al.* (1989) reported a patient who had suffered neonatal hypothermia and acidosis, and who developed flexor spasms from the age of 7 weeks. These seizures were described as flexion of the head and extremities lasting approximately 30 s and occurring 5–6 times a day. The EEG was diffusely slow with multifocal spikes. This case illustrates the difficulties encountered when dealing with reports involving inborn errors of metabolism. The term "infantile spasms" seems to have been used in an excessively broad way, and this helps to confuse the nosological definitions.

The suggestion that *pyridoxine deficiency* may be involved in some patients with infantile spasms (Cochrane, 1959; French *et al.*, 1965) has been critically reviewed by Jeavons and Bower (1974), who pointed to the conflicting results obtained with typtophane metabolism investigations in epileptic children (Hughes *et al.*, 1967; Hagberg *et al.*, 1966) and concluded that, if it exists at all, pyridoxine deficiency must be very rare in patients with infantile spasms.

Rare cases of infantile spasms combined with *Van Boggaert–Bertrand's spongy dystrophy* (Meencke, 1985; Poser and Low, 1960), *Krabbe's disease* (Williams *et al.*, 1979; Andrews *et al.*, 1971), *Leigh's disease* (Diebler and Dulac, 1987; Kamoshita *et al.*, 1970) and *orthochromatic leukodystrophy* (Bignami *et al.*, 1966) are drawn from neuropathological series without any clinical or EEG data, and they remain therefore most unreliable. Dalla Bernardina *et al.* (1979) showed that the so-called cases of infantile spasms combined with *glycine encephalopathy* were not epileptic, but due to decerebration manifestations. Colamaria *et al.* (1989) also showed that *biotinidase deficiency* does not produce epileptic spasms, but nonepileptic massive myoclonus.

Neonatal adrenoleukodystrophy may occasionally produce West syndrome with clusters of spasms and hypsarrhythmia in a severely hypotonic patient with dysmorphia of the face and extremities of the limbs (Aubourg *et al.*, 1986).

TUMORS

Several single case reports have involved a combination of brain tumors and IS occurring in the first 2 years of life (3–15 months). Focal or generalized tonic seizures may precede the spasms (Mimaki *et al.*, 1983). Epileptic spasms are combined with typical (Ruggieri *et al.*, 1989) or modified (Mimaki *et al.*, 1983) hypsarrhythmia. The initial response to steroids (Ruggieri *et al.*, 1989) or vigabatrin (personal observation) may reveal focal EEG abnormalities, although this is not always the case (Mimaki *et al.*, 1983).

The relationship between the tumor and IS is not always clear. In patients with Aicardi syndrome, it is unlikely that papilloma of the choroid plexus plays any role in the generation of IS (Pollack *et al.*, 1983; Robinow *et al.*, 1984; de Jong *et al.*, 1976; Chevrie and Aicardi, 1984). In most cases the tumor appears to be the only pathological finding, and IS may even resolve after the tumor is removed (Mimaki *et al.*, 1983; Pedespan *et al.*, 1992; Ruggieri *et al.*, 1989; Branch and Dyken, 1979; Ashkensai and Snead, 1991). The tumor is located in various areas of the brain, including the basal ganglia (Ruggieri *et al.*,1989; Gastaut *et al.*, 1978) and the temporal (Mimaki *et al.*, 1983) and frontal (Pedespan *et al.*, 1992) cortex. The tumor could be an ependymoma (Ruggieri *et al.*, 1989), glioma (Ruggieri *et al.*, 1989), ganglioglioma (Gabriel, 1983) or choroid plexus papilloma (Pollack *et al.*, 1983; Robinow *et al.*, 1984; de Jong *et al.*, 1976; Branch and Dyken, 1979).

POSTNATAL ANOXIC – ISCHEMIC ENCEPHALOPATHY

Several conditions may produce postnatal anoxic–ischemic encephalopathy. They share a common acute clinical expression with altered level of consciousness and status epilepticus (SE).

Near-miss sudden infant death, also called *apparent life-threatening event* (ALTE), has recently been recognized as a frequently overlooked cause of SE in young infants, aged 2–4 months. In one series, it accounted for 11/63 cases of infantile SE (Aubourg *et al.*, 1985). The SE consisted of repeated unilateral seizures or generalized tonic fits, with EEGs showing rhythmic slow spikes or slow spikes and waves of 2–3 Hz alternately over both hemispheres, mainly over the parieto-occipital regions. The duration of SE ranged from 1 h to 4 days, and CT showed watershed ischemic areas of edema, mainly in the parieto-occipital regions, evolving to diffuse cortical atrophy or multicystic encephalomalacia. It is usually the retrospective analysis that reveals earlier transitory respiratory failure with cyanosis, hypotonia and unresponsiveness 36 h to 4 days prior to the onset of SE.

Two patients in this series developed epilepsy after the episode of SE. They suffered from IS at 5 and 6 months, respectively, 3 months after the episode of SE, combined with severe psychomotor retardation and a focal motor defect. In both instances, the clinical and EEG characteristics of IS were the same as those encountered in patients with neonatal anoxic–ischemic encephalopathy (see Chapter 18). In both cases, steroids helped to resolve the IS. It is interesting to note that the lesions predominated in the parieto-occipital areas, according to both EEG and CT findings, as is often the case in patients with IS (Cusmai *et al.*, 1988).

Hrachovy *et al.* (1987) reported two patients who after an episode of near-drowning developed a vegetative state and tetraparesis, but no seizure in the acute stage. Three months later, in the second and third year of life, respectively, they exhibited IS with modified hypsarrhythmia. Following steroid treatment, epilepsy resolved in only one of the patients.

TRAUMA

In the early series, trauma was reported as a cause of IS. However, its incidence has varied greatly in the largest of the series: 0% in Bamburg and Mattes (1959), 10% in Kellaway (1959), 7% in Millichap *et al.* (1962) and 0.9% in Gastaut *et al.* (1964b). Like perinatal anoxia, there is surely a tendency to overestimate the frequency of trauma. This is evidenced by reports of patients with subdural hematoma by Millichap *et al.* (1962) and Gastaut *et al.* (1964b). However, no study has yet devoted itself to this specific type of brain damage and the characteristics of IS following trauma.

21

Cryptogenic/Idiopathic West Syndrome

O. DULAC, P. PLOUIN

DEFINITIONS

The combination of epileptic spasms and an EEG pattern of hypsarrhythmia occurring in infants is designated as West syndrome (WS) and can be due to a variety of brain lesions. Apart from these symptomatic cases, a sizable number of patients with WS – from 15% (Matsumoto *et al.*, 1981b) to 32% (Kellaway *et al.*, 1983) – have a normal developmental course prior to onset of the disease and have no clinical or radiological evidence of brain lesions or other etiological factors. They were classically designated as either idiopathic (Jeavons and Bower, 1964) or cryptogenic (Gastaut *et al.*, 1964b). According to these authors, both terms meant that there was no evident cause of the disease. However, as indicated later in the classification of epilepsies and epileptic syndromes of the International League Against Epilepsy (1989), both terms are not precisely synonymous when applied to epilepsy.

The term "cryptogenic", from the Greek κρυπτός, γένος (hidden origin), relates to cases in which the cause cannot be identified. This is in contrast to symptomatic cases for which etiology can be precisely determined, or in which there is evidence of brain damage. Table 21.1 shows the various definitions given for the term cryptogenic when applied to WS. The major goal in cryptogenic cases is to identify the hidden lesion, its topography and its nature.

The term "idiopathic", from the Greek ἴδιος, πάθος (disease produced by itself, and which has no other cause than itself) relates to cases without any brain damage: the condition is purely functional. It develops at a specific age and leaves no sequelae. Although the term idiopathic has applied to WS in the past, the cases referred to were in fact a combination of patients that would meet the present definition of combined idiopathic and cryptogenic WS (Jeavons and Bower, 1964). The presently more restricted definition of the term idiopathic was considered by the Commission on Classification and Terminology of the International League against Epilepsy (1989). According to this classification, WS is not supposed to be idiopathic and all cases are considered as either symptomatic or cryptogenic. However, several patients with WS have been reported who benefit from spontaneous disappearance of epilepsy and complete recovery of mental development (Bachman, 1981; Dulac *et al.*, 1986a; Hrachovy *et al.*, 1991).

A review of the published literature and our own cases shows that idiopathic WS (IWS) does exist and that it may be recognized based upon a number of clinical and electroencephalographic (EEG) characteristics, from the onset of the disease.

FREQUENCY

Given the variability of definitions of the terms "cryptogenic" and "idiopathic" in previous series, it is not surprising that the proportion of cases with favorable outcome has varied (Table 21.2). Based on present knowledge, the combination of cryptogenic and idiopathic cases includes patients with *normal*

Table 21.1 Definitions of cryptogenic infantile spasms or West syndrome

Author(s)	Definition
Kellaway *et al.* (1983)	No cause can be defined
Chugani *et al.* (1990)	No etiological diagnosis can be made
Aicardi and Chevrie (1978)	No cause and normal development before onset
Pollack *et al.* (1979)	Normal development prior to onset of seizures and absence of a probable etiology
Matsumoto *et al.* (1981a)	Uneventful life with normal development until onset of spasms; no etiology
Lombroso (1983a)	No antecedent, neurological disorder, and normal development until onset of the syndrome
Hrachovy (1983)	No known associated etiology, normal development prior to onset of spasms, and normal CT scan
Commission (1989)	Lack of previous signs of brain damage and of known etiology

Table 21.2 Outcome in cryptogenic infantile spasms or West syndrome

Author(s)	Proportion	Favorable
Cavazzuti (1973)	41%	34%
Jeavons and Bower (1973)	52%	33%
Gibbs (1976)	53%	21%
Fejerman and Medina (1977)	31%	44%
Chevrie and Aicardi (1978)	46%	42%
Ohtahara (1980)	44%	48%
Pinsard (1981)	31%	58%
Riikonen (1982)	15%	44%
Singer *et al.* (1982)	28%	40%

development prior to the occurrence of WS, symmetric spasms, no historical, clinical, EEG or radiological evidence of brain lesion, and no recognizable cause. Cryptogenic cases later exhibit evidence of persistent brain dysfunction, whereas idiopathic cases recover completely.

It is difficult to determine the respective frequency of cryptogenic and idiopathic cases thus defined. Indeed, it is often quite difficult to determine precisely whether mental development was normal prior to onset of spasms, particularly when the latter occurred early. Hypsarrhythmia may have preceded the first spasms and therefore contributed to delayed cognitive development. On the other hand, it is difficult to ascertain retrospectively normal development for 4 to 5-months-old infants, based on historical data, and confronted with patients who have experienced loss of psychomotor abilities. Reaching out for objects prior to onset of spasms is a reliable criterium for normal early development (Dulac *et al.*, 1986a), but this does not apply to the youngest patients (less than 4 months at onset of spasms). The characteristics of seizures are another clue: the occurrence of focal seizures before first spasms, the asymmetry of spasms and the recording of focal discharges all indicate focal cortical involvement. Asymmetry of spasms may involve eye or head deviation, and video recording is therefore required.

Based on this definition in nonselected series, Vigevano *et al.* (1993) found 4 cryptogenic and 27 idiopathic WS cases in a series of 103 patients with infantile spasms. The respective figures were 15 and 30 in 223 cases in one series of Dulac *et al.* (1993a).

DIAGNOSTIC CRITERIA AND FOLLOW-UP

The first step is to exclude symptomatic cases (see Chapter 13). The next step is to recognize the patients likely to suffer from "hidden" brain lesions.

Cryptogenic West Syndrome

Interictal and ictal EEG, neuropsychological investigation and functional imaging can detect patients who are likely to harbor brain lesions not visualized by conventional neuroradiological investigations. Both focal discharges and interictal EEG abnormalities suggest focal cortical involvement.

The characteristics of ictal events are a major clue to the diagnosis. During a cluster of spasms, EEG may demonstrate a focal cortical discharge that seems to drive the series of spasms (see Chapter 4), and hypsarrhythmia does not recur between consecutive spasms (Bour *et al.*, 1986; Donat and Wright, 1991a). Usually, however, no focal discharge can be recorded during a cluster, and hypsarrhythmia does not occur between spasms (Figs 21.1 and 21.2), and thus the whole cluster seems to consist of a single seizure. Indeed, parents may notice that before the cluster the infant modifies his mood and behavior as if he

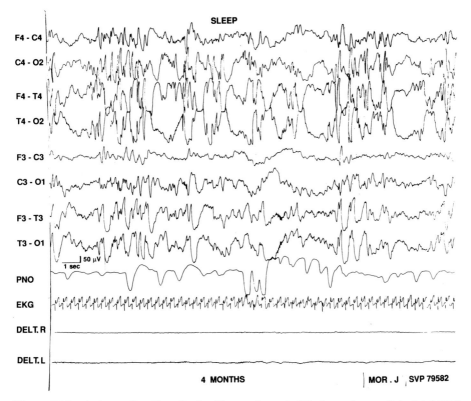

Figure 21.1   A 4-month-old patient with cryptogenic West syndrome. Interictal EEG shows a slow waves focus on the right temporal area. In the second year of life, the patient developed right temporal partial complex seizures.

was "preparing" for the cluster, a sort of aura too often overlooked by the medical staff. During the cluster, spasms occur at a high rate, every 5–10 s. The recording of such clusters and of focal discharges requires prolonged monitoring for which ambulatory systems have proved very useful (Plouin *et al.*, 1993; see also Chapter 5): 12 h recordings are usually sufficient to record a cluster.

Focal interictal EEG abnormalities can be shown either by reducing the amplitude of the tracing (Fig. 21.3) or by intravenous administration of diazepam: 0.5 mg every 20 s until hypsarrhythmia disappears, without exceeding 0.5 mg/kg. The persistence of hypsarrhythmia and the appearance of a clear spike and slow wave focus (Fig. 21.4) both indicate an unfavorable outcome (Dulac *et al.*, 1993a).

Neuropsychological investigation may demonstrate, from the onset, selective dysfunction corresponding to the topography of interictal EEG abnormalities (Jambaqué *et al.*, 1989, 1991, 1993; see also Chapter 7). Loss of eye tracking and babbling are correlated with posterior or left temporal involvement respectively, and asymmetry of spontaneous grasping movements may also be observed.

Magnetic resonance imaging (MRI) does help in some cases to detect malformations overlooked by CT scan, provided the examination is performed after the age of 2 years, once myelinization is sufficient. The border between white and gray matter is blurred, but this may be overlooked before adequate myelinization, once gray–white demarcation has become more apparent on MRI (Van Bogaert *et al.*, 1993). Sequences such as inversion recovery and thin slices may be more sensitive (see Chapter 10).

However, in patients with very frequent focal seizures or with persistent generalized epilepsy, it may be unwise to wait until the end of the second year of life to take specific therapeutic decisions such as focal surgery (Chugani *et al.*, 1990, 1993). Functional imaging may be of great help earlier in life. Brain damage "hidden" to conventional neuroradiological investigations has been demonstrated with positron emission tomography (PET) in an increasing number of patients for whom focal brain resection revealed cortical dysplasia (Chugani *et al.*, 1990, 1993; see also Chapter 23). Both single photon emission computed tomography (SPECT) and positron emission tomography (PET) may detect abnormal cortical areas in the cerebral hemispheres. Abnormal areas may be single or multiple and disseminated in both hemispheres.

Steroid treatment is effective in most cases of cryptogenic WS, with the disappearance of spasms and hypsarrhythmia, and an improvement in cognitive function. Very few cases resistent to steroids respond favorably to conventional antiepileptic drugs, valproate, nitrazepam or even vigabatrin to which

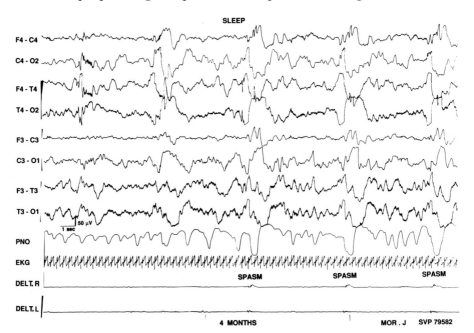

Figure 21.2 The same patient as in Fig. 21.1. A cluster of spasms without recurrence of hypsarrhythmia between consecutive spasms.

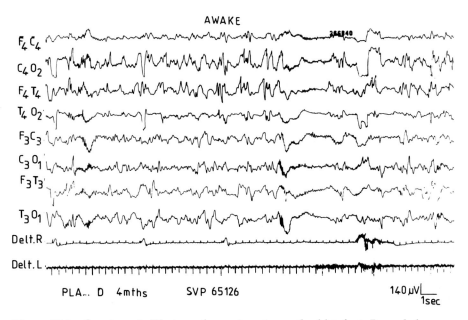

Figure 21.3 Cryptogenic West syndrome in a 4-month-old infant. Recorded spasm. The reduction in the amplitude of the tracing shows a right hemisphere spike and slow wave focus.

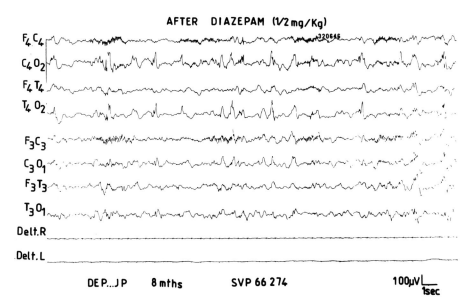

Figure 21.4 Cryptogenic West syndrome. Administration of diazepam shows a right occipital spike focus.

less than 25% give a lasting response when resistent to steroids (Chiron *et al.*, 1990a). Surgical resection is obviously an alternative when functional imaging demonstrates unifocal abnormalities. The classical strategy applied to focal epilepsy is valid in such cases, even though interictal spikes are recorded over both hemispheres: ictal discharges are recorded from the hypoperfused or hypometabolic area, and both seizures and hypsarrhythmia disappear after focal resection (Chugani *et al.*, 1990, 1993).

In unoperated cases, outcome is characterized by persistence of epilepsy in over 50% of children and by delay of mental development together with behavior disorder in most cases. It is not possible from the literature to determine precisely the frequency of sequelae, given the gathering together of all nonsymptomatic cases in a single group. In our series (Dulac *et al.*, 1993a), 10 of 15 patients suffered persistent epilepsy, 7 partial and 3 generalized. Partial epilepsy occurred at 5 months to 4 years (mean 2 years) of age and consisted of complex partial seizures with an occipital or temporal EEG focus, corresponding to the focus identified at onset of the disease. In a small number of patients, simple partial seizures with a Rolandic focus can occur. Generalized epilepsy consists of relapse of spasms and/or the occurrence of tonic seizures. Hypsarrythmia becomes atypical with increasing synchrony of both hemispheres, thus ending in a slow spike-wave pattern; combined with tonic seizures, it produces Lennox-Gastaut syndrome. Interictal EEG demonstrates in those cases a frontal or frontotemporal predominance of spikes, usually not detected at onset of the disease.

Various types of mental and behavior disorders have been reported: global mental retardation, autistic features, speech delay with hyperkinesia, and visual disorders. They are correlated with the topography of EEG and functional imaging foci (Jambaqué *et al.*, 1993). Jambaqué *et al.* (1989) found a correlation between subscores of the Brunet-Lézine test battery at onset of WS and those on follow-up.

Functional imaging during follow-up shows persistence of areas of hypoperfusion or hypometabolism detected at onset of the disease, with the same topography (Chiron *et al.*, 1993). However, in the study by Chiron *et al.* (1993) the size of hypoperfused areas increased when the hypsarrhythmic pattern disappeared.

Therefore, clinical observation, EEG, neuropsychological investigation and functional imaging help to demonstrate that focal cortical lesions precede the onset of cryptogenic WS and that they produce the complete pattern of hypsarrhythmia, of later epilepsy and of mental sequelae following recovery from WS. A number of issues remain open to further investigation. What proportion of patients with cryptogenic WS have focal abnormalities on functional imaging? Can focal lesions be overlooked on functional imaging performed at onset of the disease, as a consequence of hypsarrhythmia that increases cortical perfusion (Chiron *et al.*, 1993)? What proportion of patients with such focal abnormalities have histologically disclosable brain lesions? Does early steroid or conventional antiepileptic drug treatment reduce the risk of later intractability? To what extent does the epilepsy, particularly hypsarr-hythmia, contribute to worsen mental development and behavior transiently and over the long term?

Very few cases have undergone neuropathological investigation. In patients with focal lesions, cortical dysplasia with abnormal cortical layers, thickened cortex and giant neurons, together with heterotopias and abnormal glial cells have been reported (Chugani *et al.*, 1990; Van Bogaert *et al.*, 1993; see also Chapter 9). More widespread lesions have been reported (Meencke *et al.*, 1985), but their pathological significance remains to be demonstrated (see Chapter 9).

Idiopathic West Syndrome

There is some evidence that there are patients without brain lesions who recover completely after a disease characterized by a self-limited course (Bachman, 1981; Dulac *et al.*, 1986a; Hrachovy *et al.*, 1991). Vigevano *et al.* (1993) identified 27 children with idiopathic WS and followed them to the age of 2–13 years (mean 7.5 years) after steroid treatment. IQ at last visit ranged from 90 to 120.

Recognition of these patients among nonsymptomatic cases at the onset of the disease may appear as a challenge. However, since the study of cryptogenic cases shows that EEG, neuropathology and functional imaging demonstrate cortical lesions not disclosed by conventional neuroimaging, we hypothesized in a preliminary study that by means of the same investigations, lack of indirect evidence of cortical lesions associated with excellent outcome would indicate idiopathic cases (Dulac *et al.*, 1986a).

Normal development prior to spasms proved to be the most difficult to determine. This series comprised 14 patients with favorable outcome, and 12 had reached out for objects prior to onset, compared to 2 of 10 in the unfavorable group. All patients in the favorable group had acquired smiling and eye-tracking before the disease. Loss of acquired milestones was mild in the favorable group, since only one patient lost eye-tracking and two stopped smiling compared with six of nine patients for both instances in the unfavorable group.

EEG demonstrated symmetrical hypsarrhythmia (Fig. 21.5) with no spike or slow wave focus after intravenous diazepam. All the recorded clusters of spasms comprised the reappearance of hypsarrhythmia between consecutive spasms (Figs 21.6 and 21.7), thus suggesting that each spasm was a single seizure in contrast with the whole cluster being a single seizure for the cryptogenic or symptomatic cases.

Subsequently, we reviewed 45 nonsymptomatic patients followed from onset, throughout treatment and for at least 2 years (range 2 years to 10 years 3 months, mean 4 years 5 months) (Dulac *et al.*, 1993a). Thirty patients had complete recovery. For these 30 patients, development had been normal until onset ranging from 3 to 7 months (median 6 months), with a single exception at

11 months, and the spasms were symmetrical. Interictal EEGs showed asymmetry in three cases. Diazepam administration performed in 23 cases produced complete disappearance of spikes in 15 patients, a spike focus in 4 cases and no effect in 4 cases. Recorded clusters of spasms showed the reappearance of hypsarrhythmia between consecutive spasms in all cases except one. Ten patients underwent neuropsychological investigation and none demonstrated mental retardation or selective cognitive disorders. The treatment schedule varied, including steroids for 15–30 days, and/or valproate.

On follow-up, the Developmental Quotient ranged from 75 to 126, only one patient scoring less than 80 and no patient suffered epileptic seizures following treatment. Functional imaging by SPECT was performed in eight patients and it showed no focal cortical defect in six of them.

Thus, from the EEG point of view, the disappearance of spikes after intravenous diazepam seems the most specific, and the reappearance of hypsarrhythmia between consecutive spasms seems to be the most sensitive criterion for the diagnosis of idiopathic West syndrome (IWS). The latter criteria is dependent upon the cluster being recorded, which requires a 12–14 h recording (Plouin *et al.*, 1993).

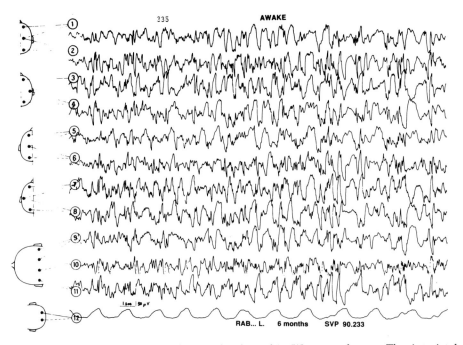

Figure 21.5 A 6-month-old infant with idiopathic West syndrome. The interictal tracing shows symmetrical hypsarrhythmia which is continuous when awake. The patient recovered completely after 2 weeks of hydrocortisone treatment.

GENETICS

The term "generalized idiopathic epilepsy" is usually applied to patients who combine generalized seizures such as tonico–clonic seizures, absences and/or massive myoclonus, and bursts of generalized spike waves on interictal EEG. This combination is supposed to indicate a genetic predisposition. This could also be the case for WS. Very few cases of familial recurrence of WS in siblings have been reported (Cotte-Ritaud and Delafin, 1965; Dulac *et al.*, 1993b). The genetic linking of cryptogenic/idiopathic WS to other idiopathic epileptic syndromes has been suggested since Matsumoto *et al.* (1981b) found an increased incidence of idiopathic epilepsy in relatives and Vigevano *et al.* (1993) an increased incidence of febrile seizures. In Vigevano's series of 27 patients with IWS, 9 had a family history of simple febrile convulsions, and 7 a family history of an idiopathic epilepsy. Five patients exhibited photoconvulsive response after the age of 5 years, and four a centrotemporal spike wave focus. Therefore, in 17 of 27 patients, the authors felt that there was a personal or familial EEG trait of "idiopathic epilepsy". However, in febrile convulsions, an increased incidence of spike waves has also been demonstrated, although this condition is not genetically linked to idiopathic epilepsy. However, in our series, there was no difference between cryptogenic and idiopathic cases in terms of familial incidence of epilepsy (Dulac *et al.*, 1993b; see also Chapter 14).

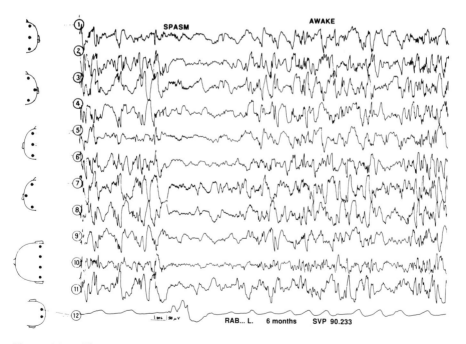

Figure 21.6 The same patient as in Fig. 21.5. Recorded spasm followed by the recurrence of hypsarrhythmia.

CONCLUSIONS

Nonsymptomatic WS patients can be split into two groups that can be reliably recognized from the very onset on the basis of EEG and neurophysiology. "Cryptogenic" cases have "hidden" lesions. Cases with resistent epilepsy and single lesions best detected by functional imaging are candidates for surgical resection (see Chapter 23). "Idiopathic" cases, without any brain lesion, experience complete, including mental, recovery. The practical implications of the nosological breakdown of epilepsies among older age groups are great,

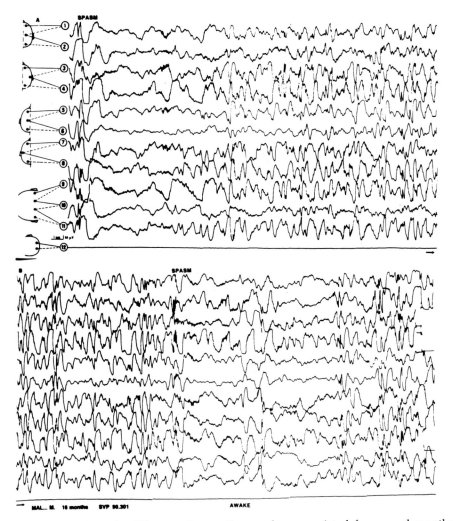

Figure 21.7 Idiopathic West syndrome. Spasms have persisted for several months without major deterioration. Note that the hypsarrhythmic tracing recurs between consecutive spasms of a cluster. Complete recovery after steroid treatment.

both in terms of treatment and prognosis. For epilepsies such as WS, which usually have a very severe mental outcome, it is most important to reassure parents of a benign course whenever the characteristics of IWS are evident. All our patients with IWS who were recognized early responded to a short course and moderate dose of hydrocortisone. It is therefore likely that these patients are usually overtreated with conventional treatment schedules, at high risk of severe and avoidable side-effects.

22

Medical Treatment

O.C. SNEAD, C. CHIRON

INTRODUCTION

The clinical entity of infantile spasms has been known since it was first eloquently described by West in 1841; however, the underlying pathogenetic mechanisms involved in this disorder elude us to this day. Therefore, the current medical treatment of infantile spasms is empiric at best, since it is based on no theoretical underpinning of knowledge either of the disease or mechanism of action of the multiplicity of drugs used in this disorder.

There is little disagreement about the desired goals of treatment of a child with infantile spasms, namely seizure control and an improved intellectual outcome. However, there is little agreement on the means to the first end, or whether the second can even be achieved.

There are only a few accepted caveats regarding the medical treatment of infantile spasms. First, the cumulative spontaneous remission rate over the first 12 months of seizures is about 25% (Hrachovy *et al.*, 1991). Second, seizures are almost always intractable to treatment with standard anticonvulsant drugs, with a possible exception of benzodiazepines and valproic acid. Third, either ACTH or oral steroid therapy should result in a significant reduction of seizures in 50–65% of patients. Fourth, natural ACTH is preferable to the synthetic form of the drug, since the former seems to have fewer side-effects (Snead, 1989). Fifth, there is probably an inverse relationship between response to treatment and age, with younger patients responding better (Millichap and Bickford, 1962; Willoughby *et al.*, 1966). Finally, the ultimate prognosis in these patients is dismal for most and depends heavily on the etiology of the spasm, the pre-existing neurological and developmental status, the presence or absence of other seizures, and the age of the patient at the onset of seizures (Pollack *et al.*, 1979; Nolte *et al.*, 1988; Riikonen, 1982; Dulac *et al.*, 1986a; Favata *et al.*, 1987). Although some feel that a short treatment lag time should be included in this list (Riikonen, 1982; Lombroso, 1983a; Matsumoto *et al.*, 1981a,b; Fois *et al.*, 1984), recent prospective data from Glaze *et al.* (1988) suggest that time from diagnosis to treatment makes no difference in the ultimate prognosis in these patients.

In summary, the child with the best prognosis is older than 3 months but less than 12 months of age, neurologically normal at the onset of the spasms, has no other kind of seizures, does not lose visual following during the course of the seizures, and lacks a demonstrable etiology for the spasms.

The controversial questions concerning the treatment of infantile spasms outnumber those which engender agreement. First, which is the most effective therapy: ACTH, oral steroids, valproic acid, benzodiazepines, a combination of some or all of these, or some other treatment, e.g. pyridoxine? Second, does it make a difference in the ultimate outcome whether the patient is treated early or late with regard to the onset of these spasms? Third, does it make any difference in the outcome in a patient with pre-existing mental retardation and an abnormal brain whether the spasms are treated at all? Fourth, what is the optimal dosage of these drugs? And, finally, how long should the patient be treated, once the spasms are brought under control? The last two questions are particularly compelling with regard to ACTH and oral steroids.

One should say at the outset that no definitive answer to any one of these questions is to be found in the literature, and only the first two have been addressed in any detail. Various reports of the efficacy of different treatment regimens and relation of therapy to outcome are difficult to compare because no standard treatment regimen has been used.

In the remainder of this chapter, I will attempt to provide a review of the various therapies used in the treatment of infantile spasms from the most to the least commonly used.

ACTH AND STEROIDS

The effect of oral steroids on the convulsive state was reported in 1942 when McQuarrie *et al.* observed that deoxycorticosterone made seizures worse. Hoefer and Glaser (1950) subsequently demonstrated that both ACTH and cortisone were associated with EEG slowing clinically. There was some debate in the late 1940s and early 1950s concerning the effect of these compounds on cerebral excitability, with some authors (Dorfman *et al.*, 1951; Wayne, 1954) expressing concern that ACTH might be proconvulsant in adult seizure patients, while others (Friedlander and Rottgers, 1951; Pine *et al.*, 1951) reached the opposite conclusion, namely that ACTH and cortisone treatment were associated with improvement of the EEG towards normal.

The initial report of therapeutic efficacy of ACTH therapy in childhood seizures appeared in 1950, when Klein and Livingston described a beneficial effect of ACTH treatment in four of six children ranging in age from 4.5 to 16 years who were suffering from a variety of seizure types intractable to standard medical therapy. Eight years later, Sorel and Dusaucy-Bauloye (1958) reported a dramatic response to ACTH therapy in a series of children with infantile spasms. These patients showed normalization of behavior, control of seizures, and an improvement in the EEG after treatment with the drug. This finding was confirmed the following year (Dumermuth, 1959; Gastaut *et al.*, 1959; Stamps *et al.*, 1959), and the benefit of oral steroids in this condition was also established (Dumermuth, 1959; Low, 1958). Since those reports in the late 1950s, a confusing array of studies concerning the use of oral steroids and/or ACTH in infantile spasms have been published. Most were uncontrolled and retrospective and all used different dosage regimens (for reviews, see Jeavons and Bower, 1964; Lacy and Penry, 1976; Holmes, 1987; Aicardi, 1986a,b).

To date, only two authors (Lombroso, 1983a; Glaze *et al.*, 1988) have looked carefully and prospectively at the cryptogenic group, those children who are normal at the onset of the spasms and in whom no etiology can be found. Since this is the group with the best prognosis (Pollack *et al.*, 1979; Lombroso, 1983a; Lacy and Penry, 1976), it is the most important one in which to define a standard treatment regimen. Although some authors have shown neither a difference in efficacy between ACTH or oral steroids nor a long-term benefit in treating spasms (Riikonen, 1982; Jeavons and Bower, 1964), the most compelling evidence for this point of view is to be found in the study reported by Hrachovy *et al.* (1983). In this double-blind study, patients were randomized to either 20 units ACTH/day plus prednisone placebo or prednisone 2 mg/kg/day plus ACTH placebo for 2 weeks. If seizure control was achieved, a 1-week taper was carried out; if not, the patient was crossed over to the other regimen. There was neither a difference in the response rate between the two groups, nor a relation between the duration of spasms before treatment and outcome. An all-or-none treatment response was observed. No attempt was made either to control for other anticonvulsant drugs or to analyze the cryptogenic group separately in the initial study.

The evidence in favor of early ACTH treatment of infantile spasms comes from several prospective open trials, two of which were published by Hrachovy *et al.* (1979, 1980) prior to the study described above. In another open trial, Snead *et al.* (1983, 1989) achieved control of spasms in 90% of patients with ACTH in a dose standardized for surface area (150 units/m^2/day) *vs* 40% with prednisone (2 mg/kg/day). However, the studies of Snead *et al.* addressed only the issue of seizure control and not developmental outcome in treated patients.

These are two published prospective studies of outcome in patients with cryptogenic spasms. Recently, Glaze *et al.* (1988) examined outcome prospectively in a number of patients with infantile spasms. Not surprisingly, it was found that the cryptogenic group ($n = 8$) had a better outcome than the symptomatic patients, with 38% of the former group being normal after the spasms. However, no significant correlation between treatment lag and outcome was observed in either the cryptogenic or symptomatic groups of patients. To put it another way, it made no difference how long the patients went untreated in terms of developmental outcome. Although these results are at odds with various retrospective studies, including those of Singer *et al.* (1980, 1982), Matsumoto *et al.* (1981a,b), Jeavons *et al.* (1973), Riikonen (1982, 1984b) and Fois *et al.* (1984, 1987), one might discount the difference since Glaze *et al.* (1988) conducted a prospective study involving relatively small numbers of patients. However, it is more difficult to reconcile the data of Glaze *et al.* with those of Lombroso (1983a), who performed a 6-year prospective follow-up study of a much larger group of 72 patients with cryptogenic spasms. Lombroso used a dose of ACTH standardized for body surface area (110 units/m²/day) and found no difference in the short term between ACTH and prednisone 2 mg/kg/day; however, he observed that ACTH was superior in the cryptogenic group of patients over the long term with regard to a better developmental outcome and decreased frequency of other seizure types. In addition, in this same study, Lombroso demonstrated a relationship between treatment lag and outcome. Those infants begun on ACTH therapy within 1 month of onset of spasms fared better than those in whom ACTH therapy was delayed ($P < 0.01$) in terms of both developmental outcome and seizures.

The other bone of contention among those who write about the treatment of infantile spasms concerns the optimal dose of ACTH to use. On the one hand, there is little disagreement that the side-effects of ACTH alluded to below are primarily dose-dependent (Ito *et al.*, 1983; Renier and Le Coultre, 1989); however, some feel that children with infantile spasms respond better to a high dose of ACTH. The main proponents of this point of view are Snead *et al.* (1983, 1989b), who have shown that infantile spasms are controllable in up to 90% of children if one uses an initial starting dose of 150 units/m². As mentioned above, Lombroso (1983a) used 110 IU/m² in his prospective study. Other authors who have used a dose of ACTH based on body weight or surface area are Fois *et al.* (1987) and Ito *et al.* (1990). These authors do not believe that there is an advantage that accrues from high-dose ACTH (Fois *et al.*, 1984; Jeavons *et al.*, 1973; Riikonen, 1984b).

The optimal duration of treatment with ACTH, or for that matter with oral steroids, is also unknown. There are no published studies which have compared in an organized fashion various time-courses of treatment. Obviously, it would be preferable if one were able to use very short courses of ACTH treatment and indeed the randomized studies referred to above (Hrachovy *et al.*, 1979, 1980, 1983) used a very short course of treatment, but did not include that as a variable in the study.

Although there is a clear lack of consensus for the best way to treat this disorder, an aggressive approach in which high-dose ACTH is used in *all* patients as soon as the diagnosis is made is suggested for two reasons. First, in the retarded child who develops spasms, one can never be sure that the retardation and incidence of later debilitating seizures will not be made worse if the spasms are allowed to continue unabated. When this reasoning is applied to the cryptogenic group of patients, the evidence is more compelling (Chiron *et al.*, 1991). Therefore, the literature does not seem to support specific indications for one type of symptomatic case (e.g. cerebral malformations) *vs* another (e.g. postnatally acquired static encephalopathies) *vs* the cryptogenic type, even though Schlumberger and Dulac (in press) suggests a better outcome in children with perinatally acquired disorders of the brain (see Chapter 18) than those with congenital anomalies (see Chapters 15 and 16), with the exception of neurofibromatosis type-1 (see Chapter 17) and Down syndrome (see Chapter 20). Second, Farwell *et al.* (1984) and Farata *et al.* (1987) have had a good success rate with over 300 children with the regimen described below.

If the decision is made to use ACTH in the treatment of infantile spasms, the child should be admitted to hospital in order to begin the ACTH, monitor blood pressure, urine and electrolytes, and to teach the parents to give the injection, measure urine glucose three times daily with Chemstix, and recognize spasms so they can keep an accurate seizure calendar. In addition, any diagnostic work-up indicated by clinical circumstances is carried out during this hospitalization. An endocrine profile, complete blood count (CBC), urinalysis, electrolytes, baseline renal function, calcium, phosphorus and serum glucose are obtained prior to starting the ACTH. The drug is not begun if any of these studies are abnormal.

The recommended initial dose of ACTH is 150 units/m^2/day of ACTH gel, 80 units/ml i.m. in two divided doses for 1 week. In week 2, the dose is 75 units/m^2/day in one daily dose for 1 week. In week 3, the dose is 75 units/m^2 every other day for 1 week. Over the next 9 weeks, the ACTH is gradually tapered. The lot number of the ACTH gel is carefully recorded. Usually, a treatment response is seen within the first 7 days, but if no response is seen in 2 weeks the lot is changed.

The patient is discharged on day 3 of therapy and arrangements are made for daily blood pressure measurement in the first week, then three times weekly after that. If hypertension occurs, attempts are made to control it with salt restriction and diuretic therapy rather than stopping the ACTH. The patient is followed in the outpatient clinic weekly for the first month and then biweekly. A waking and sleeping EEG is obtained at 1, 2 and 4 weeks after the start of ACTH to determine the treatment response. It has been suggested (Dyken *et al.*, 1985; Glaze *et al.*, 1988) that the only way to determine such a therapeutic response is by re-monitoring the patient because the parents do not recognize the spasms. However, it seems that since the treatment response is all-or-none (Dyken *et al.*, 1985; Glaze *et al.*, 1988), a positive treatment response is suggested when parents trained to recognize spasms say that there are no seizures in a child in whom the waking and sleeping EEG has normalized.

Using this regimen, a high relapse rate (50%) during the tapering period has been reported, particularly in symptomatic patients. When this occurs, the dose may be increased to the previously effective dose for 2 weeks and then another taper begun. If the seizures continue in the face of such an increased dose, the dose may be increased to 150 units/m^2/day and the regimen begun again.

If one wishes to use prednisone because of the ease of oral administration and the lower incidence of serious side-effects, the same pretreatment laboratory evaluation is recommended. However, no initial hospitalization is required for the institution of prednisone therapy. The initial dose is 3 mg/kg/day in four divided does for 2 weeks, followed by a 10-week taper. The reason for the multiple daily dose regimen is that children treated with the high-dose ACTH protocol have been shown to have sustained elevations of plasma cortisol rather than the usual peaks and valleys (Snead *et al.*, 1989; Favata *et al.*, 1987). Because of the short half-life of prednisone, the best way to produce a sustained plasma level of the steroid is to give frequent daily doses.

There is also limited experience with the use of a combination of hydrocortisone and valproate (Schlumberger and Dulac, in press) in the treatment of infantile spasms. Schlumberger and Dulac reported 90% control in cryptogenic patients and 65% in symptomatic patients. The hydrocortisone was tapered within 2 weeks of cessation of seizures, but if the seizures persisted, tetracosactrin was given for 2 weeks and then the hydrocortisone tapered over 1 month.

ACTH and steroids are dangerous drugs, particularly at these high doses. However, the morbidity and mortality reported by Riikonen and Donner (1980) with ACTH seem exceptionally high, perhaps because synthetic ACTH was used. The side-effects are more frequent and pronounced with ACTH than steroids. Virtually all children will develop cushingoid features. Many will show extreme irritability early in the course, and a few will develop hypertension. One should be constantly alert for sepsis, glucosuria, metabolic abnormalities involving electrolytes, calcium and phosphorus (Riikonen *et al.*, 1986; Rausch, 1984; Hanefeld *et al.*, 1984), and congestive heart failure (Alpert, 1984; Tacke *et al.*, 1983). An additional side-effect of ACTH is cerebral ventriculomegaly (Deonna and Voumard, 1979; Langenstein *et al.*, 1979; Maekawa *et al.*, 1980; Lyen *et al.*, 1979; Howitz *et al.*, 1990; Glaze *et al.*, 1986; Konishi *et al.*, 1992), which is not always reversible (Glaze *et al.*, 1986) and which has the potential to lead to subdural hematoma (Hara *et al.*, 1981; Okuno *et al.*, 1980). The etiology of the apparent cerebral atrophy is obscure, but this phenomenon points up the importance of doing diagnostic computerized tomographic (CT) scans in children with infantile spasms prior to initiation of ACTH. Hypothalamic-pituitary or adrenocortical dysfunction can occur as a result of ACTH therapy (Rao and Willis, 1987; Ross, 1986), so one must always use caution when withdrawing these children from ACTH. It has been suggested that while tapering ACTH one should monitor the levels of cortisol and treat any medical stress with high-dose steroids (Perheentupa *et al.*, 1986). Treatment with either ACTH or steroids can lead to immunosuppression, which may be associated with a large number of infectious complications, perhaps due to impairment of the polymorphonuclear leukocyte function (Colleselli *et al.*, 1986). The practical ramifications of this side-effect is that both ACTH and steroids are contraindicated in the face of a serious bacterial or viral infection such as varicella. Finally, rarely, ACTH can make seizures worse (Rutledge *et al.*, 1989; Kanayama *et al.*, 1989).

The mechanism of action of ACTH and steroids in the treatment of infantile spasms is unknown. One of the major reasons for this lack of knowledge is that there is no known animal model for this type of seizure. Until such a model is found, the anticonvulsant mechanism of action of ACTH and steroids can only be speculated upon (Dazord, 1983; Riikonen, 1983; Snead and Simonato, 1991).

If one accepts the point of view that there is no difference in efficacy between ACTH and oral steroids, it follows that the mechanism of action of ACTH might relate to an effect of cortisol on the brain, mediated perhaps by steroid receptors in the central nervous system (McEwen *et al.*, 1986; Carson-Jurica *et al.*, 1990). Corticosteroids have been shown to reduce the excitability of hippocampal pyramidal cells *in vitro* (Vidal *et al.*, 1986), or they could be selectively neurotoxic (Sapolsky *et al.*, 1984) to the excess of excitatory glutaminergic neurons, which is unique to the developing brain (Greenamyre *et al.*, 1987).

Alternatively, there is the possibility that ACTH exerts its anticonvulsant effects in infantile spasms through an extra-adrenal mechanism. In support of this hypothesis are the data cited above, which suggest that ACTH is more effective than steroids in the treatment of infantile spasms as well as reports that ACTH is effective against infantile spasms in adrenal suppressed patients (Crosley *et al.*, 1980; Farwell *et al.*, 1984; Willig *et al.*, 1977). Although it is difficult to conceive how ACTH would cross the blood–brain barrier after systemic administration, the peptide has protean effects on the brain which are independent of its effect on the adrenal cortex. There are now substantial electrophysiological data to support a direct effect of ACTH on the electrical activity of the brain (Olpe and Jones, 1982; Van Delft and Kitay, 1972), an activity that resides in fragments of the peptide that are devoid of corticotrophic activity (Urban *et al.*, 1974; Urban and DeWeid, 1976). However, therapeutic trials of these fragments in children with seizures have shown no antiepileptic activity against infantile spasms (Pentella *et al.*, 1982; Willig and Lagenstein, 1980, 1982).

ACTH in brain is intimately associated with endogenous opiate peptides (Akil *et al.*, 1984; Axelrod and Reisine, 1984; Watson *et al.*, 1978), some of which have potent epileptogenic properties (Snead and Bearden, 1982). Theoretically, ACTH could suppress seizure activity by acting via these opiatergic systems. Alternatively, corticotrophin-releasing factor (CRF), another peptide which is quite epileptogenic (Ehlers *et al.*, 1983; Marrosu *et al.*, 1988; Baram and Schulz, 1991), might play a role in the pathogenesis of infantile spasms (Snead, 1986; 1987a,b; Baram, 1993). If so, both ACTH and cortisol could act by inhibiting CRF release. ACTH also has the ability to increase GABAergic tone (Kendall *et al.*, 1982), a property shared by corticosteroids (Majewska *et al.*, 1985, 1986). Such an effect would be expected to raise the seizure threshold. The latter data may explain why the benzodiazepine, nitrazepam, is reported to have an efficacy equal to that of ACTH against infantile spasm (see below).

The therapeutic effect of ACTH could be mediated through adrenal steroids other than cortisol. Glaser (1953) suggested that mineralocorticoids might be important in this regard and, more recently, Riikonen and Perheentupta *et al.* (1986) have reported that ACTH responders may be identified by high serum dehydroepiandrosterone/androstenedione ratios.

A final possibility is that there are other peptides in the ACTH gel which may play a role in the therapeutic effect observed. The commercial ACTH gel used in the USA is a porcine pituitary extract which may well contain many other peptides. Conceivably one or more of these, such as dynorphin (Garant and Gale, 1985; Tortella *et al.*, 1985), could contribute to the anticonvulsant effect.

BENZODIAZEPINES

The benzodiazepines that have been reported to be effective in the treatment of infantile spasms are clonazepam, nitrazepam, chlorazepate and clobazam. Clonazepam has been reported to be of some use in the treatment of infantile spasms but is less effective than ACTH (Farrell, 1986; O'Donohoe and Paes, 1977; Vasella *et al.*, 1973; Carson and Gilden, 1968; Tatzer *et al.*, 1987; Kotlarek *et al.*, 1985) and would not be considered to be the drug of choice in the treatment of infantile spasm. Similarly, there are a few data to suggest that both chlorazepate (Mimaki *et al.*, 1984) and clobazam (Farrell, 1986; Robertson, 1986) might be effective, but there are no prospective controlled trials in this regard. However, there is good evidence that the benzodiazepine, nitrazepam, might be effective in infantile spasms (Farrell, 1986; Carson, 1968; Schmidt, 1983; Baruzzi *et al.*, 1989). Dreifuss *et al.* (1986a) have reported a controlled study in which 52 patients were enroled in a 4 week randomized, multicenter study comparing nitrazepam and corticotrophin in the treatment of infantile spasms. Both treatments resulted in a statistically significant reduction in spasm frequency from baseline, but the difference between treatments was not significant. Hence nitrazepam would seem to be the benzodiazepine of choice in the treatment of infantile spasms. Unfortunately, nitrazepam is not available for general use in the USA.

A major limitation in the use of benzodiazepines is related to their side-effects, which include excess sedation, increased bronchopulmonary secretions, and the development of tolerance to any antiepileptic effects they might have (Farrell, 1986). The initial dose of clonazepam is 0.01–0.03 mg/kg/day in two or three doses. The dosage should be increased by 0.25–0.5 mg every 3 days until a maintenance dose of 0.1–0.3 mg/kg is reached with a maximum daily dose not exceeding 6 mg. The dose of nitrazepam is 0.5–1 mg/kg/day. An additional problem with the benzodiazepines, perhaps more with nitrazepam than the others, is their propensity to thicken bronchial secretions. This presents a problem when dealing with a severely handicapped child.

VALPROIC ACID

Since the discovery that valproic acid had antiepileptic properties, this compound has proven to be a very effective, albeit somewhat toxic, broad-spectrum antiepileptic drug (Pinder *et al.*, 1977; Bruni and Wilder, 1979; Simon and Penry, 1975; Browne, 1980; Gram *et al.*, 1985). This drug has been reported to be effective in 20–45% of children with infantile spasms (Siemes *et al.*, 1988;

Bachman, 1982; Snead, 1987b; Pavone *et al.*, 1981; Dulac *et al.*, 1982, 1986b; Bourgeois, 1989; Ramsey, 1984; Dreifuss, 1983b; Chadwick, 1988; Murphy, 1988). In a prospective study of 22 children with infantile spasms, Siemes *et al.* (1988) reported that valproic acid in doses ranging from 45 to 100 mg/kg resulted in seizure control in 65% of children within 3 months of starting therapy and 73% of patients after 1 year. The mean plasma level of valproic acid maintained in this study was 113 mg/ml, but we are not told whether this was peak or trough. Dyken *et al.* (1985) have demonstrated that valproic acid may be effective in some children who have failed a therapeutic trial of ACTH or oral steroids.

The major limitation to the use of valproic acid in the treatment of infantile spasms is the potential for very toxic side-effects. There are many of these (Kingsley *et al.*, 1980; Schmidt, 1984; Jeavons, 1984), but the most serious are hepatotoxicity (Zimmerman and Ishak, 1982; Powell-Jackson *et al.*, 1984; Itoh *et al.*, 1982; Suchy *et al.*, 1975) and pancreatitis (Parker *et al.*, 1981; Wyllie *et al.*, 1984), both of which can be life-threatening. The frequency of fatal hepatotoxicity with valproic acid therapy is estimated worldwide to be between 1:10,000 and 1:50,000 treated patients (Scheffner *et al.*, 1988; Dreifuss and Santilli, 1986), with the risk factors being polytherapy and age below 2 years. Since patients with infantile spasms are below 2 years of age, by definition they are always at risk for this complication of valproic acid therapy. Scheffner *et al.* (1988) have calculated the risk of hepatoxic side-effects of valproic acid at 1:5000 patients. Moreover, these authors have been unable to confirm the risk factors of polytherapy or age. In view of these data, if one elects to try valproic acid in the treatment of infantile spasms, it should be the only drug used and liver function studies should be obtained prior to administering the drug and frequently during its use.

VIGABATRIN

Among the new antiepileptic drugs, vigabatrin (gamma vinyl GABA, VGB) is the most promising for the treatment of infantile spasms (IS). It is an irreversible inhibitor of GABA transaminase, an enzyme that increases GABA in the brain, and has been shown to have good antiepileptic efficacy in refractory partial seizures and partial epilepsy in adults (Gram *et al.*, 1983) and in children (Luna *et al.*, 1989b). A pilot multicenter open study with children has suggested that VGB might also be useful in refractory epilepsies with generalized seizures, such as West syndrome (Livingston *et al.*, 1989). A further open study, specifically addressing infantile spasms, reported impressive results in 70 patients refractory to other antiepileptic drugs including steroids (Chiron *et al.*, 1991). There was greater than 50% reduction in IS frequency in 68% of the patients treated and complete cessation in 43%. The effect was observed very rapidly, within the first week of treatment, and maintained in the long term in 55% of responders. Infants tolerated the drug well, 25% showing side-effects which were generally moderate, and transient, most often drowsiness or excitability.

Because of its striking efficacy and better tolerability than steroids and benzodiazepines, vigabatrin has recently been proposed as first line therapy in IS (Appleton, 1992). Three preliminary studies with vigabatrin as first line monotherapy for IS have been reported, involving 4 (Buti *et al.*, 1991), 15 (Appleton and Monteil-Viecca, 1992) and 6 (Vles *et al.*, 1993) patients who were followed for up to 12 months. At follow-up 50% of patients showed complete absence of IS but half of the responders later relapsed (Appleton, 1993).

Further data are required to support the use of vigabatrin as first line therapy in IS, since all open studies to date have been performed in selected patients who were nonresponders to steroids, and it may not be appropriate to apply these results to untreated patients. In addition, VGB in these studies was an add-on drug and the results may be different with monotherapy; further studies are required to determine whether VGB is more efficient when given as mono- or polytherapy.

In addition, VGB efficacy seems to differ according to the etiology of IS (Chiron *et al.*, 1991); the results are better in symptomatic than in cryptogenic IS (Fig. 23.1), and the best results are achieved in tuberous sclerosis: 12 of 14 patients with tuberous sclerosis became seizure-free when VGB was added to previous treatment, and there were no relapses over at least the next 5 years. In cryptogenic IS, only one-third of the patients became free of spasms and 60% relapsed (Lortie *et al.*, 1993b). Tuberous sclerosis would seem, therefore, to be the best indication for VGB, particularly since steroids give poor results (see Chapter 16). A prospective randomized study is required to validate the results of the open studies.

Follow-up of patients treated with VGB has shown that 40% of those with IS due to tuberous sclerosis exhibited partial seizures, whereas epileptic spasms were fully controlled. Although some patients still exhibit seizures, cognitive and behavioral parameters improved dramatically (Jambaqué, 1992). Such a special effect of VGB is unexplained but there is growing evidence that, in tuberous sclerosis, a cluster of spasms could consist of a particular type of secondary generalization from a focal discharge involving the area of major tubers (see Chapter 16). The change in seizure pattern from spasms to focal seizures would support this hypothesis if VGB prevents secondary generalization. Although partial seizures were associated with psychomotor improvement, such patients may experience transient worsening of their condition; episodes of focal status epilepticus were observed in 6 of 32 patients in one series (Nabout, unpublished).

The appropriate dose of VGB still remains to be defined, though 100–150 mg/kg/day has proved to be both well tolerated and effective within a few days (Chiron *et al.*, 1991). Smaller doses (40–70 mg/kg/day) have been reported as being effective but the effect took longer to appear.

In summary, the results of all open studies support the effectiveness of VGB in IS. However, further studies are needed before it can be recommended as

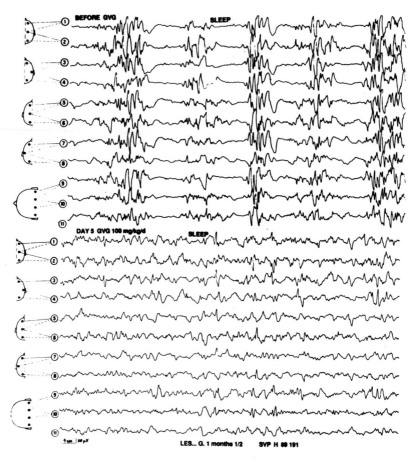

Figure 22.1 A 6-week-old boy with subcontinuous epileptic spasms and right hemisphere dysplasia. The EEG shows suppression bursts during sleep. Seizures stopped within 12 h of VGB treatment.

first line therapy. Moreover, it remains to be established whether monotherapy or polytherapy is most effective, which is the appropriate dose and for which IS etiology VGB is appropriate. Its effects on developing myelin and cognitive functions in children also need further study.

MISCELLANEOUS MEDICAL TREATMENTS

Although the drugs reviewed above are the most commonly used compounds in the treatment of infantile spasms, there are other, less well-accepted, therapeutic modalities which are mentioned in the literature. All of these treatments must be considered experimental until more controlled data are available.

Pyridoxine

Some authors (Ohtsuka *et al.*, 1987; Blennow and Starck, 1986; Pietz *et al.*, 1993) have reported that the use of high doses of pyridoxal phosphate is effective in almost 40% of cryptogenic spasms, but only in 10% of symptomatic spasms. The doses used in these studies ranged from 30 to 400 mg/kg/day. The mechanism of action of pyridoxine in this regard is unknown, since the patients reported did not seem to have either pyridoxine-deficient or -dependent seizures (Korinthenberg and Schultze, 1990). Alternatively, others (Seki, 1990; Izuora and Iloeje, 1989) have shown no significant response to pyridoxine alone and have suggested (Seki, 1990) the combination of pyridoxine and low-dose ACTH.

Immunoglobulin Therapy

ACTH and steroids are generally acknowledged as the drugs of choice in the treatment of infantile spasms. Since both of these therapeutic modalities result in significant immunosuppression, there are some who feel that this might pose a possible mechanism of action through some as yet undefined psycho-neuroimmunologic pathway (Su *et al.*, 1988). An additional rationale for this hypothesis may be found in data which suggest an increased incidence of humoral immune deficiencies among patients with chronic epilepsy (Schwartz *et al.*, 1989; van Rijckevorsel *et al.*, 1986). There have been a few small series of patients who have been treated with various regimens of intravenous immune globulin (Schwartz *et al.*, 1989; van Rijckevorsel *et al.*, 1986; Sterio *et al.*, 1990). Ariizumi *et al.* (1987) report dramatic improvement in six patients with crypto-genic spasms but only one of five patients with symptomatic spasms treated with intravenous immunoglobulin.

Thyrotropin-releasing Hormone

The use of thyrotropin-releasing hormone (TRH) is based on a reported clinical correlation between ACTH-induced suppression of thyroxine and clinical response (Izumi and Fukuyama, 1984). In addition, a TRH analog has been reported to be effective in the treatment of other forms of myoclonic seizures (Matsuishi *et al.*, 1983). Matsuishi *et al.* (1983) reported some improvement in seizure control in two patients with West syndrome treated with the TRH analog DN-1417. Matsumoto *et al.* (1987) carried out a study in which ACTH and TRH treatment were compared in infantile spasms. These authors reported seizure control in 53% of patients treated with TRH *vs* 75% of those treated with ACTH. The dose of TRH-t was 0.5–1 mg, given either intra-venously or intramuscularly. The side-effects of the TRH therapy were negligible. Subsequently, the same group of authors related a positive response rate to TRH to elevated basel prolactin levels (Matsumoto *et al.*, 1989). However, others have been unable to show elevated prolactin levels in infantile spasms (Snead *et al.*, 1989).

Other Therapies

Other medical treatments for infantile spasms which have been found not to be effective include short-acting barbiturates (Riikonen, 1984b; Riikonen *et al.*, 1988), pyretotherapy induced by typhoid vaccine (Garciade de Alba *et al.*, 1984), serotonergic compounds (Hrachovy *et al.*, 1988a, 1989) and naloxone (Nalin *et al.*, 1988).

SUMMARY

ACTH and oral corticosteroids are generally considered to be the drugs of choice for infantile spasms. However, there is still confusion and uncertainty concerning the optimal dose, best duration of therapy, and effectiveness of ACTH relative to oral steroids, as well as the long-term benefit of either of these modes of therapy in this disorder. Moreover, the mechanism of action of these compounds in infantile spasms is not known. Where available, nitrazepam may be an acceptable alternative to steroid therapy because of the apparent lower incidence of side-effects, although this drug is not without risks. The use of clonazepam in infantile spasms is limited because of its sedative side-effects. In those patients who do not respond to steroid therapy or who develop unacceptable side-effects, valproic acid is a viable alternative. However, children who receive valproic acid for infantile spasms must be monitored carefully for hepatotoxicity. Therapies on the horizon which may come to have a place in the therapeutic armamentarium for infantile spasms include thyrotropin-releasing hormone analogs.

23

Surgical Treatment

H.T. CHUGANI, J.-M. PINARD

A number of studies have indicated that the long-term prognosis for cognitive development in West syndrome is poor. In a prospective study, Glaze *et al.* (1988) found that only 38% of cryptogenic cases fit into the category of normal cognitive outcome or mild retardation; the prognosis was even worse in symptomatic cases, of which only 5% had such an outcome. These figures were similar to those obtained in previous retrospective studies (Jeavons *et al.*, 1973; Riikonen, 1982). As a result of this overall poor outcome in West syndrome, there has been a general readiness on the part of both physicians and parents to explore alternative treatment approaches.

In this chapter, we review the surgical management of West syndrome. The success of epilepsy surgery is due largely to the identification of discrete epileptogenic foci that at least lateralize to one hemisphere. With rapid advances in neuroimaging technology, there has been increasing awareness that some cases of West syndrome are associated with focal cerebral abnormalities of diverse etiology. Following sporadic reports of improved outcome due to the surgical excision of focal structural and metabolic lesions in West syndrome, there has been considerable interest in exploring surgical options in those infants whose seizures remain refractory to medical management.

ANATOMICAL LESIONS

Branch and Dyken (1979) were the first to suggest that excision of an anatomical lesion can result in cessation of infantile spasms. They reported a 7-month-old infant with infantile spasms, developmental delay and hypsarrhythmia in whom surgical excision of a choroid plexus papilloma of the left lateral ventricle detected by computed tomography (CT) resulted in alleviation of infantile spasms and normal development. Since that report, there have been a number of cases in which surgical removal of anatomical lesions defined by CT or magnetic resonance imaging (MRI) have been effective in controlling infantile spasms. The lesions have included temporal lobe astrocytoma (Mimaki *et al.*, 1983), anaplastic ependymoma (Ruggieri *et al.*, 1989) and porencephalic cyst (Uthman *et al.*, 1991). In one series of 10 infants, neurosurgical uncapping of porencephalic cysts and ventricular system fenestration resulted in cessation of spasms (Palm *et al.*, 1988). Surgical resection of a ganglioglioma associated with intractable partial epilepsy several years after infantile spasms had ceased has also been reported (Gabriel, 1980; Askenasi and Snead, 1991). Finally, a number of unoperated structural lesions associated with infantile spasms have been detected with neuroimaging; these have included calcified basal ganglia tumor (Gastaut *et al.*, 1978) and angiomatous, cortical dysplastic and porencephalic lesions (Jellinger, 1987; Cusmai *et al.*, 1988).

In one series of 23 infants with West syndrome undergoing resective surgery, 7 showed a lesion that was readily apparent on MRI; 2 others had evidence of focal atrophy without a discrete lesion (Chugani *et al.*, 1993). The lesions included focal pachygyria, choroid plexus cysts, porencephaly, hemimegalencephaly, heterotopias and hamartomas.

Carrazana *et al.* (1993) reported four patients with West syndrome and structural lesions who benefited from surgical resection. The two patients who had frontal resections showed gliosis with calcification and cortical dysplasia, respectively, in the pathological specimens. Two other children underwent hemispherectomies; one of these had Sturge-Weber syndrome and the other showed hemispheric dysgenesis in the resected brain tissue. All surgical cases had good outcomes.

The generally favorable results from surgical resection of anatomical lesions associated with infantile spasms, together with the observation that the presence of an anatomical lesion is associated with a low IQ if it is not resected (Favata *et al.*, 1987), surgical intervention should be considered as soon as it is recognized that the spasms are medically refractory in order to avoid the onset of an epileptic encephalopathy. An unresolved issue at the present time is whether infants with anatomical lesions on CT or MRI who are seizure-free on medication should also be considered for surgery. At present, the policy in most epilepsy surgery centers is not to operate on such infants unless their seizures fail to respond to pharmacological intervention.

Some authors have suggested that a macroscopic focal or lateralized structural brain lesion can often be predicted by focal features of hypsarrhythmia, ictal EEGs or the spasms themselves (Donat *et al.*, 1991). Others have found a relationship between focal delta activity in hypsarrhythmia and the presence of focal structural lesions (Parmeggiani *et al.*, 1990).

It should be pointed out that the mere presence of an anatomical lesion in West syndrome does not necessarily indicate a favorable outcome following surgical resection. In some cases, the underlying diagnosis itself may dictate a poor outcome. Poor surgical outcomes in lesional cases have included an infant with tuberous sclerosis and one with bilateral choroid plexus cysts (Chugani *et al.*, 1993).

METABOLIC LESIONS

In 1990, five infants with West syndrome who showed focal areas of decreased cortical glucose metabolism on positron emission tomography (PET) without corresponding structural abnormalities on anatomical neuroimaging were reported (Chugani *et al.*, 1990). Surface EEG in four of the infants had shown hypsarrhythmia at some time in the patients' courses, but at other times indicated localized or lateralized abnormalities which corresponded to the hypometabolic zones delineated by PET. The epilepsy was medically refractory in all five infants. As a result, four of the five infants underwent focal cortical resections guided by the localization of glucose hypometabolism on the PET scans. Intraoperatively, electrocorticography (ECoG) was performed in order to further guide the extent of resection. There was as excellent correlation between metabolic localization and localization of epileptogenic cortex from intraoperative ECoG in each of the four surgical cases. Following cortical resection, there was both a cessation of seizures and an improvement on cognitive development. Neuropathological examination of resected tissue in each case showed evidence of cortical dysplasia (Chugani *et al.*, 1990).

In an extension of the original series, Chugani *et al.* (1993) reported 23 infants and children with West syndrome who were treated surgically, 15 of whom had cortical resection and 8 had hemispherectomy. Infantile spasms were present at the time of surgery in 17 of the 23 patients; in 6, spasms had evolved

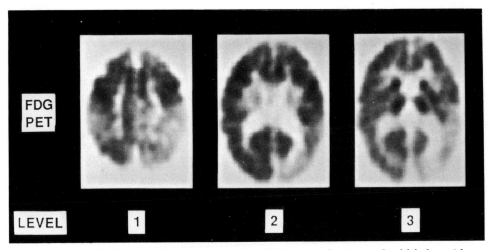

Figure 23.1 Positron emission tomography (PET) scan of a 6-month-old baby with infantile spasms, showing a large area of decreased glucose metabolism in the left parieto-occipito-temporal region, corresponding to EEG localization of epileptogenicity. Following surgical resection of this area, seizures have improved. However, the child continues to have some seizures and is markedly delayed developmentally. In retrospect, there also appears to be an area of hypometabolism in the right parietal cortex (seen in level 1).

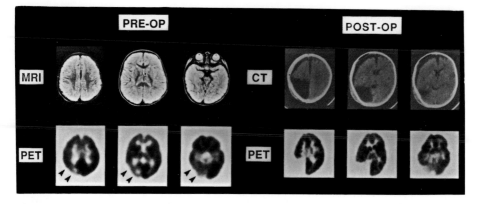

Figure 23.2 Pre- and postoperative PET, magnetic resonance imaging (MRI) and computed tomography (CT) scans of a 13-month-old patient with intractable infantile spasms. Preoperative PET showed decreased right parieto-occipital glucose metabolism, despite normal MRI scan. The area of abnormality on intraoperative electrocorticography matched the PET focus, and was documented to be dysplastic cortex. The postoperative scans illustrate that the extent of resection could be predicted by the zone of PET hypometabolism.

to other seizure types (partial, atonic) during surgical evaluation. Patients with a remote history of infantile spasms were excluded from this study. All 23 patients showed lateralized or localized abnormalities of cerebral glucose utilization on PET scanning; in 14 of these, PET was the *only* neuroimaging modality to identify the epileptogenic cortex. When this occurred, neuropathological examination of resected brain tissue typically showed malformative and dysplastic cortical lesions (Vinters *et al.*, 1992).

Focal interictal and/or ictal electrographic abnormalities were present in all 23 patients, and corresponded well with localization from neuroimaging. None of the patients were subjected to chronic invasive electrographic monitoring with intracranial electrodes. At follow-up (range 4–67 months, mean 28.3 months), 15 children were seizure-free, 3 had 90% seizure control, 1 had 75% seizure control, and 4 failed to benefit from surgery with respect to seizure frequency (Chugani *et al.*, 1993).

The postsurgical outcome can be quite good in some children with infantile spasms, particularly when the epileptogenic area is visualized only by PET. One child, with a follow-up period of 62 months, was not only developing normally but had been placed in a program for "gifted" children in school (Chugani *et al.*, 1993). A number of other children with PET-defined foci and considerable follow-up periods were doing reasonably well, but continued to exhibit some degree of developmental delay. It is not clear why these children had not achieved completely normal development. Longer follow-up will be required to evaluate the full impact of surgical intervention in these children.

There appeared to be a correlation between poor surgical result (persistence of seizures and poor developmental outcome) and the presence of additional small areas of mild hypometabolism distant from the surgical area (Fig. 23.1). Because these additional metabolic foci did not correspond to any electrographic abnormality at the time of presurgical evaluation, their significance was not clear and did not preclude a surgical decision. Only recently is it becoming evident that useful prognostic information can be derived by evaluating the pattern of glucose utilization distant from the surgical site (Chugani *et al.*, 1993).

INVASIVE ELECTROGRAPHIC MONITORING

The approach that has been taken in the majority of infants with West syndrome being operated on has been to rely on localization by anatomical (CT, MRI) and functional (PET) neuroimaging, surface EEG and intraoperative ECoG (Chugani *et al.*, 1990, 1993). It has been shown that the spatial distribution of abnormality on electrocorticography is in excellent agreement with the distribution of functional impairment on PET (Olson *et al.*, 1990; Fig. 23.2).

In some instances, when the potential surgical resection is at or very close to the sensorimotor region, and significant hemiparesis is not present, it will be necessary to perform chronic invasive electrographic monitoring. The necessity for invasive monitoring should be carefully justified in each case. When this approach is taken, chronic invasive monitoring should not be required in more than about 8–10% of potential surgical candidates with West syndrome.

Chronic intracranial monitoring, on the other hand, requires a separate surgical procedure solely for the placement of subdural or epidural grid electrodes, and is not without risk in the small infant. Complications have included wound infections, seen in 17% of cases, and transient encephalopathy due to increased intracranial pressure (Wyllie *et al.*, 1988). Furthermore, since the electrodes are kept in place for an average of 17 days (Wyllie *et al.*, 1988), the financial burden of the procedure is considerable.

RECOMMENDATIONS FOR SURGICAL EVALUATION

It is becoming increasingly clear that, in carefully selected cases of West syndrome, surgical resection of epileptogenic cortex can result in seizure control and improved developmental outcome. At present, it is recommended that selection criteria for surgical treatment include:

1. *Intractability of seizures.* The infant's seizures should be refractory to all medical management. These are reviewed in Chapter 22. In addition, new anticonvulsants approved for clinical trials in West syndrome should also be tried.
2. *Focal features on EEG.* Focal abnormalities should be present on interictal and/ or ictal EEGs of potential surgical candidates. These usually include various

combinations of focal slowing, focal attenuation of beta activity, focal decreased amplitude, lateralized electrodecrements during sleep, sleep spindle asymmetries, abnormal sodium thiopental activation patterns and focal epileptiform activity. The median nerve somatosensory evoked potentials test can be very useful in determining whether the primary sensorimotor region is affected by showing the presence or absence of latency and amplitude changes in the thalamocortical potentials.

3. *Focal abnormalities on neuroimaging*. All infants should show either an anatomical (CT/MRI) or functional (FDG-PET/SPECT) lesion. To our knowledge, not a single patient with normal CT, MRI and PET/SPECT scans have been operated upon for West syndrome. Convergence between clinical, EEG and neuroimaging localizations is an important prerequisite to surgery.

ANTERIOR AND TOTAL CALLOSOTOMY

Corpus callosum section was introduced in 1940 by Van Wagenen and Herren in adults. Since that time, callostomy has been performed in many types of

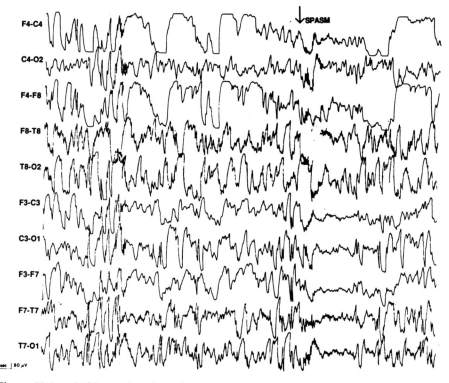

Figure 23.3a At 20 months of age, before surgery, awake, hypsarrhythmia and series of bilateral asymmetrical spasms associated with bilateral rapid rythms on EEG tracing.

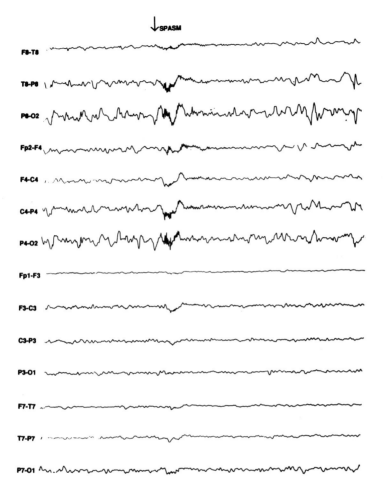

F8-T8

T8-P8

P8-O2

Fp2-F4

F4-C4

C4-P4

P4-O2

Fp1-F3

F3-C3

C3-P3

P3-O1

F7-T7

T7-P7

P7-O1

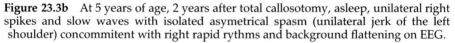

Figure 23.3b At 5 years of age, 2 years after total callosotomy, asleep, unilateral right spikes and slow waves with isolated asymetrical spasm (unilateral jerk of the left shoulder) concommitent with right rapid rythms and background flattening on EEG.

epilepsy, including Lennox-Gastaut syndrome, and multifocal or bifrontal epilepsy. In children, few results have been reported (Lussenhop *et al.*, 1970; Geoffroy *et al.*, 1983; Nordgren *et al.*, 1991). West syndrome refractory to any drugs is associated with a particularly poor prognosis. When spasms persist for 5 years or more, follow-up of children with West syndrome demonstrated that 55–60% of them remain epileptic with Lennox-Gastaut syndrome, other secondary generalized or multifocal epilepsy (Aicardi, 1986a). Mental retardation is observed in 71–81% of children (Dulac and Plouin, 1993). This poor prognosis of West syndrome, some success of callosotomy in Lennox-Gastaut syndrome and in secondary generalized epilepsy, and the link between these generalized epilepsies and West syndrome (Ohtahara, 1978), were strong arguments to attempt callosotomy in West syndrome.

In the Paris Pediatric Epilepsy Surgery Group, we performed anterior and total callosotomy in 12 children (4 girls and 8 boys), aged 1.5–14.3 years, with either persistent West syndrome (6 children) or other generalized epilepsies following West syndrome (6 children) (Pinard *et al.*, 1992, 1993). All of them had had infantile spasms that began in the first year of life: West syndrome was symptomatic without lesion (4 children) or cryptogenic (8 children). However, 11 children among the 12 had cortical abnormalities on SPECT. Thus, most of the cases could be considered as symptomatic, with multiple cortical abnormalities. Anterior callosotomy failed to improve seizures and spasms frequency in 11 children. Callosotomy was completed for these 11 children, 7 of whom showed improved seizure frequency and improved attention and behavioral skills. Among the 8 improved children, 7 still had spasms or other associated seizures but they became unilateral, much less violent episodes, with a reduction in the number of falls. Thus, injuries were eliminated or greatly reduced. One child has become seizure-free. EEG abnormalities, and hypsarrhythmia, evolved into unilateral and more focal foci in 11 children (Fig. 23.3a,b). Even though callosotomy is not a curative procedure of West syndrome, it can be an alternative when focal resection is not possible.

After total callosotomy, unilateral hypsarrhythmia with unilateral jerk of the left shoulder is seen, concomitant with rapid rhythms and background flattening (Fig. 23.3a,b).

24

Epilogue

H.T. CHUGANI

In this volume we have attempted to deal with the many advances that have occurred in the past two decades with respect to the diagnosis and management of infantile spasms. For the most part, these advances have been a direct result of technological breakthroughs in the biochemical, pharmacological and neuroimaging fields, although increasing clinical recognition and more sophisticated analytical methods have also played an important role toward progress in this disorder. As we approach the mid-portion of the "Decade of the Brain", which is already witnessing exponential advances in the neurosciences, we can expect a further and significant impact of this new knowledge on our concepts and approach to infantile spasms. It may be worthwhile, at this time, to anticipate some of the relevant areas that are likely to show progress during the remainder of this decade.

Human genome project. The rapid advances in gene mapping that are occurring on almost a weekly basis will undoubtedly have an impact on our understanding of the genetic basis of infantile spasms and the many conditions associated with this type of seizure. It is reasonable to anticipate that in the not too distant future, genetic testing in a child with, for example, tuberous sclerosis might actually indicate whether infantile spasms will become manifest. Genetic testing might also indicate with certainty whether a particular infant has the benign idiopathic form of spasms.

Molecular biology. Increasing sophistication in molecular biology techniques will continue to shed light on the aberrations of brain development associated with infantile spasms. As more brain tissue becomes available from surgical resections, neuroscientists will have a unique opportunity to apply new *in vitro* techniques to the study of cell migration and differentiation, and their relation to spasms.

Pharmacology. The development of new drugs effective in the treatment of spasms will continue to occur. In recent years, we have already seen the addition of vigabatrin to the pharmacological armamentarium of physicians involved in the treatment of spasms. A number of other drugs are showing promising results in the suppression of spasms and are being tested. It is important in this regard to differentiate between suppression of spasms and ultimate cognitive outcome. Because there is generally a poor correlation between the two, further work needs to be done in order to ensure that both goals (seizure control and normal neurological status) are met.

Neuroimaging. It is clear from this volume that advances in both structural and functional neuroimaging have been of vital importance in the identification of gross and microscopic brain lesions associated with infantile spasms. This, in turn, has led to the novel treatment of surgical resection for intractable spasms (see below). Further development of functional neuroimaging techniques, in particular, will allow the *in vivo* study of neurotransmitter mechanisms involved in the generation and propagation of spasms. A better understanding of these mechanisms will allow specific drugs to be designed for the medical treatment of spasms.

Surgical treatment. At present, the surgical treatment of intractable spasms is being performed in only a few centers and is still somewhat controversial. Both anatomical and functional neuroimaging are important for patient selection. With further experience, improved selection criteria for surgery will be developed. Finally, a better understanding of the relationship between developmental brain plasticity and epilepsy will guide the timing of surgery in order to ensure maximal recovery of function.

Animal model. Although a number of investigators are attempting to develop an animal model of infantile spasms, there is currently no suitable model. A successful and reliable model of infantile spasms would enable investigators to perform both *in vitro* and *in vivo* studies in the laboratory aimed at elucidating the pathophysiology of spasms, and to provide a means of screening new drugs developed for the treatment of spasms.

This text has shown what the general direction of future research into infantile spasms should be. We await with great enthusiasm further progress in this area.

References

Abraham A, Manho M. (1977) Disseminated herpesvirus hominis 2 infection following drug overdose. *Arch Intern Med* **137**, 1198–1200.

Ackermann RF, Moshé SL, Albala BJ. (1989) Restriction of enhanced ^{14}C-2-deoxyglucose utilization to rhinencephalic structures in immature amygdala-kindled rats. *Exp Neurol* **104**, 73–81.

Ackermann, RF, Sperber EF, Haas K, Moshé SL. (1990) Anatomical substrates of severe kindled limbic seizures in immature rats. A radiolabeled deoxyglucose and glucose study. *Epilepsia* **31**, 676.

Adams C, Hwang P, Gilday DL. *et al.* (1992) Comparison of SPECT, EEG, CT, MRI and pathology in partial epilepsy. *Pediatr Neurol* **8**, 97–103.

Agrawal HC, Davison AN. (1973) Myelination and aminoacid imbalance in the developing brain. In: Himwich W. (ed.), *Biochemistry of the Developing Brain*. New York: Dekker, pp. 143–168.

Aicardi J. (1980) Aicardi syndrome in a male infant (letter). *J Pediatr* **97**, 1040–1141.

Aicardi J. (1981) Myoclonic epilepsies. *Res Clin Forums* **2**, 47–59.

Aicardi J. (1985) Early myoclonic encephalopathy. In: Roger J. *et al.* (eds), *Epileptic Syndromes in Infancy, Childhood and Adolescence*. London: John Libbey Eurotext, pp. 12–22.

Aicardi J. (1986a) *Epilepsy in Children*. New York: Raven Press, pp. 17–38.

Aicardi J. (1986b) Treatment of infantile spasms. In: Schmidt D, Morselli PL. (eds), *Intractable Epilepsy: Clinical and Experimental Aspects*. New York: Raven Press, pp. 147–156.

Aicardi J. (1988) Sindrome de Lennox-Gastaut. In: Fejerman N, Medina CS. (eds), *Convulsiones en la Infancia*. Buenos Aires: El Ateneo, pp. 148–156.

Aicardi J. (1991a) Secondary bilateral synchrony in patients with partial epileptogenic lesions. In: Ohtahara S, Roger J. (eds), *New Trends in Pediatric Epileptology*. Japan: Okayama University, pp. 37–46.

Aicardi J, (1991b) The agyria-pachygyria complex: A spectrum of cortical malformations. *Brain Dev* **13**, 1–8.

Aicardi J. (1992) Early myoclonic encephalopathy (neonatal myoclonic encephalopathy). In: Roger J. *et al.* (eds), *Epileptic Syndromes in Infancy, Childhood and Adolescence*, 2nd edn. London: John Libbey Eurotext.

Aicardi J, Chevrie JJ. (1971) Myoclonic epilepsies of childhood. *Neuropädiatrie* **3**, 177–190.

Aicardi J, Chevrie JJ. (1978) Les spasmes infantiles. *Arch Fr Pédiatr* **35**, 1015–1023.

Aicardi J, Chevrie JJ. (1981) Les epilepsies du nourrisson en dehors des syndromes de West et de Lennox-Gastaut. *Rev EEG Neurophysiol* **11**, 412–418.

Aicardi J, Gomes AL. (1989) The myoclonic epilepsies of childhood. *Cleveland Clin J Med* **56** (Suppl. I): 534–539.

Aicardi J, Chevrie JJ, Rousselie F. (1969) Le syndrome spasmes en flexion, agénésie calleuse, anomalies choriorétiniennes. *Arch Fr Pédiatr* **26**, 1103–1120.

Akil H, Watson ST, Young G. *et al.* (1984) Endogenous opioids: biology and function. *Ann Rev Neurosci* **7**: 223–255.

Albala BJ, Moshé SL, Okada R. (1984) Kainic-acid-induced seizures: a developmental study. *Dev Brain Res* **13**, 139–148.

Alford C, Stagno S, Pass R, Britt W. (1990) Congenital and perinatal cytomegalovirus infection. *Rev Infect Dis* **12** (Suppl. 7): 745–753.

Alpert BS. (1984) Steroid-induced hypertrophic cardiomyopathy in an infant. *Pediatr Cardiol* **5**: 117–118.

Al-Rajeh S, Abomelha A, Awada A, Bademosi O, Ismail H. (1991) Epilepsy and other convulsive disorders in Saudi Arabia: a prospective study of 1,000 consecutive cases. *Acta Neurol Scand* **82**, 341–345.

Altman K, Shewmon DA. (1990) Local paroxysmal fast activity: significance interictally and in infantile spasms. (abstract) *Epilepsia* **31**, 623.

Alvarez LA, Shinnar S, Moshé SL. (1987) Infantile spasms due to unilateral cerebral infarcts. *Pediatrics* **79**, 1024–1026.

American Academy of Pediatrics (AAP). (1991) The relationship between pertussis vaccine and brain damage: Reassessment. *AAP News* **7**, 18–19.

Andermann F, Keene DL, Andermann E, Quesney LF. (1980) Startle disease or hyperekplexia. Further delineation of the syndrome. *Brain* **103**, 985–997.

Andrews JM, Cancilla PA, Grippo J, Menkes JM. (1971) Globoid cell leukodystrophy (Krabbe's disease). *Neurology* **21**, 337–352.

Angelini L, Rumi V, Lamperti E, Nardocci N. (1988) Transient paroxysmal dystonia in infancy. *Neuropediatrics* **19**, 171–174.

Applegate CD, Burchfiel JL. (1990) Evidence for a norepinephrine-dependent brain-stem substrate in the development of kindling antagonism. *Epilepsy Res* **6**, 23–32.

Appleton ER. (1993) The role of vigabatrin in the management of infantile epileptic syndromes. *Neurology* **43** (Suppl. 5) S21–S23.

Appleton RE, Monteil-Viecca F. (1992) Vigabatrin in infantile spasms. Why add-on? *Lancet* 341, 962.

Araki Y, Mori S, Kanoh M. *et al.* (1987) Congenital hemicerebral arterial ectasia complicating unilateral megalencephaly. *Br J Radiol* **60**, 395–400.

Ardinger HH, Bell WE. (1986) Hypomelanosis or Ito. *Arch Neurol* **43**, 848–850.

Ariizumi M, Baba K, Hibio S. *et al.* (1987) Immunoglobulin therapy in the West syndrome. *Brain Dev* **9**, 422–425.

Asal B, Moro E. (1925) Uber bösartige Nickkrämpfe im führen Kindersalter. *Jahrbuch für Kinderheilkunde* **107**, 1–17.

Ashkenasi A, Snead OC III. (1989) Infantile spasms secondary to ganglioglioma: a nine-year follow-up. (abstract) *Epilepsia* **30**, 737.

Ashkenasi A, Snead OC. III (1991) Infantile spasms secondary to a brain tumor. *J Child Neurol* **6**, 180–182.

Aubourg P, Dulac O, Plouin P, Diebler C. (1985) Infantile status epilepticus as a complication of "near miss" *Dev Med Child Neurol* **27**, 40–48.

Aubourg P, Scotto J, Rocchiciio F, Feldmann-Pautrat D, Robain O. (1986) Neonatal adrenoleucodystrophy. *J Neurol Neurosurg Psychiatr* **49**, 77–86.

Aurelius E, Johansson B, Sköldenberg B, Staland Å, Forsgren M. (1991) Rapid diagnosis of herpes simplex encephalitis by nested polymerase chain reaction assay of cerebrospinal fluid. *Lancet* **337**, 189–192.

Avrahmi E, Harel S, Jurgenson U. *et al.* (1985) Computed tomographic demonstration of brain changes in Incontinentia Pigmenti. *Am J Dis Child* **139**, 372–374.

Axelrod J, Reisine TD. (1984) Stress hormones: their interaction and regulation. *Science* **224**: 452–459.

Bachman DS. (1981) Spontaneous remission of infantile spasms with hypsarrhythmia. *Arch Neurol* **38**, 785.

Bachman DS. (1982) Use of valproic acid in treatment of infantile spasms. *Arch Neurol* **39**, 49–52.

Backer LE. (1991) Synaptic dysgenesis. *Can J Neurol Sci* **18**, 170–180.

Baird HW, Borofsky LG. (1957) Infantile myoclonic seizures. *J Pediatr* **50**, 332–339.

Bale J. (1984) Human cytomegalovirus infection and disorders of the nervous system. *Arch Neurol* **41**, 310–320.

Bamburg P and Matthes A. (1959) *Anfälle in Kindesalter.* Basel, New York: Karger.

Baram TZ. (1993) Pathophysiology of massive infantile spasms: perspective on the putative role of brain adrenal axis. *Ann Neurol* **33**, 231–236.

Baram TZ, Schultz L. (1991) Corticotropin-releasing hormone is a rapid and potent convulsant in the infant rat. *Dev Brain Res* **61**, 97–101.

Barkovich AJ. (1990) Phakomatoses. In: *Pediatric Neuroimaging*. New York: Raven Press, pp. 123–147.

Barkovich AJ and Chuang SH. (1990) Unilateral megalencephaly: Correlation of MR imaging and pathologic characteristics. *AJNR* **11**, 523–531.

Barkovich AJ, Koch TK, Carrol CL. (1991) The spectrum of lissencephaly: Report of ten patients analyzed by magnetic resonance imaging. *Ann Neurol* **30**, 139–146.

Barnes H. (1873) Eclampsia nutans or the nodding convulsions of infancy. *Liverpool and Manchester Med Surg Reports* **145**, 54.

Barth PG. (1987) Disorders of neuronal migration. *Can J Neurol Sci* **14**, 1–16.

Bartholini G, Scatton B, Zivkovic KG. *et al.* (1985) GABA receptor agonists as a new therapeutic class. In: Bartholini G. *et al.* (eds), *Epilepsy and GABA Receptor Agonists*. New York: Raven Press, pp. 1–30.

Baruzzi A, Michelucci R, Tassinari CA. (1989) Nitrazepam. In: Levy RH. *et al.* (eds), *Antiepileptic Drugs*. New York: Raven Press, pp. 785–804.

Bear DM, Levin K, Blumer D, Chetham D, Ryder J. (1982) Interictal behaviour in hospitalised temporal lobe epileptics: Relationship to idiopathic psychiatric syndromes. *J Neurol Neurosurg Psychiat* **45**, 481–488.

Beaumanoir A. (1973) Les spasmes infantiles avec hypsarrythmie. In: Lugaresi E, Pazzaglia P, Tassinari CA. (eds), *Evolution and Prognosis of Epilepsies*. Bologna: Aulo Gaggi.

Bebin EM, Gomez MR, Hirschorn KA, Shephard CV. (1990) Tuberectomy and hamartectomy for intractable seizures in tuberous sclerosis. *Ann Neurol* **28**, 435.

Bellman MH, Ross EM, Miller DL. (1983) Infantile spasms and pertussis immunisation. *Lancet* **i**, 1031–1034.

Beltramino JC. (1987) Mioclonías benignas de la infancia temprana o mioclonías de Fejerman. *Arch Arg Pediatr* **85**, 119–24.

Bender BL, Yunis EJ. (1980) Central nervous system pathology of tuberous sclerosis in children. *Ultrastruct Pathol* **1**, 287–299.

Berbel P, Innocenti GM. (1988) The development of the corpus callosum in cats: A light- and electron-microscopic study. *J Comp Neurol* **276**, 132–156.

Bialek R, Haverkamp FA, Fichsel, H. (1990) Epstein-Barr virus infection as a cause of infantile spasms. *Lancet* **i**, 425.

Bignami A, Zappella M, Benedetti P. (1964) Infantile spasms with hypsarrhythmia. A pathological study. *Helv Paediatr Acta* **4**, 326–342.

Bignami A, Maccagnani F, Zappella M, Tingey AH. (1966) Familial infantile spasms and hypsarrhythmia associated with leucodystrophy. *J Neurol Neurosurg Psychiat* **29**, 129–134.

Bignami A, Palladini G, Zappella M. (1968) Unilateral megalencephaly with nerve cell hypertrophy. An anatomical and quantitative histochemical study. *Brain Res* **9**, 103–114.

Billette de Villemeur T, Chiron C, Robain O. (1992) Unlayered polymicrogyria and agenesis of the corpus callosum: A relevant association? *Acta Neuropathol* **83**, 265–270.

Blennow G. (1985) Benign infantile nocturnal myoclonus. *Acta Paediatr Scand* **74**, 505–507.

Blennow G, Starck L. (1986) High dose B6 treatment in infantile spasms. *Neuropediatrics* **17**, 7–10.

Blue ME, Parnavelas JG. (1983) The formation and maturation of synapses in the visual cortex of the rat. II. Quantitative analysis. *J Neurcytol* **12**, 697–712.

Blume WT, Pillay M. (1985) Electrographic and clinical correlates of secondary bilateral synchrony. *Epilepsia* **26**, 636–641.

Bobele GB, Bodensteiner JB. (1990) Infantile spasms in neurologic clinics: *Pediatr Neurol* **8**, 633–645.

Bordarier C, Robain O, Rethoré M-O, Dulac O, Dhellemes C. (1986) Inverted neurons in agyria. A Golgi study of a case with abnormal chromosome 17. *Hum Genet* **73**, 374–378.

Bour F, Chiron C, Dulac O, Plouin P. (1986) Caractères électrocliniques des crises dans le syndrome d'Alcardi. *Rev EEG Neurophysiol Clin* **16**, 341–353.

Bourgeois B. (1989) Valproic acid: Clinical use. In: Levy RH *et al.* (eds), *Antiepileptic Drugs*. New York: Raven Press, pp. 643–652.

Bovolin P., Memo M, Costa E, Grayson DR. (1990) Differential expression of GABA$_A$ receptor subunits in primary neuronal and glial cell cultures. *Soc Neurosci Abstracts* **16**, 75.

Bower BD, Jeavons PM. (1967) The "Happy puppet" syndrome. *Arch Dis Child* **42**, 298–303.

Bowery NG, Hill DR, Hudson AL. (1983) Characteristics of GABA$_B$ receptor binding sites on rat whole brain synaptic membranes. *Br J Pharmacol* **78**, 191–206.

Bowery NG, Price GW, Hudson AL, Hill DR, Wilkin GP. (1984) GABA receptor multiplicity. Visualization of different receptor types in the mammalian CNS. *Neuropharm* **23**, 219–231.

Bowery NG, Hudson AL, Price GW. (1987) GABA$_A$ and GABA$_B$ receptor site distribution in the rat central nervous system. *Neuroscience* **20**, 365–383.

Boyd SG, Harden A, Egger J, Pampiglione G. (1986) Progressive neuronal degeneration of childhood with liver disease (Alper's disease): characteristic neurophysiological features. *Neuropediatrics* **17**, 75–80.

Brady RJ, Smith KL, Swann JW. (1991) Calcium modulation of the N-methyl-D-aspartate (NMDA) response and electrographic seizures in immature hippocampus. *Neurosci Lett* **124**, 92–96.

Branch CE, Dyken PR. (1979) Choroid plexus papilloma and infantile spasms. *Ann Neurol* **5**, 302–304.

Bridge EM. (1949) *Epilepsy and Convulsive Disorders In Children*. New York, Toronto, London: MacGraw Hill.

Brown DA. (1979) Extrasynaptic GABA systems. *Trends Neurosci* **2**, 271–273.

Brown JK, Livingston J. (1985) The malignant epilepsies of childhood: West's syndrome and the Lennox-Gastaut syndrome. In: Ross E, Reynolds E. (eds), *Paediatric Perspectives on Epilepsy*. New York: Wiley, pp. 29–39.

Brown LL, Sperber EF, Moshé SL. (1991) Nigral gamma-vinyl GABA and seizures in developing animals: mapping of the nigral efferents with deoxyglucose. *Epilepsia* **32**, 33.

Browne TR. (1986) Valproic acid. *N Engl J Med* **302**, 661–666.

Browning RA. (1985) Role of the brain-stem reticular formation in tonic-clonic seizures: lesion and pharmacological studies. *Fed Proc* **44**, 2425–2431.

Bruni J, Wilder BJ. (1979) Valproic acid. Review of a new antiepileptic drug. *Arch Neurol* **36**, 393–398.

Buchanan D. (1946) Convulsions in infancy and childhood. *Med Clin North Am* **30**, 163–172.

Burchfiel, JL, Applegate, CD. (1989) Stepwise progression of kindling: perspectives from the kindling antagonism model. In: Cain DP, Teskey D. (eds), *Neuroscience and Biobehavioral Reviews*. New York: Pergamon, pp. 289–308.

Burnham WM. (1985) Core mechanisms in generalized convulsions. *Fed Proc* **44**, 2442–2445.

Buti D, Lini M, Bardini R, Marvulli I, Tromboni P, Nencioli L. (1991) Early treatment of infantile spasms with vigabatrin monotherapy: results in 4 patients (abstract). *Epilepsia* **32**, 89.

Campistol J, Prats JM, Garaizar L. (1993) Benign paroxysomal tonic upage of childhood with ataxia. A neuro-ophthalmological syndrome of familial origin? *Dev Med Child Neurol* **35**, 431–448.

Cao A, Cianchetti C, Signiorini E, Loi M, Sanna G, de Vergilis S. (1977) Agenesis of the corpus callosum, infantile spasms, spastic quadriplegia, microcephalia and severe mental retardation in three siblings. *Clin Genet* **21**, 290–296.

Caplan R, Guthrie D, Mundley P. *et al.* (1992) Non-verbal communication skills of surgically treated children with infantile spasms. *Dev Med Child Neurol* **34**, 499–506.

Carey E. (1982) The biochemistry of fetal brain development and myelination. In: Jones C. *et al.* (ed.), *Biochemical Development of the Fetus and Neonate*. Amsterdam: Elsevier Biomedical Press, pp. 287–336.

Carrazana EJ, Barlow JK, Holmes GL. (1990) Infantile spasms provoked by partial seizures. *J Epilepsy* **3**, 97–100.

Carrazana EJ, Lombroso CT, Mikati M, Helmers S, Holmes GL. (1993) Facilitation of infantile spasms by partial seizures. *Epilepsia* **34**, 97–109.

Carson M. (1968) Treatment of minor motor seizures with nitrazepam. *Dev Med Child Neurol* **10**, 772–775.

Carson JM, Gilden C. (1968) Treatment of minor motor seizures with clonazepam. *Dev Med Child Neurol* **10**, 306–310.

Carson-Jurica MA, Schrader WT, O'Malley BW. (1990) Steroid receptor family: structure and functions. *Endocr Rev* **11**, 201–220.

Cavalheiro EA, Silva DF, Turski WA. *et al.* (1987) The susceptibility of rats to pilocarpine-induced seizures is age dependent. *Dev Brain Res* **37**, 43–58.

Cavazzuti GB. (1973) Infantile spasms with hyperarrhythmia. In: Lugomas *et al.* (eds), *Evolution and Prognosis of Epilepsies*. Bologna: Aulo Gagg, pp. 109–117.

Cavazzuti GB, Ferrari P, Lalla M. (1984) Follow-up study of 482 cases with convulsive disorders in the first year of life. *Devel Med Child Neurol* **26**, 425–437.

Chadwick D. (1988) Comparison of monotherapy with valproate and other antiepileptic drugs in the treatment of seizure disorders. *Am J Med* **84**, 3–6.

Chadwick D, Harris R, Jenner, P. *et al.* (1975) Manipulation of brain serotonin in the treatment of myoclonus. *Lancet* **ii**, 434–443.

Changeux JP, Danchin A. (1976) Selective stabilization of developing synapses as a mechanism for the specification of neuronal network. *Nature* **264**, 705–712.

Chevrie JJ, Aicardi J. (1971) Le pronostic psychique des spasmes infantiles traités par l'ACTH ou les corticoïdes. *J Neurol Sci* **12**, 351–357.

Chevrie JJ, Aicardi J. (1977) Convulsive disorders in the first year of life: etiological factors. *Epilepsia* **18**, 489–498.

Chevrie JJ, Aicardi J. (1978) Convulsive disorders in the first year of life: neurological and mental outcome and mortality. *Epilepsia* **19**, 67–74.

Chevrie JJ, Aicardi J. (1984) Le syndrome d'Aicardi. *Boll Lega Ital Epilessia* **45/46**, 13–18.

Chevrie JJ, Aicardi J. (1986a) The Aicardi syndrome. *Recent Adv Epilepsy* **3**, 189–210.

Chevrie JJ, Aicardi J. (1986b) The Aicardi syndrome. In: Pedley TA, Meldum BS. *et al.* (eds), *Recent Advances in Epilepsy*, Vol. 3. Edinburgh: Churchill, Livingstone, pp. 189–210.

Chiron C, Raynaud C, Jambaque I, *et al.* (1987) 133-Xe brain SPECT imaging in cryptogenic West syndrome: Correlations between regional rCBF defects and neuropsychological disorders. *J Nucl Med* **28**, 592.

Chiron C, Raynaud C, Dulac O. *et al.* (1989a) Study of the cerebral blood flow in partial epilepsy of childhood using the SPECT method. *J Neuroradiol* **16**, 317–324.

Chiron C, Dulac O, Raynaud C, Jambaque I, Plouin P. (1989b) 133-Xe brain SPECT imaging in cryptogenic West syndrome: correlations between the regional cerebral blood flow defects and the EEG and neuropsychological findings. *Epilepsia* **30**, 654.

Chiron C, Dulac O, Luna D. (1990a) Vigabatrin in infantile spasms. *Lancet* **1**, 363-364.

Chiron C, Raynaud C, Cusmai R, Dulac O, Plouin P. (1990b) Morphological functional study in tuberous sclerosis: brain MRI/SPECT correlations. *Epilepsia* **31**, 613.

Chiron C, Dulac O, Beaumont D. *et al.* (1991) Therapeutic trial of vigabatrin in refractory infantile spasms. *J Child Neurol* **6** (Suppl. 2), S52–S59.

Chiron C, Raynaud C, Mazière B. *et al.* (1992) Changes in regional cerebral blood flow during brain maturation in children and adolescents. *J Nucl Med* **33**, 696–703.

Chiron C, Dulac O, Bulteau C. *et al.* (1993) Study of regional cerebral blood flow in West syndrome. *Epilepsia* **34**, 707–715.

Choi BH, Kudo M. (1981) Abnormal neuronal migration and gliomatosis cerebri in epidermal nevus syndrome. *Acta Neuropathol* **53**, 319–325.

Chou S. (1990) Newer methods for diagnosis of cytomegalovirus infection. *Rev Infect Dis* **12** (Suppl. 7): 727–736.

Christensen E, Melchior JC. (1960) Neuropathological findings in children with infantile spasms and hypsarrhythmia. *Dan Med Bull* **7**, 121–127.

Chugani HT. (1992) Functional brain imaging in pediatrics. *Pediat Clin North Am* **39**, 777-799.

Chugani HT, Phelps ME (1986) Maturational changes in cerebral function in infants determined by [18]FDG positron emission tomography. *Science* **231**, 840–843.

Chugani HT, Mazziotta JC, Engel J Jr, Phelps ME. (1984) Positron emission tomography with 18F-2-fluorodeoxyglucose in infantile spasms. *Ann Neurol* **16**, 376–377.

Chugani HT, Phelps ME, Mazziotta JC. (1987) Positron emission tomography study of human brain functional development. *Ann Neurol* **22**, 487–497.

Chugani HT, Shields WD, Shewmon DA. *et al.* (1990) Infantile spasms I: PET identifies focal cortical dysgenesis in cryptogenic cases for surgical treatment. *Ann Neurol* **27**, 406–413.

Chugani HT, Shewmon DA, Sankar R. *et al.* (1992) Infantile spasms: II. Lenticular nuclei and brainstem activation on positron emission tomography. *Ann Neurol* **31**, 212–219.

Chugani HT, Shewmon DA, Shields WD. *et al.* (1993) Surgery for intractable infantile spasms: Neuroimaging perspectives. *Epilepsia* **34**, 764–771.

Cochrane WA. (1959) The syndrome of infantile spasms and progressive mental deterioration related to aminoacid and pyridoxine metabolism. *Proc IXth Int Congr Paediatrics.*

Colamaria V, Lombardi A, Capovilla G, Bondavalli S, Dalla Bernardina B. (1982) Caratteri electroclinici della sindrome di Menkes. *Boll Lega It Epil* **39**, 195–196.

Colamaria V, Burlina AB, Gaburro D, Pajno-Ferrara F. *et al.* (1989) Biotine-response infantile encephalopathy: EEG polygraphic study of a case. *Epilepsia* **30**, 573–578.

Coleman M. (1971) Infantile spasms associated with 5-hydroxytryptophan administration in patients with Down's syndrome. *Neurology* **21**, 911–919.

Coleman M, Boulin D, Davis M. (1971) Serotonine abnormalities in the infantile spasms syndrome. *Neurology* **21**, 421.

Colleselli P, Milani M, Drigo P. *et al.* (1986) Impairment of polymorphonuclear leucocyte function during therapy with synthetic ACTH in children affected by epileptic encephalopathies. *Acta Paediatr Scand* **75**, 159–163.

Commission on Classification and Terminology of the International League Against Epilepsy. (1981) Proposal for revised clinical and electroencephalographic classification of epileptic seizures. *Epilepsia* **22**, 489–501.

Commission on Classification and Terminology of the International League Against Epilepsy. (1985) Proposal for Classification of Epilepsies and Epileptic Syndromes. *Epilepsia* **26**, 268–278.

Commission on Classification and Termination of the International League Against Epilepsy. (1989) Proposal for revised classification of epilepsies and epileptic syndromes. *Epilepsia* **30**, 389–399.

Commission on Pediatric Epilepsy of the International League against Epilepsy (1992) Workshop on infantile spasms. *Epilepsia* **3**, 195.

Committee on Safety of Medicines and the Joint Committee on Vaccination and Immunisation. (1981) *Whooping Cough*. Department of Health and Social Security. London: Her Majesty's Stationery Office.

Corcoran ME, Weiss GK. (1990) Noradrenaline and kindling revisited. In: Wada JA. (ed.), *Kindling* Vol. 4. New York: Plenum Press, pp. 141–153.

Corcoran ME, Urstad H, McCaughran JAJ, Wada JA. (1976) Frontal lobe and kindling in the rat. In: Wada JA (ed.), *Kindling*. New York: Raven Press, pp. 214–225.

Coriat LF, Fejerman N. (1963) Infantile spasms in children with triosomy 21. *Semin Med Pediatr* **15**, 493–500.

Cotte-Ritaud MR, Delafin J. (1965) Présentation d'une observation familiale de maladie des spasmes en flexion avec hypsarythmie. *Rev Neurol* **112**, 301–303.

Coulter D, Allen R. (1982) Benign neonatal sleep myoclonus. *Arch Neurol* **39**, 191.

Cowan LD, Hudson LS. (1991) The epidemiology and natural history of infantile spasms. *J Child Neurol* **6**, 355–364.

Cowan L, Bodensteiner J, Leviton A. *et al.* (1989) Prevalence of the epilepsies in children and adolescents. *Epilepsia* **30**, 94–106.

Crichton JU. (1966) Infantile spasms and skin anomalies. *Dev Med Child Neurol* **8**, 273–278.

Crichton JU. (1968) Infantile spasms in children of low birth weight. *Dev Med Child Neurol* **10**, 36–41.

Critchley M, Earl CJC. (1932) Tuberous sclerosis and allied conditions. *Brain* **55**, 311–346.

Crome L. (1956) Pachygyria. *J Path Bact* **71**, 335–352.

Crosley CJ, Richman RA, Thorpy MJ. (1980) Evidence for cortisol-independent anticonvulsant activity of adrenocorticotrophic hormone in infantile spasms. *Ann Neurol* **8**, 220.

Curatolo P. (1991) Epilepsy in tuberous sclerosis. In: Ohtahara S, Roger J. (eds), *New Trends in Pediatric Epileptology*. Okayama: Okayama University Medical School, pp. 86–93.

Curatolo P. (1994) Vigabatrin for refractory partial seizures in children with tuberous sclerosis. *Neuropediatrics* **25**, 55.

Curatolo P, Cusmai R. (1987a) The value of MRI in tuberous sclerosis. *Neuropediatrics* **18**, 34–35.

Curatolo P, Cusmai R. (1987b) Autism and infantile spasms in children with tuberous sclerosis. *Dev Med Chil Neurol* **29**, 550–551.

Curatolo P, Cusmai R. (1988) MRI in Bourneville disease: relationships with EEG findings. *Neurophysiol Clin* **18**, 149–157.

Curatolo P, Libutti G, Dallapiccola B. (1980) Aicardi syndrome in a male infant. *J Pediatr* **96**, 286.

Curatolo P, Pelliccia A, Cotroneo E. (1982) Prognostic significance of CT findings in West syndrome. In: Akimoto H. *et al.* (eds), *Advances in Epileptology: XIII Epilepsy International Symposium.* New York: Raven Press, pp. 191–194.

Curatolo P, Libutti G, Brinchi V. (1983) Infantile spasms and the CHARGE association. *Dev Med Child Neurol* **25**, 367–369.

Curatolo P, Cusmai R, Pruna D, Giannoli G. (1987) Multiple variable prediction of outcome following West syndrome. In: Wolf P. *et al.* (eds), *Advances in Epileptology* Vol. 16. New York: Raven Press, pp. 185–190.

Curatolo P, Cusmai R, Cortesi F. *et al.* (1991) Neuropsychiatric aspects of tuberous sclerosis. *Ann New York Acad Sci* **61**, 8–16.

Cusmai R, Dulac O, Diebler C. (1988) Lésions focales dans les spasmes infantiles. *Neurophysiol Clin* **18**, 235–241.

Cusmai R, Chiron C, Curatolo P, Dulac O, Tran-Dinh S. (1990a) Topographic comparative study of magnetic resonance imaging and electroencephalography in 34 children with tuberous sclerosis. *Epilepsia* **31**, 747–755.

Cusmai R, Curatolo P, Mangano S, Cheminal R, Echenne B. (1990b) Hemimegalencephaly and neurofibromatosis. *Neuropediatrics* **21**, 179–182.

Cusmai R, Ricci S, Pinard JM, Plouin P, Fariello G, Dulac O. (1993) West syndrome due to perinatal insults. *Epilepsia* **34**, 738–742.

Cutler PD, Cherry SR, Hoffman EJ. *et al.* (1992) Design features and performance of a PET system for animal research. *J Nucl Med* **33**, 595–604.

Dabbagh O, Swaiman KF. (1988) Cockayne syndrome: MRI correlates of hypomyelination. *Pediatr Neurol* **4**, 113–116.

Dalla Bernardina B. (1989) Biotine-response infantile encephalopathy: EEG polygraphic study of a case. *Epilepsia* **30**, 573–578.

Dalla Bernardina B. (1992) Le epilessie dei primi tre anni di vita. In: *Manuale Italiano di Epilettologia, a cura della Lega Italiana contro l'Epilessia*, pp. 365–419.

Dalla Bernardina B. (1993) L'EEG nelle convulsioni e nelle epilessie dei primi anni di vita. In: *Le Epilessie Oggi.* Paris: Masson, pp. 41–76.

Dalla Bernardina B, Aicardi J, Goutières F, Plouin P. (1979) Glycine encephalopathy. *Neuropediatrie* **10**, 209–225.

Dalla Bernardina B, Dulac O, Fejerman N. *et al.* (1983) Early myoclonic epileptic encephalopathy. *Eur J Pediatr* **140**, 248–252.

Dalla Bernardina B. *et al.* (1984) Epileptic syndromes and cerebral malformations in infancy: multicentric study. *Boll Lega Ital Epil* **45/46**, 65–67.

Dalla Bernardina B, Trevisan E, Colamaria V, Magaudda A. (1985) Myoclonic epilepsy ("myoclonic status") in non-progressive encephalopathies. In: Roger J. *et al.* (eds), *Epileptic Syndromes in Infancy, Childhood and Adolescence.* London: John Libbey Eurotext.

Dalla Bernardina B, Zullini E, Fontana E. *et al.* (1992a) Angelman's syndrome: EEG and polygraphic study of 8 cases. *Boll Lega It Epil* **79/80**, 257–259.

Dalla Bernardina B, Sgro V, Fontana E, Colamaria V, La Selva L. (1992b) Idiopathic partial epilepsies in children. In: Roger J. *et al.* (eds), *Epileptic Syndromes in Infancy Childhood and Adolescence*, 2nd edn. London: John Libbey Eurotext, pp. 173–188.

Dalla Bernardina B, Fontana E, Sgro V, Colamaria V, Elia M. (1992c) Myoclonic epilepsy (Myoclonic status) in fixed encephalopathies. In: Roger J. *et al.* (eds), *Epileptic Syndromes in Infancy Childhood and Adolescence*, 2nd edn. London: John Libbey Eurotext, pp. 89–96.

Dalla Bernardina B, Perez A, Fontana E. *et al.* (1993) Epilessie infantili e disturbi della migrazione neuronale: studio elettroclinico di 62 casi. *Boll Lega It Epil* **84**.

Davison AN. (1970) The biochemistry of the myelin sheath. In: Davison AN, Peters A. (eds), *Myelination.* Springfield Illinois: C.C. Thomas, pp. 80–161.

Dazord A. (1983) Mécanisme d'action de l'ACTH. *Ann Endocrinol* **44**, 15–28.

Defiore CH, Turner BB. (1983) [^{3}H] Corticosterone binding in the caudate-putamen. *Brain Res* **278**, 93–101.

Dehay C, Horsburgh G, Berland M, Killackey H, Kennedy H. (1991) The effects of bilateral enucleation in the primate fetus on the parcellation of visual cortex. *Dev Brain Res* **62**, 137–141.

de Jong JGY, Delleman, JW, Houben M, Manschot WA, de Minjer A, Mol J, Slooff JL. (1976) Agenesis of the corpus callosum, infantile spasms, ocular anomalies (Aicardi's syndrome): clinical and pathologic findings. *Neurology* **26**, 1152–1158.

Dekaban A. (1965) Large defects in cerebral hemisphere associated with cortical dysgenesis. *J Neuropathol Exp Neurol* **24**, 512–530.

Delgado-Escueta AV, Greenberg DA, Treiman L. *et al.* (1989) Mapping the gene for myoclonic epilepsy. *Epilepsia* **30** (Suppl. 4): S8–S18.

DeMeyer W. (1967) Ontogenesis of the rat corticospinal tract. *Arch Neurol* **16**, 203–211.

Denays R, Rubinstein M, Ham H, Piepsz A, Noel P. (1988) Single photon emission computed tomography in seizure disorders. *Arch Dis Child* **63**, 1184–1188.

Denays R, Ham HR, Tondeur M, Piepsz A, Noël P. (1992) Detection of bilateral and symmetrical anomalies in Tc-99m HMPAO brain SPECT studies. *J Nucl Med* **33**, 485–490.

Deonna TW, Martin D. (1981) Benign paroxysmal torticollis in infancy. *Arch Dis Child* **56**, 956–959.

Deonna T, Voumard C. (1979) Reversible cerebral atrophy and corticotrophin. *Lancet* **ii**, 207.

Deonna TW, Ziegler AL, Nielsen J. (1991) Transient idiopathic dystonia in infancy. *Neuropediatrics* **22**, 220–224.

Deonna T, Ziegler AL, Moura-Serra J, Innocenti G. (1993) Autistic regression in relation to limbic pathology and epilepsy: report of two cases. *Dev Med Child Neurol* **35**, 166–176.

De Recondo J, Hagueneau M. (1972) Neuropathologic survey of the phakomatosis and allied disorders. In: Vinken PJ, Bruyn GW. (eds), *Handbook of Clinical Neurology: The Phakomatoses*, Vol. 14. North Holland: Amsterdam, pp. 19–71.

De Rosa MJ, Secor DL, Barsom M, Fisher RS, Vinters HV. (1992) Neuropathologic findings in surgically treated hemimegalencephaly: immunohistochemical, morphometric, and ultrastructural study. *Acta Neuropathol* **84**, 250–260.

Descroizilles. (1886) Du vertige épileptique et du tic de Salaam chez les enfants. *Sem Med* **5**, 29–30.

De Volder A, Bol A, Michel C, Congneau M, Goffinet A. (1987) Brain glucose metabolism in children with the autistic syndrome: positron tomography analysis. *Brain Dev* **9**, 581–587.

Dhellemmes C, Girard S, Dulac O. *et al.* (1988) Agyria-pachygyria and Miller-Dieker syndrome: clinical, genetic and chromosome studies. *Hum Genet* **79**, 163–167.

Diebler C, Dulac O. (1987) *Pediatric Neurology and Neuroradiology. Cerebral and Cranial Diseases.* Berlin: Springer-Verlag, pp. 1–408.

Diebler C, Dulac O. (1990) *Neurologie et Neuroradiologie Infantiles. Maladies du Cerveau et du Crâne.* Berlin: Springer-Verlag, pp. 1–454.

Diebler C, Dusser H, Dulac O. (1985) Congenital toxoplasmosis. *Neuroradiology* **27**, 125–130.

Dietrich RB, Bradley WG, Zaragoza IVEJ. *et al.* (1988) MR evaluation of early myelination patterns in normal and developmentally delayed infants. *AJNR* **9**, 69–76.

Dobyns WB, Stratton RF, Greenberg F. (1984) Syndromes with lissencephaly. I: Miller-Dieker and Norman-Roberts syndromes and isolated lissencephaly. *Am J Med Genet* **18**, 509–526.

Donat JF, Wright FS. (1989) "Absence" seizures in patients who have infantile spasms. (abstract) *Neurology* **39** (Suppl. 1); 214.

Donat JF, Wright FS. (1991a) Simultaneous infantile spasms and partial seizures. *J Child Neurol* **6**, 246–250.

Donat JF, Wright FS. (1991b) Unusual variants of infantile spasms. *J Child Neurol* **6**, 313–318.

Donat JF, Wright FS. (1991c) Mixed seizure disorder in West syndrome. (abstract) *Electroencephalogr Clin Neurophysiol* **79**, 28P.

Donat JF, Wright FS. (1991d) Seizures in series: similarities between seizures of the West and Lennox-Gastaut syndromes. *Epilepsia* **32**, 504–509.

Donat JF, Wright FS. (1992) Myoclonic seizures and infantile spasms. (abstract) *Epilepsia* **33** (Suppl. 3), 6.

Donat JF, Lo WD, Wright FS. (1991) Significance of focal features in West syndrome. (abstract) *Epilepsia* **32** (Suppl. 3), 83.

Dongier S, Charles C, Chabert F. (1964) Sémiologie psychiatrique et psychométrique. In: Gastaut H. *et al.* (eds), *L'Encéphalopathie Myoclonique Infantile avec Hypsarythmie (Syndrome de West).* Paris: Masson.

Dooley JM, Andermann F. (1989) Startle disease or hyperekplexia. Adolescent onset and response to valproate. *Pediatr Neurol* **5**, 126–127.

Doose H, Gerken H, Morstmann T, Völzke E. (1970) Centrencephalic myoclonic-astatic petit mal. *Neuropediatrics* **2**, 59–78.

Doose H, Ritter K, Völzke E. (1983) EEG longitudinal studies in febrile convulsions. Genetic aspects. *Neuropediatrics* **14**, 81–87.

Dorfman A, Apter NS, Smull, K, Bergenstal DM, Richter RB. (1951) Status epilepticus coincident with the use of pituitary adrenocorticotrophic hormone; report of three cases. *J Am Med Assoc* **146**, 25–29.

Dravet C, Bureau M. (1981) L'epilepsie myoclonique bénigne du nourrisson. *Rev EEG Neurophysiol* **11**, 438–444.

Dravet C, Roger J, Bureau M, Dalla Bernardina B. (1982) Myoclonic epilepsies in childhood. In: Akimoto H. *et al*. (eds), *Advances in Epileptology: XIIIth Epilepsy International Symposium*, New York: Raven Press, pp. 135–140.

Dravet C, Giraud N, Bureau M, Roger J. (1986) Benign myoclonus of early infancy or benign non-epileptic infantile spasms. *Neuropediatrics* **17**, 33–38.

Dravet C, Catani C, Bureau M, Roger J. (1989) Partial epilepsies in infancy: a study of 40 cases. *Epilepsia* **30**, 807–812.

Dreifuss FE. (1983a) Infantile spasms. In: John Wright and PSG. (eds), *Pediatric Epileptology: Classification and Management of Seizures in the Child*. Boston: Little Brown and Co., pp. 97–108.

Dreifuss FE. (1983b) How to use valproate. In: Morselli PO, Pipenger CE, Penry JK. (eds), *Antiepileptic Drug Therapy in Pediatrics*. New York: Raven Press, pp. 219–228.

Dreifuss FE, Santilli N. (1986) Valproic acid hepatic fatalities: analysis of US cases. *Neurology* **36** (Suppl. 1), 175.

Dreifuss F, Farwell J, Holmes G. *et al*. (1986) Infantile spasms. Comparative trial of nitrazepam and corticotropin. *Arch Neurol* **43**, 1107–1110.

Druckman R, Chao D. (1955) Massive spasms in infancy and childhood. *Epilepsia* **4**, 61–72.

Druckman R, Chao D, Alvord EC Jr. (1959) A case of atonic cerebral diplegia with lissencephaly. *Neurology* **9**, 806–814.

Duffner PK, Cohen ME. (1975) Infantile spasms associated with histidinemia. *Neurology* **25**, 195–197.

Dulac O, Plouin P. (1993) Infantile spasms and West syndrome. In: Wyllie E. (ed.), *The Treatment of Epilepsies*. Philadelphia: Lea & Febinger, pp. 464–491.

Dulac O, Schlumberger E. (1993) Treatment of West syndrome. In: Wylie E. (ed.), *The Treatment of Epilepsy; Principles and Practice*. Philadelphia: Lea & Febiger, pp. 595–603.

Dulac O, Steru D, Rey E, Arthuis M. (1982) Monothérapie par le valproate de sodium dans les épilepsies de l'enfant. *Arch Fr Pediatr* **39**, 347–353.

Dulac O, Plouin P, Perulli L, Motte J. (1983a) L'épilepsie dans l'agyrie-pachygyrie classique. *Rev EEG Neurophysiol Clin* **13**, 232–239.

Dulac O, Lemaitre A, Aubourg P. (1983b) Epilepsies dans les syndromes neurocutanés. In: *Journées Parisiennes de Pédiatrie*. Paris: Flammarion, pp. 77–84.

Dulac O, Lemaitre A, Plouin P. (1984) The Bourneville syndrome: clinical and EEG features of epilepsy in the first year of life. *Boll Lega Ital Epil* **45/46**, 39–42.

Dulac O, Plouin P, Jambaqué I, Motte J. (1986a) Spasmes infantiles épileptiques bénins. *Rev EEG Neurophysiol Clin* **16**, 371–382.

Dulac O, Steru D, Rey E, Perret A, Arthuis M. (1986b) Sodium valproate monotherapy in childhood epilepsy. *Brain Dev* **8**, 47–52.

Dulac O, Raynaud C, Chiron C. *et al*. (1987a) Etude du débit sanguin cérébral dans le syndrome de West idiopathique: corrélations avec les données électroencéphalographiques. *Rev EEG Neurophysiol Clin* **17**, 169–182.

Dulac O, Chiron C, Jambaqué I, Plouin P, Raynaud C. (1987b) Infantile spasms. *Prog Clin Neurosci (Neurological Society of India)* **2**, 97–109.

Dulac O, Chiron C, Jambaqué I, Plouin P, Raynaud C. (1987c) Les spasmes infantiles. *Ann Pediatr (Paris)* **34**, 183–191.

Dulac O, Plouin P, Jambaqué I. (1993a) Predicting favorable outcome in idiopathic West syndrome. *Epilepsia* **34**, 747–756.

Dulac O, Feingold J, Plouin P. *et al*. (1993b) Genetic predisposition to West syndrome. *Epilepsia* **34**, 732–737.

Dumermuth G. (1959) Über die Blitz-Nick-Salaam-Krämpfe und ihre Behandlung mit ACTH und Hydrocortison. *Mitteilung Helv Ped Acta* **14**, 250–270.

Dumermuth G. (1961) Ueber das Syndrom der Blitz-Nick-Salaam-Krämpfe und seine Behandlung mit ACTH und Hydrocortison. II. Zwischenbalanz. *Helv Pediatr Acta* **6**, 244–266.

Dumermuth G. (1966) Epilepsie maligne de la 1ère enfance. *Med Hyg* **478**, 729–732.

Duong T, De Rosa MJ, Poukens V, Vinters HV, Fisher RS. Neuronal cyto-skeletal abnormalities in human cerebral cortical dysplasia. *Acta Neuropathol* (in press).

Dvorák K, Feit J, Juránková Z. (1978) Experimentally induced focal microgyria and status verrucosus deforms in rats, pathogenesis and interrelation. Histological and autoradiographical study. *Acta Neuropathol* **44**, 121–129.

Dyken PR, DuRant RH, Minden DB, King DW. (1985) Short term effects of valproate on infantile spasms. *Ped Neurol* **1**, 34–37.

Eayrs JT, Goodhead B. (1959) Postnatal development of the cerebral cortex in the rat. *J Anat* **93**, 385–402.

Echenne B, Rivier F. (1992) Benign paroxysmal tonic upward gaze. *Pediatr Neurol* **8**, 154–155.

Echenne B, Parayre-Chanez M, Clot J, Baldy-Mouliner M. (1987) Treatment of infantile spasms with intravenous gamma-globulins. *Neuropediatrics* **18**, 126.

Eeg-Olofsson O, Sidenvall R. (1992) Epidemiological studies in infantile spasms. (abstract) *6th Congress of the International Child Neurology Association*, Buenos Aires, 8–13 November 1992.

Egli M, Mothersill I, O'Kane M, O'Kane F. (1985) The axial spasm—the predominant type of drop seizure in patients with secondary generalized epilepsy. *Epilepsia* **26**, 401–415.

Ehlers CL, Henriksen SJ, Wang M. *et al.* (1983) Corticotrophin releasing factor produces increase in brain excitability and convulsive seizures in rats. *Brain Res* **278**, 332–336.

Ellenberg JH, Hirtz DG, Nelson KB. (1984) Age at onset of seizures in young children. *Ann Neurol* **15**, 127–34.

Engel J Jr. (1984) The use of positron emission tomographic scanning in epilepsy. *Ann Neurol* **15**, S181–S191.

Engel J, Brown WJ, Kuhl D. *et al.* (1982) Pathological findings underlying temporal lobe hypometabolism in partial epilepsy. *Ann Neurol* **12**, 518–528.

Enjolras O, Riché MC. (1990) *Hemangiomes et Malformations Vasculaires Superficielles.* New York, Paris: McGraw Hill, pp. 72–73.

Enna SJ. (1988) GABA$_A$ receptors. In: Squires RF. (ed), *GABA and Benzodiazepine Receptors.* Boca Raton Florida: CRC Press, pp. 91–106.

Fariello RG, Chun RWM, Doro JM, Buncic JR, Prichard JS. (1977) EEG Recognition of Aicardi's syndrome. *Arch Neurol* **34**, 563–566.

Farkas-Bargeton E, Diebler MF, Rosenberg B, Wehrle R. (1984) Histochemical changes of the developing human cerebral neocortex. *Neuropediatrics* **15**, 82–91.

Farrell K. (1986) Benzodiazepines in the treatment of children with epilepsy. *Epilepsia* **27** (Suppl. 1), S45–S51.

Farrell MA, De Rosa MJ, Curran JG. *et al.* (1992) Neuropathologic findings in cortical resections (including hemispherectomies) performed for the treatment of intractable childhood epilepsy. *Acta Neuropathol* **83**, 246–259.

Farwell J, Milstein J, Opheim K, Smith E, Glass S. (1984) Adrenocorticotropic hormone controls infantile spasms independently of cortisol stimulation. *Epilepsia* **25**, 605–608.

Favata I, Leuzzi V, Curatolo M. (1987) Mental outcome in West syndrome: Prognostic value of some clinical factors. *J Ment Defic Res* **31**, 9–15.

Feinberg AP, Leahy WR. (1977) Infantile spasms: Case report of sex-linked inheritance. *Dev Med Child Neurol* **19**, 524–526.

Fejerman N. (1972) Resultados del tratamiento de 114 casos de epilepsia en flexión generalizada. In: *Agravio Encefálico del Recién Nacido.* Montevideo: Delta, pp. 24–29.

Fejerman N. (1977) Mioclonías benignas de la infancia temprana. Comunicación preliminar. Actas IV jornadas rioplatenses de neurología infantil, 1976. Neuropediatría latinoamericana. Montevideo: Delta, pp. 131–134.

Fejerman N. (1980) Myoclonies bénignes du nourrisson. Réunion de la societé de neurologie infantile, Luxembourg.

Fejerman N. (1984) Mioclonías benignas de la infancia temprana. *An Esp Ped* **21**, 725–731.

Fejerman N. (1991a) Myoclonus and epilepsies. In: Ohtahara S, Roger J. (eds), *New Trends in Pediatric Epileptology*. Japan: Okayama University, pp. 94–110.

Fejerman N. (1991b) Myoclonus and epilepsies in children. *Rev Neurol* 147, 782–797.

Fejerman N, Medina CS, (1977) *Convulsiones en la Infancia*, 1st edn. Buenos Aires: Editorial Ergon.

Fejerman N, Medina CS. (1986) *Convulsiones en la Infancia*, 2nd edn. Buenos Aires: El Ateneo.

Fejerman N, Medina CS. (1988) Hiperekplexia. In: Fejerman N, Fernandez Alvarez E. (eds), *Neurología Pediátrica*. Buenos Aires: El Ateneo.

Feldman RA, Schwarz JF. (1968) Possible association between cytomegalovirus infection and infantile spasms. *Lancet* i, 180–181.

Féré C. (1883) Le tic de Salaam, les salutations névropathiques. *Le progrès médical* 11, 970–971.

Ferraz FG, Dubois B, Lebecq MF, Fontaine G. (1986) Le syndrome de West. Etude clinique, therapeutique et pronostique. A propos de 66 observations. *Arch Fr Pediatr* 43: 321–326.

Ferrer I, Cusi MV, Liarte A, Campistol J. (1986) A Golgi study of the polymicrogyric cortex in Aicardi syndrome. *Brain Dev* 8, 518–525.

Finkelstein H. (1938) *Lehrubuch der Saüglings-Krankheiten*. Amsterdam: Elsevier.

Fleiszar KA, Daniel WL, Imrey PB. (1977) Genetic study of infantile spasms with hypsarrhythmia. *Epilepsia* 18, 55–62.

Fois A, Malandrini F, Balestri P, Giorgi D. (1984) Infantile spasms—long term results of ACTH treatment. *Eur J Pediatr* 142, 51–55.

Fois A, Malandrini F, Mostardini R. (1987) Further observations on the treatment of infantile spasms with corticotropin. *Brain Dev* 99, 82.

Fowler JS, Wolf AP. (1986) Positron emitter-labeled compounds: Priorities and problems. *In*; Phelps ME, Mazziotta JC, Schelbert HR. (eds), *Positron Emission Tomography and Autoradiography: Principles and Applications for the Brain and Heart*. New York: Raven Press, pp. 391–450.

French JH, Grueter BB, Druckman R, O'Brien D. (1965) Pyridoxine and infantile myoclonic seizures. *Neurology* 15, 101–113.

Friede RL. (1989) *Developmental Neuropathology*, 2nd ed. Berlin: Springer-Verlag.

Friedlander WJ, Rottgers E. (1951) The effects of cortisone on the electroencephalograph. *Electroencephalogr Clin Neurophysiol* 3, 311–320.

Frost JD, Hrachovy RA, Kellaway P. (1978) Quantitative analysis and characterization of infantile spasms. *Epilepsia* 19, 273–282.

Fukuyama F, Tsuchiya S. (1979) A study on Sturge Weber syndrome. Report of a case associated with infantile spasms and electroencephalographic evolution in five cases. *Eur Neurol* 18, 194–204.

Fukuyama Y. (1960) Studies on the etiolgy and pathogenesis of flexor spasms. *Adv Neurol Sci (Tokyo)* 4, 861–867.

Fukuyama Y, Miyao M, Ishizu T, Maruyama H. (1979a) Developmental changes in normal cranial measurements by computed tomography. *Dev Med Child Neurol* 21, 425–432.

Fukuyama, Y, Shionaga A, Iida Y. (1979b) Polygraphic study during whole night sleep in infantile spasms. *Eur Neurol* 18, 302–311.

Fusco L, Vigevano F. (1993) Ictal clinical electroencephalographic findings of spasms in West syndrome. *Epilepsia* 34, 671–678.

Futagi Y, Abe J, Ohtani K, Okamoto N. (1988) Cerebral blood flow during ACTH therapy: especially diurnal changes within the first week of therapy. *Brain Dev* 10, 164–168.

Gabriel YH. (1980) Unilateral hemispheric ganglioglioma with infantile spasms. *Ann Neurol* 7, 287–288.

Gaily EK, Shewmon DA. (1992) Asymmetric infantile spasms. (abstract) *Epilepsia* 33 (Suppl. 3), 6.

Gaily EK, Shewmon DA. Relationship between behavior and EEG in asymmetric and/or asynchronous infantile spasms. (abstract) Western EEG Society, Las Vegas, NV, 11 February 1993. *Electroencephalogr Clin Neurophysiol* (in press).

Gale K. (1985) Mechanisms of seizure control mediated by gamma-aminobutyric acid: role of the substantia nigra. *Fed Proc* 44, 2414–2424.

Gale K. (1989) GABA in epilepsy: the pharmacologic basis. *Epilepsia* 30, S1–S11.

Galletti F, Brinciotti M, Emanuelli O. (1989) Familial occurrence of benign myoclonus of early infancy. *Epilepsia* 30, 579–581.

Ganji S, Titton AC, Happel L, Marino S. (1987) Hypsarrhythmia—infantile spasms in near-drowning: clinical, EEG, CT scan and evoked potential studies. *Clin Electroencephalogr* **18**, 180–176.

Garcia Alvarez M, Caraballo R, Fejerman N. (1992) West syndrome and gelastic seizures in a child with hypothalamic hamartoma. (abstract) *Epilepsia* **32** (Suppl. 1), 4.

Garcia de Alba GO, Garcia AR, Crespo FV. (1984) Pyretotherapy as treatment in West's syndrome. *Clin Electroencephalogr* **15**, 140–144.

Garcia de Alba GO, Gamboa Marrufo JD, Valencia Mayoral P, Delgadillo JF. (1989) Development of West syndrome in a patient with Reye syndrome: A case study. *Clin Electroencephalogr* **20**, 86–90.

Garant DS, Gale K. (1985) Infusion of opiates into substantia nigra protects against maximal electroshock seizures in rats. *J Pharmacol Exp Ther* **234**, 45–48.

Garant DS, Sperber EF, Moshé SL. (1992) The density of $GABA_B$ binding sites is selectively increased in the substantia nigra of rat pups. *Eur J Pharmacol* **214**, 75–79.

Gastaut H, Poirier F. (1964) Historique. In: Gastaut H. *et al.* (eds), *L'Encéphalopathie Myoclonique Infantile avec Hypsarythmie (Syndrome de West)*. Paris: Masson.

Gastaut H, Rémond A. (1952) Etude électroencéphalographique des myoclonies. *Rev Neurol* **86**, 596–609.

Gastaut H, Villeneuve A. (1967) The startle disease or hyperekplexia. Pathological surprise reaction. *J Neurol Sci* **5**, 523–542.

Gastaut H, Zifkin B. (1988) Secondary bilateral synchrony and Lennox-Gastaut syndrome. In: *Lennox-Gastaut syndrome*. New York: A.R. Liss Inc, pp. 221–242.

Gastaut H, Satfiel J, Raybaud C, Pitot M, Meynadier AA. (1959) A propos du traitement par l'ACTH des encéphalities myoclonique de la première enfance avec dysrythmie majeure—(Hypsarythmie). *Pediatrie* **15**, 35–45.

Gastaut H, Roger A, Régis H, Ouhachi S. (1964a) Sémiologie électrographique. In: Gastaut H. *et al.* (ed.), *L'Encéphalopathie Myoclonique Infantile avec Hypsarythmie (Syndrome de West)*. Paris: Masson.

Gastaut H, Soulayrol R, Roger J, Pinsard N. (eds) (1964b) *L'Encéphalopathie Myoclonique Infantile avec Hypsarythmie (Syndrome de West)*. Paris: Masson.

Gastaut H, Broughton R, Tassinari CA, Roger J. (1974) Unilateral epileptic siezures. In: Vinken PJ, Bruyn GW. (eds), *Handbook of Clinical Neurology, The Epilepsies*. New York: Elsevier, pp. 235–245.

Gastaut H, Gastaut JL, Regis H. *et al.* (1978) Computerized tomography in the study of West's syndrome. *Dev Med Child Neurol* **20**, 21–27.

Gastaut H, Pinsard N, Raybaud C, Aicardi J, Zifkin B. (1987) Lissencephaly (agyria-pachygyria): Clinical findings and serial EEG studies. *Dev Med Child Neurol* **29**, 167–180.

Gatrad AR. (1976) Dystonic reactions to metoclopramide. *Dev Med Child Neurol* **18**, 767–769.

Geoffroy G, Lassonde M, Delisle F. *et al.* (1983) Corpus callosotomy for control of intractable epilepsy in children. *Neurology* **33**, 891–897.

Gibbs FA, Gibbs EL. (1952) *Atlas of Electroencephalography: Epilepsy*, Vol II. Cambridge, Mass: Addison-Wesley, p. 2.

Gibbs FA, Gibbs EL. (1976) Follow-up of ACTH-treated and untreated cases of hypsarrhythmia. *Clin Electroencephalogr* **7**, 149–157.

Giraud N. (1982) Les spasmes infantiles bénins non epileptiques. These Faculté de Medicine, Marseille.

Glaser GH. (1953) On the relationship between adrenal cortical activity and the convulsive state. *Epilepsia* **2**, 7–14.

Glaze DG, Hrachovy RA, Frost JD, Zion TE, Bryan RN. (1986) Computed tomography in infantile spasms: effects of hormonal therapy. *Pediatr Neurol* **2**, 23–27.

Glaze DG, Hrachovy RA, Frost JD, Kellaway P, Zion TE. (1988) Prospective study of outcome of infants with infantile spasms treated during controlled studies of ACTH and prednisone. *J Pediatr* **112**, 389–396.

Gobbi G, Dravet C, Bureau M, Giovanardi Rossi P, Roger J. (1982) Les spasmes bénins du nourrisson (Syndrome de Lombroso et Fejerman) *Boll Lega It Epil* **39** (Suppl.), S17.

Gobbi G, Bruno L, Pini A, Rossi PG, Tassinari CA. (1987) Periodic spasms: an unclassified type of epileptic seizure in childhood. *Dev Med Child Neurol* **29**, 766–775.

Gobbi G, Pini A, Parmeggiani A. *et al.* (1989) Periodic spasms: an unclassified type of epileptic seizure in childhood. (abstract) *Epilepsia* **30**, 691.

Gobbi G, Parmeggiani A, Pini A, Tassinari CA. (1991a) Periodic spasms: a particular type of infantile spasm. (abstract) *Epilepsia* **32**, 17.

Gobbi G, Parmeggiani A, Pini A, Tassinari CA. (1991b) Periodic spasm. A particular type of infantile spasms. In: Ohtahara S, Roger J. (eds), *New Trends in Pediatric Epileptology*. Okayama, Japan: Okayama University, Medical School.

Goddard GV, McIntyre DC, Leech CK. (1969) A permanent change in brain function resulting from daily electrical stimulation. *Exp Neurol* **25**, 295–330.

Gomez MR. (1979) *Tuberous Sclerosis*. New York: Raven Press.

Gomez MR. (1988) Neurologic and psychiatric features. In: Gomez MR. (ed.), *Tuberous Sclerosis*. Raven Press, New York, pp. 21–36.

Gomibuchi K, Ochiai Y, Kanraku S, Maekawa K. (1990) Infantile spasms and gelastic seizures due to hypothalamic hamartoma. *No To Hattatsu* **22**, 392–394.

Gottlieb A, Keydor I, Epstein HT (1977) Rodent brain growth stages. An analytical review. *Biol Neonate* **32**, 166–176.

Goutières F, Aicardi J. (1971) Spasmes en flexion et agyrie cérébrale. *Cah Epilepsie* **3**, 105–112.

Gram L, Lyon BB, Dam M. (1983) Gamma-vinyl GABA: A single-blind trial in patients with epilepsy. *Acta Neurol Scand* **68**, 34–39.

Gram L, Drachmann Bentson K. (1985) Valproate: an updated review. *Acta Neurol Scand* **72**, 129–139.

Granström M-L, Leinikki P, Santavuori P, Pettay O. (1977) Perinatal cytomegalovirus infection in man. *Arch Dis Child* **52**, 354–359.

Greenamyre T, Penny JB, Young AB. *et al.* (1987) Evidence for transient perinatal glutaminergic innervation of globus pallidus. *J Neurosci* **7**, 1022–1030.

Guerrini R, Battaglia A, Stagi P. *et al.* (1979) *Boll Ega It Epil* **66/67**, 317–319.

Guerrini R, Battaglia A, Stagi P. *et al.* (1989) Caracteristiche elettrocliniche dell'epilessia nella sindrome di Down. *Boll Lega It Epil* **66/67**, 317–319.

Guerrini R, Genton P, Bureau M, Dravet C, Roger J. (1990) Reflex seizures are frequent in patients with Down syndrome and epilepsy. *Epilepsia* **31**, 406–417.

Guilleminault C, Elridge FL, Tiklian A, Simmons FB, Dement WC. (1975) Sleep apnea syndrome due to upper airway obstruction. *Arch Intern Med* **137**, 296–300.

Guzzetta G, Cristafulli A, Crino MI. (1993) Cognitive assessment in infants with West syndrome: how useful is it for diagnosis and prognosis? *Dev Med Child Neurol* **35**, 379–387.

Haas K, Sperber EF, Moshé SL. (1990) Kindling in developing animals: expression of severe seizures and enhanced development of bilateral foci. *Dev Brain Res* **56**, 275–280.

Hagberg, B. (ed.) (1993) *Rett Syndrome: Clinical and Biochemical Aspects*. London: MacKeith Press.

Hagberg B, Hamfelt A, Hansson O. (1966) Tryptophane load test and pyridoxal-5-phosphate in epileptic children. *Acta Paed Scand* **55**: 363–384.

Hakamada S, Watanabe K, Hara K, Miyazaki S. (1979) The evolution of electroencephalographic features in lissencephaly syndrome. *Brain Dev* **1**, 277–283.

Hanefeld F, Sperner J, Rating D, Rausch H, Kaufmann HJ. (1984) Renal and pancreatic calcification during treatment of infantile spasms with ACTH. *Lancet* **i**, 901.

Hara K, Watanabe K, Miyazaki S. *et al.* (1981) Apparent brain atrophy and subdural hematoma following ACTH therapy. *Brain Dev* **3**, 45–49.

Harris R, Pampiglione G. (1962) EEG and histopathology of eleven children with infantile spasms. *Electoenceph Clin Neurophysiol* **14**, 283.

Hattori H, Hayashi K, Okuno T. *et al.* (1985) *De novo* reciprocal translocation t (6; 14) (q 27; q 13.3) in a child with infantile spasms. *Epilepsia* **26**, 310–313.

Hauser WA, Kurland LT. (1975) The epidemiology of epilepsy in Rochester, Minnesota, 1935–1967. *Epilepsia* **16**, 1–66.

Hauser WA, Nelson KB. (1988) Epidemiology of epilepsy in children. *Cleveland Clinic J Med* **56** (Suppl. 2), S185–S194.

Hauw JJ, Perie G, Ponnette J. (1977) Les lésions cérébrales de l'incontinentia pigmenti. *Acta Neuropath (Berl)* **38**, 159–162.

Haynes RC. (1990) Adrenocorticotropic hormone; adrenocortical steroids and their synthetic analogs; inhibitors of the synthesis and actions of adrenocortical hormones. In: Goodman and Gilman (eds), *The Pharmacological Basis of Therapeutics*. New York: Pergamon Press.

Hayward JC, Titelbaum S, Clancy RR, Zimmerman RA. (1991) Lissencephaly-pachygyria associated with congenital cytomegalovirus infection. *J Child Neurol* **6**, 109–114.

Hedman K, Lappalainen M, Seppälä I, Mäkelä O. (1989) Recent primary toxoplasma infection indicated by a low avidity of specific IgG. *J Infect Dis* **159**, 736–740.

Heijbel J, Blom S, Bergfors PG. (1975) Benign epilepsy of children with centrotemporal EEG foci. A study of incidence rate in outpatient care. *Epilepsia* **16**, 657–664.

Herbst BA, Cohen MF. (1971) Linear nevus sebaceus syndrome: A neurocutaneous syndrome associated with infantile spasms. *Arch Neurol* **24**, 317–322.

Herpin T. (1867) *Des Accès Incomplets de l'Épilepsie.* Paris: Baillère.

Herrick-Davis K, Maisonneuve IM, Titeler M. (1989) Postsynaptic localization and up-regulation of serotonin 5-HT$_{1D}$ receptors in rat brain. *Brain Res* **483**, 155–157.

Heyer EJ, Nowak LM, MacDonald RL. (1981) Bicuculline: A convulsant with synaptic and nonsynaptic actions. *Neurology* **31**, 1381–1390.

Hill DR, Bowery NG. (1981) ^{3}H-baclofen and ^{3}H-GABA bind to bicuculline insensitive GABA$_B$ sites in rat brain. *Nature(Lond)* **290**, 149–152.

Hirano A, Tuazon R, Zimmerman HM. (1968) Neurofibrillary changes, granulovacuolar bodies and argentophilic globules observed in tuberous sclerosis. *Acta Neuropathol* **11**, 257–261.

Ho M, Dummer JS. (1990) Risk factors and approaches to infections in transplant recipients. In: Mandell GL, Douglas RG, Bennett JE. (eds), *Principles and Practice of Infectious Diseases*, 3rd edn. New York: Churchill Livingstone.

Hoefer PFA, Glaser GH. (1950) Effects of pituitary adrenocorticotrophic hormone therapy. Electroencephalographic and neuropsychiatric changes in 15 patients. *J Am Med Assoc* **143**, 620–624.

Hoffman EJ, Phelps ME. (1986) Positron emission tomography: Principles and quantitation. In: Phelps ME, Mazziotta JC, Schelbert HR. (eds), *Positron Emission Tomography and Autoradiography: Principles and Applications for the Brain and Heart.* New York: Raven Press, pp. 237–286.

Hoffman EJ, Phelps ME, Huang SC. *et al.* (1987) A new PET system for high-resolution 3-dimensional brain imaging. *J Nucl Med* **28**, 758–759.

Holmes GL. (1987) *Diagnosis and Management of Seizures in Children.* Philadelphia: W.B. Saunders, pp. 212–225.

Holmes GL, Russman BS. (1986) Shuddering attacks. *Am J Dis Child* **140**, 72–74.

Holmes GL, Weber DA. (1986) Effects of ACTH on seizure susceptibility in the developing brain. *Ann Neurol* **20**, 82–88.

Homan RW, Paulman RG, Devous MD. (1989) Cognitive function and regional cerebral blood flow in partial seizures. *Arch Neurol* **46**, 964–970.

Howitz P, Platz P. (1978) Infantile spasms and HLA antigens. *Arch Dis Child* **53**, 680–682.

Howitz P, Neergaard K, Pedersen H. (1990) Cranial computed tomography in infantile spasms. Primary findings related to long term mental prognosis. *Acta Paediatr Scand* **79**, 1087–1091.

Hrachovy RA, Frost JD Jr. (1986) Intensive monitoring of infantile spasms. In: Schmidt D, Morselli PL. (eds), *Intractable Epilepsy.* New York: Raven Press, pp. 87–97.

Hrachovy RA, Frost JD Jr. (1989a) Infantile spasms. *Pediat Clin N Am* **36**, 311–329.

Hrachovy RA, Frost JD Jr. (1989b) Infantile spasms: A disorder of the developing nervous system. In: Kellaway P, Noebels JL (eds), *Problems and Concepts in Developmental Neurophysiology.* Baltimore: Johns Hopkins University Press, pp. 131–147.

Hrachovy RA, Frost JD, Kellaway PR, Zion TE. (1979) A controlled study of prednisone therapy in infantile spasms. *Epilepsia* **20**, 403–407.

Hrachovy RA, Frost JD, Kellaway PR, Zion TE. (1980) A controlled study of ACTH therapy in infantile spasms. *Epilepsia* **21**, 631–636.

Hrachovy RA, Frost JD Jr, Kellaway P. (1981) Sleep characteristics in infantile spasms. *Neurology* **31**, 688–694.

Hrachovy RA, Frost JD, Kellaway PR, Zion TE. (1983) Double-blind study of ACTH vs prednisone therapy in infantile spasms. *J Pediatr* **103**, 641–645.

Hrachovy RA, Frost JD Jr, Kellaway P. (1984) Hypsarrhythmia: variations on the theme. *Epilepsia* **25**, 317–325.

Hrachovy RA, Frost JD, Gospe SM, Glaze DG. (1987) Infantile spasms following near-drowning: a report of two cases. *Epilepsia* **28**, 45–48.

Hrachovy RA, Frost JD Jr, Glaze DG. (1988a) Treatment of infantile spasms with tetrabenazine. *Epilepsia* **29**, 561–563.

Hrachovy RA, Frost JD, Pollack MS, Glaze DG. (1988b) Serologic HLA typing in infantile spasms. *Epilepsia* **29**, 817–819.

Hrachovy RA, Frost JD, Glaze DG, Rose D. (1989) Treatment of infantile spasms with methysergide, and alpha-methylparatyrosine. *Epilepsia* **30**, 607–610.

Hrachovy RA, Glaze DG, Frost JD. (1991) A retrospective study of spontaneous remission and long-term outcome in patients with infantile spasms. *Epilepsia* **32**, 212–214.

Huang SC, Phelps ME. (1986) Principles of tracer kinetic modeling in positron emission tomography and autoradiography. In: Phelps ME, Mazziotta JC, Schelbert HR. (eds), *Positron Emission Tomography and Autoradiography: Principles and Applications for the Brain and Heart.* New York: Raven Press, pp. 287–346.

Hughes JR, Long KJ. (1986) Infection as a possible etiology of hypsarrhythmia. *Clin Electroencephalography* **17**, 78–81.

Hughes PAM, Bower BD, Raine DN, Syed N. (1967) Effect of treatment on the metabolism of tryptophane in childhood epilepsy. *Arch Dis Childh* **42**, 281–289.

Humphreys P, Rosen GD, Press DM, Sherman GF, Galaburda AM. (1991) Freezing lesions of the developing rat brain: A model for cerebrocortical microgyria. *J Neuropathol Exp Neurol* **50**, 145–160.

Hunt A. (1983) Tuberous sclerosis: a survey of 97 cases. *Dev Med Child Neurol* **25**, 346–349.

Hunt A, Dennis JJ. (1987) Psychiatric disorders among children with tuberous sclerosis. *Dev Med Child Neurol* **29**, 190–198.

Hurst DL. (1990) Epidemiology of severe myoclonic epilepsy of infancy. *Epilepsia* **31**, 397–400.

Huson SI, Harper PS, Compston DAS. (1988) Van Recklinghausen neurofibromatosis. A clinical and population study in South East Wales. *Brain* **111**, 1355–1381.

Huttenlochter PR. (1974) Dendritic development in neocortex of children with mental defect and infantile spasms. *Neurology* **24**, 203–210.

Huttenlocher P. (1979) Synaptic density in human frontal cortex. Developmental changes and effects of aging. *Brain Res* **163**, 195–205.

Huttenlocher PR. (1985) *Tuberous Sclerosis. Recent Advances in Clinical Neurology.* Oxford: Raven Press.

Hwang P, Gilday DL, Adams C. *et al.* (1990) SPECT studies in epilepsy: applications to epilepsy surgery in children. *J Epilepsy* **3S**, 83–92.

Hwang P, Otsulo H, Koo B. *et al.* Infantile spasms: cerebral blood flow abnormalities correlate with EEG, neuroimaging and pathological findings (in prep).

Iadarola MJ, Gale K. (1982) Substantia nigra: site of anticonvulsant activity mediated by gamma-aminobutyric acid. *Science* **218**, 1237–1240.

Ikeno T, Shigematsu H, Miyakoshi M. *et al.* (1985) An analytic study of epileptic falls. *Epilepsia* **26**, 612–621.

Illingworth RS. (1955) Sudden mental deterioration with convulsions in infancy. *Arch Dis Childh* **30**, 529–537.

Ito M, Takao T, Oduno T, Mikawa H. (1983) Sequential CT studies of 24 children with infantile spasms on ACTH therapy. *Dev Med Child Neurol* **25**, 475–480.

Ito M, Okuno T, Fujii T. *et al.* (1990) ACTH therapy in infantile spasms: relationship between dose of ACTH and initial effect or long-term prognosis. *Pediatr Neurol* **6**, 240–244.

Itoh S, Yamada Y, Matsuo S, Sakea M, Ichioe A. (1982) Sodium valproate-induced liver injury. *Am J Gastroenterol* **77**, 875.

Iwase K, Watanabe K. (1972) A study on the changes of hypsarrhythmia during paradoxical sleep. *No to Hattatsu* **4**, 339–344.

Izumi T, Fukuyama Y. (1984) Influence of ACTH on serum hormone content and its anticonvulsant action towards infantile spasms. *Life Sci* **34**, 1023–1028.

Izuora GI, Iloeje SO. (1989) Pyridoxine therapy on Nigerian children with infantile spasms. *East Afr Med J* **66**, 525–530.

Jacquet L. (1903) *Le tic de Salaam.* Paris: Thesis, 56 pp.

Jambaqué I. (1992) Cognitive troubles in infantile spasms. *6th Congress of the ICNA.* Buenos Aires.

Jambaqué I, Dulac O. (1989a) Approche neuropsychologique des épilepsies chez l'enfant. *Epilepsies* **1**, 80–85.

Jambaqué I, Dulac O. (1989b) Syndrome frontal réversible et épilepsie frontale chez un enfant de 8 ans. *Arch Fr Pediatr* **46**, 525–529.

Jambaqué I, Dulac O, Arthuis M. (1989) Etude neuropsychologique prospective des spasmes infantiles. *J Paris Pédiatr* Flammarion.

Jambaqué I, Cusmai R, Curatolo P. *et al.* (1991) Neuropsychological aspects of tuberous sclerosis: Relation to epilepsy and MRI findings. *Dev Med Child Neurol* **33**, 698–705.

Jambaqué I, Chiron C, Dulac O, Raynaud C, Syrota A. (1993) Visual inattention in West syndrome: A neuropsychological and neurofunctional imaging study. *Epilepsia* **34**, 692–700.

Janz D, Matthes A. (1955) *Die propulsive Petit Mal Epilepsie*, Klinik und verlauf der sogennante Blitz-Nick und Salaamkrämpfe. Bibliotheca Paediatrica, Basel, New York; Karger, 60 pp.

Jeavons PM (1977) Nosological problems of myoclonic epilepsies in childhood and adolescence. *Dev Med Child Neurol* **19**, 3–8.

Jeavons PM. (1984) Non dose-related side-effects of valproate. *Epilepsia* **25**, 550–559.

Jeavons PM. (1985) West syndrome: infantile spasms. In: Roger J. *et al.* (eds), *Epileptic Syndromes in Infancy, Childhood and Adolescence*. London: John Libbey Eurotext, pp. 42–50.

Jeavons PM, Bower BD. (1964) Infantile spasms, a review of the literature and a study of 112 cases. In: *Clinics in Developmental Medicine*, no. 15. London: William Heinemann Medical Books, pp. 8–25; 82.

Jeavons PM, Bower BD. (1974) Infantile spams. In: Vinken PJ, Bruyn GW. (eds), *Handbook of Clinical Neurology*, Vol. 15. *The Epilepsies*. Amsterdam: Elsevier North Holland, pp. 219–234.

Jeavons PM, Moore JR. (1972) The EEG in "happy puppet" syndrome. *Electroenceph Clin Neurophysiol* **33**, 347–348.

Jeavons PM, Harper JR, Bower BD. (1990) Long-term prognosis of infantile spasms: A follow-up report on 112 cases. *Dev Med Child Neurol* **12**, 413–421.

Jeavons PM, Bower DM, Dimitrakoudi M. (1973) Long-term prognosis of 150 cases of "West syndrome". *Epilepsia* **14**, 153–164.

Jellinger K. (1970) Neuropathological aspects of hypsarrhythmia. *Neuropediatrie* **1**, 277–294.

Jellinger K. (1987) Neuropathological aspects of infantile spasms. *Brain Dev* **9**, 349–357.

Jeshima A, Eda I, Matsui A. *et al.* (1983) Computed tomography in Krabbe's disease: comparison with neuropathology. *Neuroradiology* **25**, 323–327.

Joels M, de Kloet ER. (1992) Control of neuronal excitability by corticosteroid hormones. *Trends Neurosci* **15**, 25–30.

de Jong JGY, Delleman JW, Houben M. *et al.* (1976) Agenesis of the corpus callosum, infantile spasms, ocular anomalies (Aicardi's syndrome): clinical and pathologic findings. *Neurology* **26**, 1152–1158.

Josephy H. (1944) Congenital agyria and defect of corpus callosum. *J Neuropath Exp Neurol* **3**, 63–68.

Kalifa GL, Chiron C, Sellier N. (1987) Hemimegalencephaly: MR imaging in five children. *Radiology* **165**, 29–33.

Kamoshita S, Mizutani I, Fukuyama Y. (1970) Leigh's subacute necrotizing encephalomyelopathy in a child with infantile spasms and hypsarrhythmia. *Dev Med Child Neurol* **12**, 430–435.

Kanayama M, Ishikawa T, Tauchi A. *et al.* (1989) ACTH-induced seizures in an infant with West syndrome. *Brain Dev* **11**, 329–331.

Kazee AM, Lapham LW, Torres CF, Wang DD. (1991) Generalized cortical dysplasia. Clinical and pathologic aspects. *Arch Neurol* **48**, 850–853.

Kellaway P. (1952) Myoclonic phenomena in infants. *EEG Clin Neurophysiol* **4**, 243.

Kellaway P. (1959) Neurologic status of patients with hypsarrhythmia. In: Gibbs FA. (ed.), *Molecules and Mental Health*. Philadelphia: J.B. Lippincott, pp. 134–149.

Kellaway P, Hrachovy RA, Frost JD Jr, Zion T. (1979) Precise characterization and quantification of infantile spasms. *Ann Neurol* **6**, 214–218.

Kellaway P, Frost JD, Hrachovy RA. (1983) Infantile spasms. In: Morselli PL. *et al.* (eds), *Antiepileptic Drug Therapy in Pediatrics*. New York: Raven Press, pp. 115–136.

Kendall B, Holland I. (1981) Benign communicating hydrocephalus in children. *Neuroradiology* **21**, 93–96.

Kendall DA, McEwen BS, Enna SJ. (1982) The influence of ACTH and corticosterone on the [³H]-GABA receptor binding in rat brain. *Brain Res* **236**, 365–374.

Khrestchatisky M, MacLennan AJ, Chiang MY. *et al.* (1989) A novel alpha subunit in rat brain GABA$_A$ receptors. *Neuron* **3**, 745–753.

King DW, Dyken PR, Spinks IL, Murvin AL. (1985a) Infantile spasms: ictal phenomena. *Pediat Neurol* **1**, 213–218.

King M, Stephenson JBP, Ziervogel M, Doyle D, Galbraith S. (1985b) Hemimegalencephaly—a case for hemispherectomy? *Neuropediatrics* **16**, 46–55.

Kingsley E, Tweedale R, Toman KG. (1980) Hepatotoxicity of sodium valproate and other anticonvulsants in rat hepatocyte cultures. *Epilepsia* **21**, 699–706.

Klawans H, Goetz C, Weiner WJ. (1973) 5-Hydroxytryptophan induced myoclonus in guinea pigs and the possible role of serotonin in infantile spasms. *Neurology* **23**, 1234–1240.

Klein R. Livingston S. (1950) The effect of adrenocorticotrophic hormone in epilepsy. *J Pediatr* **37**, 733–742.

Knauer H. (1925) Ein Beitrag zur Frage der Salaam krämpfe. *Monatschrift für Kinderheilkunde* **30**, 428.

Kohl S. (1988) Herpes simplex virus encephalitis in children. New topics in pediatric infectious disease. *Pediatr Clin N Am* **35**, 465–487.

Konishi Y, Yasujima M, Kuriyama M. *et al.* (1992) Magnetic resonance imaging in infantile spasms: effects of hormonal therapy. *Epilepsia* **33**, 304–309.

Konkol RJ, Holmes GL, Thompson JL. (1990) The effect of regional differences in noradrenergic growth patterns on juvenile kindling. *Dev Brain Res* **52**, 25–29.

Koo B, Hwang P, Logan W, Hunjan A. (1993) Infantile spasms: outcome and prognosis factors of cryptogenic and symptomatic groups. *Neurology* **43**, 2322–2327.

Korinthenberg R, Schultze C. (1990) Pyridoxine-dependent seizures. Remarks on clinical variability and pathogenesis. *Monatsschr-Kinderheilkd* **138**, 759–762.

Koskiniemi M, Ketonen L. (1981) Herpes simplex virus encephalitis: progression of lesion shown by CT. *J Neurol* **225**, 9–13.

Koskiniemi M, Vaheri A, Taskinen E. (1984) Cerebrospinal fluid alterations in herpes simplex virus encephalitis. *Rev Infect Dis* **6**, 608–618.

Kotlarek F, Deselaers M, Hotes G. (1985) How effective is the treatment schedule in children with infantile spasms? *Klin Padiatr* **197**, 21–24.

Kotte W, Künze P. (1971) Alobare Holoprosencephalie (arhinencephalie) mit medianer Lippenkiefersfalte und normalen Karyotype. *Zentral Allg Pathol* **114**, 173–184.

Kramer W. (1953) Poliodysplasia cerebri. *Acta Psychiatr Neurol Scand* **28**, 413–427.

Kriegstein AR, Suppes T, Prince DA. (1987) Cellular and synaptic physiology and epileptogenesis of the developing rat neocortical neurons in vitro. *Dev Brain Res* **34**, 161–171.

Kuriyama M, Shigematsu Y, Konishi Y. *et al.* (1988) Septo-optic dysplasia with infantile spasms. *Pediatr Neurol* **4**, 62–65.

Kurokawa T, Goya N, Fukuyama Y. *et al.* (1980) West syndrome and Lennox-Gastaut syndrome: a survey of natural history. *Pediatrics* **65**, 81–88.

Kurokawa T, Sasaki H, Hanai T. *et al.* (1981) Linear nevus sebaceus syndrome. Report of a case with Lennox-Gastaut syndrome following infantile spasms. *Arch Neurol* **38**, 375–377.

Kuzniecky R, Andermann F, Tampieri D. *et al.* (1989) Bilateral central macrogyria: epilepsy, pseudobulbar palsy and mental retardation—a recognizable neuronal migration disorder. *Ann Neurol* **25**, 547–554.

Kuzniecky R, Garcia JH, Faught E, Morawetz RB. (1991a) Cortical dysplasia in temporal lobe epilepsy: Magnetic resonance imaging correlations. *Ann Neurol* **29**, 293–298.

Kuzniecky R, Andermann F, Guerrini R. (1991b) Congenital bilateral perisylvian syndrome: a new recognizable entity. *Epilepsia* **32** (Suppl. 1), 16 (abstract).

Lacy JR, Penry JK. (1976) *Infantile Spasms.* New York: Raven Press.

Lance JW (1977) Familiar paroxysmal dystonic choreoathetosis and its differentiation from related syndromes. *Ann Neurol* **2**, 285.

Langenstein I, Willig RP, Kuehn D. (1979) Cranial computed tomography (CCT) findings in children with ACTH and dexamethasone: first results. *Neuropediatrics* **10**, 370–384.

Larregue M, Lauret P, Beauvais P, Bressieux JM. (1977) Dermo-neuro-hypsarythmie. Association d'une dermatose congenitale et d'une hypsarythmie. A propos de 9 cas. *Ann Dermatol Venerol* **104**, 26–31.

Larson HJ. (1969) *Introduction to Probability Theory and Statistical Inference.* Monterey, California: John Wiley & Sons.

Lassen NA. (1985) Cerebral blood flow tomography with xenon-133. *Semin Nucl Med* **15**, 347–356.

Laurie DJ, Seeburg PH, Wisden W. (1992) The distribution of 13 GABA$_A$ receptor subunit mRNAs in the rat brain. II. Olfactory bulb and cerebellum. *J Neurosci* **12**, 1063–1076.

Lederer M. (1926) Betrage zur Kenntnis der Nickkrämpfe. *Jahrbuch für kinderheilkunde* **31**, 113–275.

Lee S, Murata R, Matsuura S. (1989) The developmental study of hippocampal kindling. *Epilepsia* **30**, 266–270.

Lennox W. (1966) *Epilepsy and Related Disorders.* London: Churchill Livingstone.

Lennox WG, Davis JP. (1950) Clinical correlates of the fast and slow spike-wave encephalogram. *Pediatrics* **4**, 626–644.

Leppert M, Anderson VE, Quattlebaum T. *et al.* (1989) Benign familial neonatal convulsions linked to genetic markers on chromosome 20. *Nature* **337**, 647–648.

Lerman P. (1969) Hypsarrhythmia. (abstract) *Electroencephalogr Clin Neurophysiol* **27**, 216.

Lerman P, Kivity S. (1982) The efficacy of corticotropin in primary infantile spasms. *J Pediatr* **101**, 294–296.

Levin S, Robinson RO, Aicardi J, Hoare RD. (1984) Computed tomography appearances in the linear sebaceous naevus syndrome. *Neuroradiology* **26**, 469–472.

Levitan ES, Blair LAC, Dionne VE, Barnard EA. (1988a) Biophysical and pharmacological properties of cloned GABA$_A$ receptor subunits expressed in xenopus oocytes. *Neuron* **1**, 773–781.

Levitan ES, Schofield PR, Burt DR. *et al.* (1988b) Structural and functional basis for GABA$_A$ receptor heterogeneity. *Nature* **335**, 76–79.

Leyh F, Loewel R. (1973) Ein Fall von Schimmelpennig-Fuerstein-Mim Syndrom mit allmaelicher Kataraktentwicklung. *Z Hautkr* **48**, 695–698.

Livingston JH, Beaumont D, Arzimanoglou A, Aicardi J. (1989) Vigabatrin in the treatment of epilepsy in children. *Br J Clin Pharmacol* **27**, S109–S112.

Loiseau P, Legroux HM, Grimond P, Du Pasquier P, Henry P. (1974) Taxometric classification of myoclonic epilepsies. *Epilepsia* **15**, 1–11.

Loiseau J, Loiseau P, Guyot M. *et al.* (1990) Survey of seizure disorders in the French southwest. I. Incidence of epileptic syndromes. *Epilepsia* **31**, 391–396.

Loiseau P, Duche B, Loiseau J. (1991) Classification of epilepsies and epileptic syndromes in two different samples of patients. *Epilepsia* **32**, 303–309.

Lombroso CT. (1982) Differentiation of seizures in newborns and in early infancy. In: Morselli PL, Pippinger CE, Penry JK. (eds), *Antiepileptic Drug Therapy in Pediatrics.* New York: Raven Press, pp. 85–102.

Lombroso CT. (1983a) A prospective study of infantile spasms: Clinical and therapeutic correlations. *Epilepsia* **24**, 135–158.

Lombroso CT. (1983b) Prognosis in neonatal seizures. In: Delgado-Escueta AV. *et al.* (eds), *Advance in Neurology.* New York: Raven Press, *Status Epilepticus* **34**, 101–113.

Lombroso CT. (1990) Early myoclonic encephalopathy, early infantile encephalopathy and benign and severe infantile myoclonic epilepsies: a critical review and personal contributions. *J Clin Neurophysiol* **7**, 380–408.

Lombroso CT, Erba G. (1982) Myoclonic seizures: considerations in taxonomy. In: Akimoto *et al.* (eds), *Advances in Epileptology: XIIIth Epilepsy International Symposium.* New York: Raven Press, 129–134.

Lombroso CT, Fejerman N. (1977) Benign myoclonus of early infancy. *Ann Neurol* **1**, 138–143.

Lortie A, Plouin P, Pinard JM, Dulac O. (1993a) Occipital epilepsy in neonates and infants. In: Andermann F. *et al.* (eds), *Occipital Seizures and Epilepsy in Children.* London: John Libbey Eurotext, pp. 121–132.

Lortie A, Chiron C, Mumford J, Dulac O. (1993b) The potential for increasing seizure frequency, relapse, and appearance of new seizure types with vigabatrin. *Neurology* **43**, S24–S27.

Lou H, Henriksen L, Bruhn P. (1990) Focal cerebral dysfunction in developmental learning disabilities. *Lancet* **335**, 8–11.

Lovejoy FH, Boyle WE. (1973) Linear nevus sebaceus syndrome: report of two cases and a review of the literature. *Pediatrics* **52**, 382–387.

Low NL. (1958) Infantile spasms with mental retardation: I. treatment with cortisone and adrenocorticotropin. *Pediatrics* **22**, 1165–1169.

Ludwig B. (1987) Review: neuroradiological aspects of infantile spasms. *Brain Dev* **9**, 358–360.

Luna D, Chiron C, Pajot N. *et al.* (1988) Epidemiologie des epilepsies de l'enfant dans le departement de l'Oise. *Ligue Française contre l'Épilepsie*. John Libbey Eurotext, pp. 41–53.

Luna D, Dulac O, Plouin P. (1989a) Ictal characteristics of cryptogenic partial epilepsies in infancy. *Epilepsia* **30**, 827–832.

Luna D, Dulac O, Pajot N, Beaumont D. (1989b) Vigabatrin in the treatment of childhood epilepsies: A single-blind placebo-controlled study. *Epilepsia*, **30**, 430–437.

Lussenhop A, De la Cruz T, Fenichel G. (1970) Surgical disconnection of cerebral hemispheres for intractable seizures. *J Am Med Assoc* **213**, 1630–1636.

Lyen KR, Holland IM, Lyen YC. (1979) Reversible cerebral atrophy in infantile spasms caused by corticotropin. *Lancet* **2**, 237–238.

Lyon G, Gastaut H. (1985) Considerations on the significance attributed to unusual cerebral histological findings recently described in eight patients with primary generalized epilepsy. *Epilepsia* **26**, 365–367.

McBride MC, Kemper TL. (1982) Pathogenesis of four-layered microgyric cortex in man. *Acta Neuropathol* **57**, 93–98.

McDonald JW, Johnston MV. (1990) Physiological pathophysiological roles of excitatory aminoacids during central nervous system development. *Brain Res Rev* **15**, 41–70.

McEwen BS, DeKloet ER, Rostene W. (1986) Adrenal steroid receptors and actions in the nervous system. *Physiol Rev* **66**, 1122–1187.

McIntyre DC. (1981) Catecholamine involvement in amygdala kindling of the rat. In: Wada JA. (ed.), *Kindling*, Vol. 2. New York: Raven Press, pp. 67–79.

McIntyre DC, Rajalla J, Edson N. (1987) Suppression of amygdala kindling with short interstimulus intervals: effect of norepinephrine depletion. *Exp Neurol* **95**, 391–402.

McQuarrie I, Anderson JA, Ziegler RR. (1942) Observations on the antagonistic effects of posterior pituitary and cortico-adrenal hormones in the epileptic subject. *J Clin Endocrinol* **2**, 406–410.

McShane, Finn JP, Hall-Craggs MA, Hammer O, Harper J. (1990) Neonatal hemangiomatosis presenting as infantile spasms. *Neuropediatrics* **22**, 211–212.

Maekawa K, Ohta H, Tamai I. (1980) Transient brain shrinkage in infantile spasms after ACTH treatment. Report of two cases. *Neuropadiatrie* **11**, 80–84.

Maheshwari MC, Jeavons PM. (1975) The prognostic implications of suppression-burst activity in the EEG in infancy. *Epilepsia* **16**, 127–131.

Majewska MD, Bisserbe JC, Eskay RL. (1985) Glucocorticoids are modulators of $GABA_a$ receptors in brain. *Brain Res* **339**, 178–182.

Majewska MD, Harrison TL, Schwartz RD, Barker JD, Paul SM. (1986) Steroid hormone metabolites and barbiturate-like modulators of the GABA receptor. *Science* **232**, 1004–1008.

Malamud N. (1966) Neuropathology of phenylketonuria. *J Neuropathol Exp Neurol* **25**, 254–268.

Marchal G, Andermann F, Tampieri D. *et al.* (1989) Generalized cortical dysplasia manifested by diffusely thick cerebral cortex. *Arch Neurol* **46**, 430–434.

Marchand L, De Ajuriaguerra J. (1948) *Les Épilepsies, Leurs Formes Cliniques, Leur Traitement*. Paris: Desclée de Brouwer.

Marciani MG, Gigli GL, Orlandi L. (1992) Long follow-up of tuberous sclerosis treated with vigabatrin. *Lancet* **34**, 1554.

Marciniak M, Dambska M, Wisczor-Adamczyk B. (1971) Neuropathologic changes in the syndrome of infantile spasms. *Neuropathol Pol* **9**, 211–218.

Maremmani C, Rossi G, Bonuccelli U, Murri L. (1991) Descriptive epidemiologic study of epilepsy syndromes in a district of northwest Tuscany, Italy. *Epilepsia* **32**, 294–298.

Marin Palida M. (1975) Abnormal neuronal differentiation (functional maturation) in mental retardation. *Birth Defects* **9**, 133–153.

Marrosu F, Fratta W, Carcangiu P, Giagheddu M, Gessa GL. (1988) Localized epileptiform activity induced by murine CRF in rats. *Epilepsia* **29**, 369–373.

Marseille Consensus Group. (1990) Classification of PME and related disorders. *Ann Neurol* **28**, 113–116.

Martin F. (1964) Physiopathogénie. In: Gastaut H. *et al. L'Encéphalopathie Myoclonique Infantile avec Hypsarythmie (Syndrome de West).. Paris: Masson.*

Martin G, Loiseau P, Bottin JJ. *(1961) Encephalopathie chronique avec hypsarhythmie, séquelle d'une anoxie néonatale. Arch Franc Pediat* **18**, 609–619.

Martin Blazquez JL, Fijo Lopez Viota J, Alonso Luengo O. *et al.* (1988) Sebaceous nevus of Jadassohn associated with infantile spasms. *An Esp Pediatr* **28**, 266–268.

Matsuishi T, Yano E, Inanaga K. *et al.* (1983) A pilot study on the anticonvulsive effects of a thyrotropin-releasing hormone analog in intractable epilepsy. *Brain Dev* **5**, 421–428.

Matsumoto A, Watanabe K, Negoro T. *et al.* (1981a) Long-term prognosis after infantile spasms: A statistical study of prognostic factors in 200 cases. *Dev Med Child Neurol* **23**, 51–65.

Matsumoto A, Watanabe K, Negoro T. *et al.* (1981b) Infantile spasms: Etiological factors, clinical aspects, and long-term prognosis in 200 cases. *Eur J Pediatr* **135**, 239–244.

Matsumoto A, Watanabe K, Negoro T. *et al.* (1981c) Prognostic factors of infantile spasms from the etiological viewpoint. *Brain Dev* **3**, 361–364.

Matsumoto A, Watanabe K, Jugiura M. *et al.* (1983) Prognostic factors of convulsive disorders in the first year of life. *Brain Dev* **5**, 469–473.

Matsumoto A, Kumagai T, Takeuchi T, Miyazaki S, Watanabe K. (1987) Clinical effects of thryotropin-releasing hormone for severe epilepsy in childhood: A comparative study with ACTH therapy. *Epilepsia* **28**, 49–55.

Matsumoto A, Kumagai T, Takeuchi T, Miyazaki S, Watanabe K. (1989) Factors influencing effectiveness of thryotropoin-releasing hormone therapy for severe epilepsy in childhood: significance of serum prolactin levels. *Epilepsia* **30**, 45–49.

Matsumoto A, Kumagi T, Miura K. *et al.* (1992) Epilepsy in Angelman syndrome associated with chromosome 15q deletion. *Epilepsia* **33**, 1083–1090.

Meencke HJ. (1985) Morphological aspects of aetiology and the course of infantile spasms. *Neuropediatrics* **16**, 59–66.

Meencke HJ, Gerhard C. (1985) Morphological aspects of aetiology and the course of infantile spasms (West-syndrome). *Neuropediatrics* **16**, 59–66.

Meencke HJ, Janz D. (1984) Neuropathological findings in primary generalized epilepsy: A study of eight cases. *Epilepsia* **25**, 8–21.

Melchior JC. (1971) Infantile spasms and immunisation in the first year of life. *Neuropediatrie* **3**, 3–10.

Melchior JC. (1977) Infantile spasms and early immunization against whooping cough. *Arch Dis Child* **52**, 134–137.

Menkes JH, Philippart M, Clark DB. (1964) Hereditary partial agenesis of corpus callosum. *Arch Neurol* **11**, 198–208.

Michelson HB, Butterbaugh GG. (1985) Amygdala kindling in juvenile rats following neonatal administration of 6-hydroxydopamine. *Exp Neurol* **90**, 588–593.

Midulla M, Balducci L, Iannetti P. *et al.* (1976) Infantile spasms and cytomegalovirus infection. *Lancet* **2**, 377.

Mikati MA, Feraru E, Krishnamoorthy K, Lombroso CT. (1990) Neonatal herpes simplex meningoencephalitis: EEG investigations and clinical correlates. *Neurology* **40**, 1433–1437.

Miller DL, Ross EM, Alderslade R, Bellman MH, Rawson NSB. (1981) Pertussis immunisation and serious acute neurological illness in children. *Brit Med J* **282**, 1595–1599.

Millichap JG, Bickford RG. (1962) Infantile spasms, hypsarrhythmia, and mental retardation. *J Am Med Assoc* **182**, 125–129.

Millichap JG, Bickford RG, Klass DW. *et al.* (1962) Infantile spasms, hypsarrhythmia and mental retardation. A study of etiology in 61 patients. *Epilepsia* **3**, 188–197.

Mimaki T, Ono J, Yabuuchi H. (1983) Temporal lobe astrocytoma with infantile spasms. *Ann Neurol* **14**, 695–696.

Mimaki T, Tagawa T, Ono J. *et al.* (1984) Antiepileptic effect and serum levels of chlorazepate on children with refractory seizures. *Brain Dev* **6**, 539–544.

Miyake S, Yamashita S, Yamada M. *et al.* (1986) Unilateral hemispheric neoplasm in infantile spasms. *No To Hattutsu* **18**, 316–321.

Möhler H, Malherbe P, Draguhn A, Richards JG. (1990) GABA$_A$-receptors: structural requirements and sites of gene expression in mammalian brain. *Neurochem Res* **15**, 199–207.

Molfese VJ. (1992) Neuropsychological assessment in infancy. In: Rapin I, Segalowicz SJ. (eds), *Handbook of Neuropsychology*, Vol. 6. New York: Elsevier.

Moreland DB, Glasauer FE, Egnatchik JG, Heffner RR, Alker GJ Jr. (1988) Focal cortical dysplasia. Case report. *J Neurosurg* **68**, 487–490.

Morimatsu Y, Sato J. (1983) Neuropathological studies of West syndrome. *Adv Neurolog Sci* **27**, 636–645.

Morimatsu Y, Murofushi R, Handa T, Shinohara T, Shiraki H. (1977) Pathological studies of severe physically and mentally handicapped; with special reference to four cases of infantile spasms. *Adv Neurol Sci* **16**, 465–470.

Morimoto K, Abekura M, Nii Y. *et al.* (1989) Nodding attacks (infantile spasms) associated with temporal lobe astrocytoma—case report. *Neurol Med Chir (Tokyo)* **29**, 610–613.

Moshé SL. (1981) The effects of age on the kindling phenomenon. *Dev Psychobiol* **14**, 75–81.

Moshé SL. (1987) Epileptogenesis and the immature brain. *Epilepsia* **28** (Suppl.), S3–S15.

Moshé SL. (1989) Ontogeny of seizures and substantia nigra modulation. In: Kellaway P, Noebels JF. (eds), *Problems and Concepts in Developmental Neurophysiology*. Baltimore: Johns Hopkins Press, pp. 247–262.

Moshé SL, Albala BJ. (1982) Kindling in developing rats: persistence of seizures into adulthood. *Dev Brain Res* **4**, 67–71.

Moshé SL, Albala BJ. (1983) Maturational changes in postictal refractoriness and seizure susceptibility in developing rats. *Ann Neurol* **13**, 552–557.

Moshé SL, Sperber EF. (1990) Substantia nigra-mediated control of generalized seizures. In: Gloor G. *et al.* (eds), *Generalized Epilepsy: Cellular, Molecular and Pharmacological Approaches*. Boston: Birkhauser Inc, pp. 355–367.

Moshé SL, Sharpless NS, Kaplan J. (1981) Kindling in developing rats: afterdischarge thresholds. *Brain Res* **211**, 190–195.

Moshé SL, Albala BJ, Ackermann RF, Engel JJ. (1983) Increased seizure susceptibility of the immature brain. *Dev Brain Res* **7**, 81–85.

Moshé SL, Sperber EF, Brown LL. *et al.* (1988) Experimental epilepsy: developmental aspects. *Cleveland Clinic J Med* **56** (Suppl. 1), S92–S99.

Moshé SL, Sperber EF, Haas K. (1990) Pathophysiology of experimental seizures in developing animals. In: Sillanpaa M. *et al.* (eds), *Pediatric Epilepsy*. Stroud: Wrightson Biomedical Publ. pp. 17–30.

Moshé SL, Holmes GL, Mares P. (1991) Epileptogenesis and the immature brain: Subcortical mechanisms. In: Klee MR. *et al.* (eds) *Physiology, Pharmacology and Development of Epileptic Phenomena*. Berlin: Springer, pp. 147–149.

Moshé SL, Sperber EF, Haas K, Xu S, Shinnar S. (1992) Effects of maturational process on epileptogenesis. In: Lüders H. (ed.), *Epilepsy Surgery*. New York: Raven Press, pp. 741–747.

Motte J, Billard C, Fejerman N. *et al.* (1993) Neurofibromatosis type one and West Syndrome: a relatively benign association. *Epilepsia* **34**, 723–726.

Moutard ML, Guerrini R, Parrain D. *et al.* (1994) Aspect électrophysiologiques des hétérotopies en bandes. Presented at the Société de Neurophysiologie Clinique de Langue Française, 2 March 1994.

Moynahan FJ, Wolff OH. (1967) A new neurocutaneous syndrome (skin, eye and brain) consisting of linear nevus, bilateral lipodermoid of the conjonctivae, cranial thickening, cerebral atrophy and mental retardation. *Br J Dermatol* **79**, 651–652.

Murphy JV. (1988) Valproate monotherapy in children. *Am J Med* **84**, 17–22.

Murphy MJ, Tenser, RB. (1982) Nevoid basal cell carcinoma syndrome and epilepsy. *Ann Neurol* **11**, 372–376.

Nalin A, Petraglia F, Genazzani AR, Frigieri G, Facchinetti F. (1988) Lack of clinical EEG effects of naloxone injection on infantile spasms. *Childs Nerv Syst* **4**, 365–366.

National Institutes of Health. (1982) Neurofibromatosis. *National Institutes Consensus Development Conference Statement*. Bethesda: The Institute, p. 6.

Nausieda PA, Carvey PM, Braun A. (1982) Long-term suppression of central serotonergic activity by corticosteroids: A possible model of steroid-responsive myoclonic disorders. *Neurology* **32**, 772–775.

Negoro T, Watanabe K, Matsumoto A. *et al.* (1983) Long-term follow-up study of West syndrome. Seizure types and EEG findings at age 5–10 years. *Japan J Epil* **1**, 40–45.

Nelson K. (1972) Discussion. In: Alter M, Hauser WA. (eds), *The Epidemiology of Epilepsy: A Workshop*. NINDS Monograph No. 14. Washington: US Government Printing Office, p. 78.

Neville BGR. (1972) The origin of infantile spasms: Evidence from a case of hydranencephaly. *Dev Med Child Neurol* **14**, 644–656.

Newnham W. (1849) History of four cases of eclampsia nutans or the salaam convulsions of infancy. *Br Record Obstet Med* **2**, 1. (Quoted by Zellweger).

Nieuwenhuys R. (1985) *Chemoarchitecture of the Brain*. New York: Springer-Verlag.

Nixon JR, Miller GM, Gomez MR. (1989) Cerebral tuberous sclerosis: post-mortem MRI and pathology anatomy. *Mayo Clinic Proc* **64**, 305–311.

Nolte R. (1989) Neonatal sleep myoclonus followed by myoclonic-astatic epilepsy: a case report. *Epilepsia* **30**, 844–850.

Nolte R, Christen HJ, Doerrer J. (1988) Preliminary report of a multi-center study on the West syndrome. *Brain Dev* **10**, 236–242.

Nordgren R, Reeves A, Viguera A. *et al.* (1991) Corpus callosotomy for intractable seizures in the pediatric age group. *Arch Neurol* **48**, 364–372.

Nuno K, Mihara M, Shimao S. (1990) Linear sebaceous nevus syndrome. *Dermatologica* **181**, 221–223.

Oates R, Harvey D. (1976) Congenital rubella associated with hypsarrhythmia. *Arch Dis Child* **51**, 77–79.

Obeso JA, Artieda J, Luquin MR, Vaamonde J, Martinez Lage JM (1986) Antimyoclonic action of piracetam. *Clin Neuropharmacol* **9**, 58–64.

O'Donohoe NV, Paes BA. (1977) A trial of clonazepam in the treatment of severe epilepsy in infancy and childhood. In: Penry JK (ed.), *Epilepsia: the VIIIth International Symposium*. New York: Raven Press, pp. 159–162.

Ohtahara S. (1965) Electroencephalographic studies in infantile spasms. (abstract) *Dev Med Child Neurol* **7**, 707.

Ohtahara S. (1978) Clinico-electrical delineation of epileptic encephalopathies in childhood. *Asian Med J* **21**, 7–17.

Ohtahara S. (1987) Transition between syndromes: developmental aspects of epilepsy. In: Wolf P. *et al.* (eds), *Advances in Epileptology*. New York: Raven Press. 171–174.

Ohtahara S, Ishida T, Oka E. *et al.* (1976) On the specific age-dependent epileptic syndrome. The early-infantile epileptic encephalopathy with suppression-burst. (in Japanese) *No to Hattatsu* **8**, 270–280.

Ohtahara S, Yamatoki Y, Ohtsuka Y, Oka E, Ishida T (1980) Prognosis of West syndrome with special reference to Lennox syndrome: a developmental study. In: Wada J. and Penny JK (eds), *Advances in Epileptology: the Xth Epilepsy International Symposium*. New York: Raven Press, pp. 149–154.

Ohtahara S, Ishida S, Oka E. *et al.* (1981) Epilepsy and febrile convulsions in Okayama prefecture. A neuroepidemiologic study. In: Fukuyama Y. *et al.* (ed.), *Proceedings of the IYDP Commemorative International Symposium on Developmental Disabilities*. Tokyo, Amsterdam: Elsevier, pp. 376–382.

Ohtahara S, Ohtsuka Y, Yamatogi Y, Oka E. (1987) The early-infantile epileptic encephalopathy with suppression-burst: developmental aspects. *Brain Devel* **9**, 371–376.

Ohtaki E, Yamagushi Y, Shiotsuki Y. *et al.* (1987) A case of infantile spasms due to herpes simplex type virus encephalitis. *No To Hattatsu* **19**, 502–506.

Ohtsuka Y, Ogino T, Murakami N. *et al.* (1986) Developmental aspects of epilepsy with special reference to age-dependent epileptic encephalopathy. *Japan J Psychiat Neurol* **40**, 307–313.

Ohtsuka Y, Matsuda M, Ogino T, Kobayashi K, Ohtahara S. (1987) Treatment of the West syndrome with high-dose pyridoxal phosphate. *Brain Dev* **9**, 418–421.

Ohtsuka Y, Ogino T, Amano R, Enoki H, Ohtahara S. (1989) Evolutional process from the West syndrome into the Lennox-Gastaut syndrome: A developmental study. *J Japan Epil Soc* **7**, 59–66.

Ohtsuka Y, Oka E, Terakasi T, Ohtahara S. (1993) Aicardi syndrome: a longitudinal clinical and electroencephalographic study. *Epilepsia* **34**, 627–634.

Okada R, Nagishi N, Nagaya H. (1989) The role of the nigrotegmental GABAergic pathway in the propagation of pentylenetetrazol induced seizures. *Brain Res* **480**, 383–387.

Okuno T, Ito M, Konishi Y, Yoshioka M, Nakano Y. (1980) Cerebral atrophy following ACTH therapy. *J Comput Assist Tomogr* **4**, 20–23.

Okuyama K. (1965) Neuropathological findings in eight cases of infantile spasms with hypsarrhythmia. *Dev Med Child Neurol* **7**, 707–708.

Olpe HR, Jones RSG. (1982) Excitatory effects of ACTH on noradrenergic neurons of the locus coeruleus in the rat. *Brain Res* **251**, 177–179.

Olsen RW, Bann M, Miller T. (1976) Studies on the neuropharmacological activity of bicuculline and related compounds. *Brain Res* **102**, 283–299.

Olsen RW, Greenlee D, Van Ness P, Ticku MK. (1978) Studies on the gamma-aminobutyric acid receptor/ionophore proteins in mammalian brain. In: Fonnum F. (ed.), *Amino Acids as Chemical Transmitters*. New York: Plenum Press, pp. 467–486.

Olsen RW, Snowhill EW, Wamsley JK. (1983) Autoradiographic localization of low affinity GABA receptors with ^{3}H-bicuculline methochloride. *Eur J Pharm* **99**, 247–248.

Olsen RW, McCabe RT, Walmsley JK. (1990) GABA$_A$ receptor subtypes: autoradiographic comparison of GABA$_A$, benzodiazepine, and convulsant binding sites in the rat central nervous system. *J Chem Neuroanatomy* **3**, 59–76.

Olson DM, Chugani HT, Shewmon DA, Phelps ME, Peacock WJ. (1990) Electrocorticographic confirmation of focal positron emission tomographic abnormalities in children with intractable epilepsy. *Epilepsia* **31**, 731–739.

Otsubo H, Hwanp PA, Jay V *et al.* (1993) Focal cortical dysplasia in children with localization-related epilepsy: EEG, MRI and SPECT findings. *Ped Neurol* **9**, 101–107.

Pagon RA, Graham JM, Zonana J, Si-Li Yong. (1981) Coloboma, congenital heart disease and choanal atresia with multiple anomalies: CHARGE association. *J Pediatr* **99**, 223–227.

Paladin F, Chiron C, Dulac O, Plouin P, Ponsot G. (1989) Electroencephalographic aspects of hemimegalencephaly. *Dev Med Child Neurol* **31**, 377–383.

Palm L, Blennow G, Brun A. (1986) Infantile spasms and neuronal heterotopias. A report of six cases. *Acta Paediatr Scand* **75**, 855–859.

Palm DG, Brandt M, Korinthenberg R. (1988) West syndrome and Lennox-Gastaut syndrome in children with porencephalic cysts. Long-term follow-up after neurosurgical treatment. In: Niedermeyer E, Degen R. (eds), *The Lennox-Gastaut Syndrome*. New-York: Liss, pp. 419–426.

Palmini A, Andermann F, Olivier A, Tempieri D, Robitaille Y. (1991a) Focal neuronal migration disorders and intractable partial epilepsy: Results of surgical treatment. *Ann Neurol* **30**, 750–757.

Palmini A, Andermann F, Olivier A. *et al.* (1991b) Focal neuronal migration disorders and intractable partial epilepsy: A study of 30 patients. *Ann Neurol* **30**, 741–749.

Paltiel HJ, O'Gorman AM, Merger-Villemure K. *et al.* (1987) Subacute necrotizing encephalomyelopathy (Leigh's disease): CT study. *Radiology* **162**, 115–118.

Paludan J. (1961) Autopsy findings in a child with infantile spasms and hypsarrhythmia, with a survey of the effect of ACTH. *Dan Med Bull* **8**, 128–130.

Pampiglione G. (1963) Post-anoxic encephalopathies in children. *Rev Enceph Neurophysiol* **1**, 84.

Pampiglione G, Pugh E. (1975) Infantile spasms and subsequent appearance of tuberous sclerosis syndrome. *Lancet* **ii**, 1046–1048.

Pampliglione G, Moynahan EJ. (1976) The tuberous sclerosis syndrome: clinical and EEG studies in 100 children. *J Neurol Neurosurg Psychiatr* **39**, 666–673.

Parker PH, Helinek GL, Ghishan FK, Greene HL. (1981) Recurrent pancreatitis associated with valproate acid. A case report and review of the literature. *Gastroenterology* **80**, 826–828.

Parmeggiani A, Plouin P, Dulac O. (1990) Quantification of diffuse and focal delta activity in hypsarrhythmia. *Brain Dev* **12**, 310–315.

Patry G, Lyagoubi S, Tassinari CA. (1971) Subclinical "electrical status epilepticus" induced by sleep in children. *Arch Neurol* **24**, 242–252.

Pavone L, Mollica F, Incorpora G, Pampiglione G. (1980) Infantile spasms syndrome in monozygotic twins. *Arch Dis Child* **55**, 870–872.

Pavone L, Incorpora G, La Rosa M, Livolti S, Mollica F. (1981) Treatment of infantile spasms with sodium dipropylacetic acid. *Dev Med Child Neurol* **23**, 454–461.

Pedersen H, Neergaard K, Howitz P. (1990) Cerebral computed tomography in infantile spasms. *Ugeskr Laeger* **152**, 1593–1595.

Pedespan JM, Fontan D, Pere Y, Guerin J, Guillard JM. (1992) Spasmes infantiles associés à une tumeur cérébrale. *Arch Fr Pédiatr* **49**, 887–889.

Pellock JM. (1987) Carbamazepine side effects in children and adults. *Epilepsia* **28** (Suppl. 3), S64–S70.

Pentella K, Bachman DS, Sandman CA. (1982) Trial of an ACTH 4–9 analog (ORG 2766) in children with intractable seizures. *Neuropediatrics* **13**, 59–62.

Perheentupa J, Riikonen R, Dunkel L, Simell O. (1986) Adrenocortical hyporesponsiveness after treatment with ACTH of infantile spasms. *Arch Dis Child* **61**, 750–753.

Peroutka SJ. (1988) 5-Hydroxytryptamine receptor subtypes: molecular, biochemical and physiological characterization. *TINS* **11**, 496–500.

Peterson SL, Albertson TE, Stark LG. (1981) Intertrial intervals and kindled seizures. *Exp Neurol* **71**, 144–153.

Pfeiffer J. (1963) *Morphologische Aspekts des Epilepsien*. Berlin-Göttingen-Heidelberg: Springer.

Phelps ME, Mazziotta JC. (1985) Positron emission tomography: human brain function and biochemistry. *Science* **228**, 799–809.

Pietz J, Benninger C, Schaefer H. *et al.* (1993) Treatment of infantile spasms with high dosage vitamin B6. *Epilepsia* **34**, 757–763.

Pinard JM, Delalande O, Plouin P. *et al.* (1992) Results of callosotomy in children according to etiology and epileptic syndromes. *Epilepsia* **33** (Suppl. 3), 27.

Pinard JM, Delalande O, Plouin P. *et al.* (1993) Callosotomy in West syndrome suggests a cortical origin of hypsarrhythmia. *Epilepsia* **34**, 780–787.

Pinard JM, Motte J, Brian R, Dulac O. Subcortical laminar heterotopia and lissencephaly in two families: a common autosomal dominant or x-linked gene? *J Neurol Neurosurg Psychiat* (in press).

Pinder RM, Brogden RN, Speight TM, Avery GS. (1977) Sodium valproate: a review of its pharmacologic properties and therapeutic efficacy in epilepsy. *Drugs* **13**, 81–123.

Pine I, Engle L, Schwartz TB. (1951) The electroencephalogram in ACTH and cortisone treated patients. *Electroencephalogr Clin Neurophysiol* **3**, 301–310.

Pinel JPJ, Rovner LI. (1978) Experimental epileptogenesis: kindling induced epilepsy in rats. *Exp Neurol* **58**, 190–202.

Pinsard N. (1981) Evolution à long terme du syndrome de West (à propos du 100 cas). *Gaslin* **12**, (Suppl. 1) 24–26.

Plouin P, Dulac O, Jalin C, Chiron C. (1989) Partial seizures in West Syndrome: 24 hour ambulatory EEG monitoring. *Epilepsia* **30**, 690.

Plouin P, Dulac O, Jalin C, Chiron C. (1993) Twenty-four-hour ambulatory EEG monitoring in infantile spasms. *Epilepsia* **34**, 686–691.

Pognanno JR, Edwards MK, Lee Ta. *et al.* (1988) Cranial MR imaging in neurofibromatosis. *AJ Roentgen* **151**, 381–388.

Poley JR, Dumermuth G. (1968) EEG findings in patient with phenylketonuria before and during treatment with a low phenylalanine diet and in patients with some other inborn errors of metabolism. In: Holt KS, Coffey VP. (eds), *Some Recent Advances in Inborn Errors of Metabolism*. Edinburgh: Churchill Livingston, pp. 61–69.

Pollack MA, Golden GS, Schmidt R. *et al.* (1978) Infantile spasms in Down syndrome: a report of 5 cases and review of the literature. *Ann Neurol* **3**, 406–408.

Pollack MA, Zion TE, Kellaway PR. (1979) Long term prognosis of patients with infantile spasms following ACTH therapy. *Epilepsia* **20**, 255–260.

Pollack JM, Fernandez RE, Ward JD, Ghatak NR. (1983) Choroid plexus papilloma in Aicardi's syndrome. Paper presented at the meeting of the Child Neurology Society, Williamsburg, Va, 13–15 October 1983.

Poser CM, Low NL. (1960) Autopsy findings in three cases of hypsarrhythmia (infantile spasms with mental retardation). *Acta Paediatr (Uppsala)* **49**, 695–706.

Poulter MO, Barker JL, O'Carrol A, Lolait SJ, Mahan LC. (1992) Differrential and transient expression of GABA_A receptor α-subunit mRNAs in the developing rat CNS. *J Neurosci* **12**, 2888–2900.

Pou Serradel A. (1984) Epilepsia y Neurofibromatosis. *Boll Lega It Epil* **45/46**, 47–49.

Pou Serradel A, Salez-Vasquez R. (1971) Manifestations neurologiques (centrales) et non tumorales au cours de la neurofibromatose de Recklinghausen. *Rev Neurol (Paris)* **124**, 431–437.

Powell-Jackson PR, Tredger JM, Williams R. (1984) Hepatic toxicity of sodium valproate. A review. *Gut* **25**, 673–681.

Prats JM, Garaizar C, Rua MJ, Garcia-Nieto ML, Madoz P. (1991) Infantile spasms treated with high doses of sodium valproate: initial response and follow-up. *Dev Med Child Neurol* **33**, 617–625.

Preblud S, Alford C. (1990) Rubella. In: Remington J, Klein J. (eds), *Infectious Diseases of the Fetus and Newborn Infant*, London: W.B. Saunders.

Prichard JW, Gallagher BB, Glaser GH. (1969) Experimental seizure threshold testing with flurothyl. *J Pharm Exp Ther* **166**, 170–178.

Pritchett DB, Sontheimer H, Gorman CM. *et al.* (1988) Transient expression shows ligand gating and allosteric potentiation of GABA_A receptor subunits. *Science* **242**, 1306–1308.

Probst A, Ohnacker H. (1977) Sclérose tubéreuse de Bourneville chez un prématuré. *Acta Neuropathol* **40**, 157–161.

Pueschel SM, Louis S, McKnight P. (1991) Seizure disorders in Down syndrome. *Arch Neurol* **48**, 318–320.

Purves D, Lichtman JW. (1980) Elimination of synapses in the developing nervous system. *Science* **210**, 153–157.

Quesney LF, Risinger MW, Shewmon DA. (1993) Extracranial EEG evaluation. In: Engel J Jr. (ed.), *Surgical Treatment of the Epilepsies* 2nd edn. New York: Raven Press, pp. 173–195.

Racine RJ. (1972a) Modification of seizure activity by electrical stimulation: I. after-discharge threshold. *Electroencephal Clin Neurophysiol* **32**, 269–279.

Racine RJ. (1972b) Modification of seizure activity by electrical stimulation: II. motor seizures. *Electroencephal Clin Neurophysiol* **32**, 281–294.

Radermaker J, Toga M, Guazzi G. (1964) Etude anatomopathologique. In: Gastaut H. *et al.* (eds), *L'Encéphalopathie Infantile avec Hypsarrythmie (Syndrome de West)*, Paris: Masson.

Radvanyi-Bouvet MF, de Btehman O, Monsat-Couchard M, Fazzi E. (1987) Cerebral lesions in early prematurity: EEG prognostic value in the neonatal period. *Brain Dev* **9**, 399–405.

Rakic P. (1988a) Specification of cerebral cortical areas. *Science* **241**, 170–176.

Rakic P. (1988b) Defects of neuronal migration and the pathogenesis of cortical malformations. *Prog Brain Res* **73**, 15–37.

Ramsey RE. (1984) Controlled and comparative trials with valproate: United States. *Epilepsia* (Suppl. I) **25**, S40–S43.

Rao JK, Willis J. (1987) Hypothalamo-pituitary-adrenal function in infantile spasms: effects of ACTH therapy. *J Child Neurol* **2**, 220–223.

Rausch HP. (1984) Medullary nephrocalcinosis and pancreatic calcifications demonstrated by ultrasound and CT in infants after treatment with ACTH. *Radiology* **153**, 105–107.

Rayn SG, Sherman SL, Terry JL. *et al.* (1992) Startle disease or hyperekplexia: response to clonazepam and assignment to the gene (STHE) to chromosome 5 q by linkage analysis. *Ann Neurol* **31**, 663–668.

Raynaud C, Chiron C, Maziere B. *et al.* (1990) Follow-up of regional CBF in children from birth to 18 years with Xe-133. *J Nucl Med* **31**, 892.

Reif-Lehrer L, Stemmerman MG. (1975) Monosodium glutamate intolerance in children. *N Engl J Med* **293**, 1204.

Remington J, Desmonts G. (1990) Toxoplasmosis. In: Remington J, Klein J. (eds), *Infectious Diseases of the Fetus and Newborn Infant*. London: W.B. Saunders.

Renier WO, Le-Coultre R. (1989) Selected data from childhood epilepsies. ACTH treatment and ketogenic diet: a critical evaluation. *Tijdschr-Kindergeneeskd* **57**, 81–86.

Represa A, Robain O, Tremblay E, Ben Ari Y. (1989) Hippocampal plasticity in childhood epilepsy. *Neuroscience (Letter)* **99**, 351–355.

Resnick TJ, Moshé SL, Perotta L, Chambers HJ. (1986) Benign neonatal sleep myoclonus. Relationship to sleep states. *Arch Neurol* **43**, 266–268.

Ribadeau Dumas JL, Poirier J, Escourolle R. (1973) Etude ultrastructurale des lésions cérébrales de la sclérose tubéreuse de Bourneville. A propos de deux cas. *Acta Neuropathol* **25**, 259–270.

Richman DP, Stewart RM, Caviness VS Jr. (1974) Cerebral microgyria in a 27-week fetus: An architectonic and topographic analysis. *J Neuropathol Exp Neurol* **33**, 374–384.

Richter RB. (1957) Infantile subacute necrotizing encephalopathy with predilection for the brain stem. *J Neuropathol Exp Neurol* **16**, 281–307.

Riikonen R. (1978) Cytomegalovirus infection and infantile spasms. *Dev Med Child Neurol* **20**, 570–579.

Riikonen R. (1982) A long-term follow-up study of 214 children with the syndrome of infantile spasms. *Neuropediatrics* **13**, 14–23.

Riikonen R. (1983) Infantile spasms: some new theoretical aspects. *Epilepsia* **24**, 159–168.

Riikonen R. (1984a) Infantile spasms: modern practical aspects. *Acta Paediatr Scand* **73**, 1–12.

Riikonen R. (1984b) An unusual case of recovery from infantile spasms. *Dev Med Child Neurol* **26**, 18–821.

Riikonen R, Amnell G. (1981) Psychiatric disorders in children with earlier infantile spasms. *Dev Med Child Neurol* **23**, 747–760.

Riikonen R, Donner M. (1979) Incidence and aetiology of infantile spasms from 1960 to 1976: a population study in Finland. *Dev Med Child Neurol* **21**, 333–343.

Riikonen R, Donner M. (1980) ACTH therapy in infantile spasms: Side effects. *Arch Dis Child* **55**, 664–672.

Riikonen R, Meurnan O. (1989) Long-term persistence of intrathecal viral antibody responses in postinfectious diseases of the central nervous system and in Rett syndrome. *Neuropediatrics* **20**, 215–219.

Riikonen R, Perheentupa J. (1986) Serum steroids and success of corticotropin therapy in infantile spasms. *Acta Paediatr Scand* **75**, 598–600.

Riikonen R, Simell O, Jääskeläinen J, Rapola J, Perheentupa J. (1986) Disturbed calcium and phosphate homeostasis during treatment with ACTH of infantile spasms. *Arch Dis Child* **61**, 671–676.

Riikonen R, Santavuori P, Meretojoa O. *et al.* (1988) Can barbiturate anaesthesia cure infantile spasms? *Brain Dev* **10**, 300–304.

Rintahaka PJ, Chugani HT, Messa C, Phelps ME. (1993) Hemimegalencephaly: evaluation with positron emission tomography. *Pediatr Neurol* **9**, 21–28.

Robain O, Deonna T. (1983) Pachygyria and congenital nephrosis disorder of migration and neuronal orientation. *Acta Neuropathol* **60**, 137–141.

Robain O, Dulac O (1992) Early epileptic encephalopathy with suppression bursts and olivary–dentate dysplasia. *Neuropediatrics* **23**, 162–164.

Robain O, Gorce F. (1972) Arhinencephalie. Etude clinique, anatomique et étiologique de 13 cas. *Arch Franc Péd* **29**, 861–879.

Robain O, Floquet J, Heldt N, Rozenberg F. (1988) Hemimegalencephaly: A clinicopathological study of four cases. *Neuropathol Appl Neurobiol* **14**, 125–135.

Robain O, Chiron C, Dulac O. (1989) Electron microscopic and Golgi study in a case of hemimegalencephaly. *Acta Neuropathol* **77**, 664–666.

Robertson MM. (1986) Current status of the 1,4- and 1,5-benzodiazepines in the treatment of epilepsy: the place of clobazam. *Epilepsia* **27** (Suppl. 1), S27–S41.

Robinow M, Johnson GF, Minella PA. (1984) Aicardi syndrome, papilloma of the choroid plexus, cleft lip, and cleft of the posterior palate. *J Pediatr* **104**, 404–405.

Roger J, Dravet C, Boniver C. *et al.* (1984) L'épilepsie dans la sclérose tubéreuse de Bourneville. *Boll Lega It Epil* **45**, 33–38.

Roos RA, Maaswinkel-Mooy PD, Loo EM, Kanhai HH. (1987) Congenital microcephaly, infantile spasms, psychomotor retardation and nephrotic syndrome in two sibs. *Eur J Pediatr* **146**, 532–536.

Rosemberg S, Arita FN, Campos C. *et al.* (1984) Hypamelanosis of Ito. Case report with involvement of the central nervous system and review of the literature. *Neuropediatrics* **15**, 52–55.

Ross DL. (1986) Supressed pituitary ACTH response after ACTH treatment of infantile spasms. *J Child Neurol* 1, 34–37.

Ross DL, Liwnicz BH, Chun RW, Gilbert E. (1982) Hypomelanosis of Ito. A clinicopathological study: Macrocephaly and grey matter heteropias. *Neurology* 32, 1013–1016.

Rowe C, Berkovic S, Sia B. *et al.* (1989) Localization of epileptic foci with postictal single photon emission computed tomography. *Ann Neurol* 26, 660–668.

Rubinstein M, Denays R, Ham HR. *et al.* (1989) Functional imaging of brain maturation in humans using Iodine-123 Iodoamphetamine and SPECT. *J Nucl Med* 30, 1982–1985.

Ruggieri V, Caraballo R, Fejerman N. (1989) Intracranial tumors and West syndrome. *Pediatr Neurol* 5, 327–329.

Rugtveit J. (1986) X-linked mental retardation and infantile spasms in two brothers. *Dev Med Child Neurol* 28, 543–549.

Rumsey JM, Duara R, Grady C. *et al.* (1985) Brain metabolism in autism. Resting cerebral glucose utilization rate as measured with positron emission tomography. *Arch Gen Psychiat* 42, 448–455.

Rutledge SL, Snead OC, Kelly DR. *et al.* (1986) Pyruvate carboxylase deficiency presenting with acute exacerbation after the use of ACTH for infantile spasms. *Ann Neurol* 20, 401–402.

Rutledge SL, Snead OC, Kelly DR. *et al.* (1989) Pyruvate carboxylase deficiency: Acute exacerbation after ACTH treatment of infantile spasms. *Pediatr Neurol* 5, 201–206.

Saenz-Lope E, Herranz-Tanarro FJ, Masdeu JC, Chacon Peña JR. (1984) Hyperekplexia: a syndrome of pathological startle responses. *Ann Neurol* 15, 36–41.

Sainio K, Granström M-L, Pettay O, Donner M. (1983) EEG in neonatal herpes simplex encephalitis. *Electroencephalog Clin Neurophysiol* 56, 556–561.

Salonen R, Somer M, Haltia M. *et al.* (1991) Progressive encephalopathy with edema, hypsarrhythmia, and optic atrophy (PEHO syndrome). *Clin Genet* 39, 287–293.

Sandstedt P, Kostulas V, Larsson L. (1984) Intravenous gammaglobulin for postencephalitic epilepsy. *Lancet* 17, 1154–1155.

Sapolsky RM. (1987) Glucocorticoid and hippocampal damage. *Trends Neurosci* 10, 346–349.

Sapolsky RM, Krey LC, McEwen BS. (1984) Prolonged glucocorticoid exposure reduces hippocampal neuron number: implications for aging. *J Neurosci* 5, 1222–1227.

Sarnat HB (1992) *Cerebral Dysgenesis—Embryology and Clinical Expression.* New York: Oxford University Press.

Sarrieau A, Dussaillant M, Sapolsky RM. *et al.* (1988) Glucocorticoid binding sites in human temporal cortex. *Brain Res* 442, 157–160.

Satoh J, Takeshige H, Hara H, Fukuyama Y. (1982) Brain shrinkage and subdural effusion associated with ACTH administration. *Brain Dev* 4, 13–20.

Satoh J, Mizutani T, Morimatsu Y. *et al.* (1984) Neuropathology of infantile spasms. *Brain Dev* 6, 196.

Sauvage D. (1984) *Autisme du Nourrisson et du Jeune Enfant (−3 ans.). Signes Précoces et Diagnostic.* Paris: Masson.

Schachter M. (1954) Etudes sur les rythmes du jour et du sommeil de l'enfant (spasmus nutans, tic de Salaam, jactatio capitis nocturna). *L'encéphale* 43, 173–292.

Scheffner D, Konig S, Rauterberg-Ruland I. *et al.* (1988) Fatal liver failure in 16 children with valproate therapy. *Epilepsia* 29, 530–542.

Schlumberger E, Dulac O. A restricted and elective steroid treatment schedule for West syndrome (in press).

Schlumberger E, Dulac O, Plouin P. (1992) Early infantile epileptic syndrome(s) with suppression burst, nosological considerations. In: Roger J. *et al.* (eds), *Epileptic Syndromes in Infancy, Childhood and Adolescence,* 2nd edn. London: John Libbey Eurotext, pp. 35–42.

Schmidt D. (1983) How to use benzodiazepines. In: Morselli PL, Pippenger CE, Penry JK (eds), *Antiepileptic Drug Therapy in Pediatrics.* New York: Raven Press, pp. 271–278.

Schmidt D. (1984) Adverse effects of valproate. *Epilepsia* 25, 550–559.

Schofield PR, Darlison MG, Fujita N. *et al.* (1987) Sequence and functional expression of the GABA$_A$ receptor shows a ligand-gated receptor superfamily. *Nature* 328, 221–227.

Schwartz SA, Gordon KE, Johnston MV, Goldstein GW. (1989) Use of intravenous immune globulin in the treatment of seizure disorders. *J All Clin Immunol* 84, 603–606.

Schwartzberg DG, Nakane PK. (1983) ACTH-related peptide containing neurons within the medulla oblongata of the rat. *Brain Res* 276, 351–356.

Schwartzkroin PA. (1984) Epileptogenesis in the immature CNS. In: Schwartzkroin PA, Wheal HV. (eds), *Electrophysiology of Epilepsy*. London: Academic Press, pp. 389–412.

Schwartzkroin PA, Kunkel DD, Mathers LH. (1982) Development of rabbit hippocampus; anatomy. *Dev Brain Res* **2**, 452–468.

Seki T. (1990) Combination treatment of high-dose pyridoxal phosphate and low dose ACTH on children with West syndrome and related disorders. *Jap J Psychiatr Neurol* **44**, 219–237.

Senga P, Mayanda HF, Yidika M. (1986) Infantile spasms in 2 monozygotic twins. A new case (letter). *Presse Med* **15**, 485.

Seress L, Ribak CE. (1988) The development of GABAergic neurons in the rat hippocampal formation, an immunocytochemical study. *Dev Brain Res* **44**, 197–210.

Seri S, Cerquiglini A, Cusmai R, Curatolo P. (1991) Tuberous sclerosis: relationship between topographic mapping of EEG, VEPs and MRI findings. *Neurophysiol Clin* **21**, 161–72.

Shewmon DA, Shields WD, Olson DM, Peacock WJ, Chugani HT. (1989) Multifocal independent epileptogenicity in children treated by focal cortical resection. (abstract) *Epilepsia* **30**, 660.

Shewmon DA, Shields WD, Chugani HT, Peacock WJ. (1990) Contrasts between pediatric and adult epilepsy surgery: rationale and strategy for focal resection. *J Epilepsy* **3** (Suppl. 1), 141–155.

Shields WD, Nielsen C, Buch D. *et al.* (1988) Relationship of pertussis immunization to the onset of neurologic disorders: A retrospective epidemiologic study. *J Pediatr* **113**, 801–5.

Shields WD, Shewmon DA, Chugani HT, Peacock WJ. (1990) The role of surgery in the treatment of infantile spasms. *J Epilepsy* **3** (Suppl. 1), 321–324.

Shields WD, Shewmon DA, Chugani HT, Peacock WJ. (1992) Treatment of infantile spasms: Medical or surgical? *Epilepsia* **33** (Suppl. 4), S26–S31.

Shih VE, Efron ML, Moser HW. (1969) Hyperornithinemia, hyperammonemia and homocitrullinuria: a new disorder of amino acid metabolism associated with myoclonic seizures and mental retardation. *Am J Dis Child* **117**, 83–92.

Shouse MN, King A, Langer J. *et al.* (1990) The ontogeny of feline temporal lobe epilepsy: kindling a spontaneous seizure disorder in kittens. *Dev Brain Res* **52**, 215–224.

Shouse MN, Dittes P, Langer J, Nienhuis R. (1992) The ontogeny of feline temporal lobe epilepsy, II: Stability of spontaneous sleep epilepsy in amygdala-kindled kittens. *Epilepsia* **33**, 789–798.

Siegel RE. (1988) The mRNSAs encoding GABA$_A$/benzodiazepine receptor subunits are localized in different cell populations of the bovine cerebellum. *Neuron* **1**, 579–84.

Siemes H, Spohr HL, Michael T, Nau H. (1988) Therapy of infantile spasms with valproate: results of a prospective study. *Epilepsia* **29**, 553–560.

Silverstein F, Johnston MV. (1984) Cerebrospinal fluid monoamine metabolites in patients with infantile spasms. *Neurology* **34**, 102–105.

Simon D, Penry JK. (1975) Sodium di-n-propylacetate (DPA) in the treatment of epilepsy. A review. *Epilepsia* **16**, 549–573.

Simonsson H. (1972) Incontinentia pigmenti, Bloch-Sulzberger syndrome associated with infantile spasms. *Acta Paediat Scand* **61**, 612–614.

Sinton DW, Patterson PR. (1962) Infantile spasms. A case report with clinical and pathologic correlation. *Neurology* **12**, 351–360.

Singer WD, Rabe EF, Haller JS. (1980) The effect of ACTH therapy on infantile spasms. *J Pediatr* **96**, 485–489.

Singer WD, Haller JS, Sullivan LR. *et al.* (1982) The value of neuroradiology in infantile spasms. *J Pediatr* **100**, 47–50.

Snead OC. (1986) Neuropeptides and epilepsy. *Neurol Clin* **4**, 869–875.

Snead OC. (1987a) Opiate peptides and seizures. *Rev Clin Basic Pharmacol* **6**, 329–350.

Snead OC. (1987b) The neuropharmacology of epileptic falling spells. *Clin Neuropharmacol* **10**, 205–214.

Snead, OC III. (1989) Other antiepileptic drugs: Adrenocorticotrophic hormone (ACTH). In: Levy R. *et al.* (eds), *Antiepileptic Drugs*. New York: Raven Press, pp. 905–912.

Snead OC, Bearden LJ. (1982) The epileptogenic spectrum of opiate agonists. *Neuropharmacology* **21**, 1137–1144.

Snead OC, Simonato M. (1991) Opiate peptides and seizures. In: Fisher RJ, Coyle JT. (eds), *Neurotransmitters and Epilepsy*. New York: Wiley-Liss, pp. 181–200.

Snead OC, Benton JW, Myers GJ. (1983) ACTH and prednisone in childhood seizure disorders. *Neurology* **33**, 966–970.

Snead OC, Benton JW, Hosey LC. *et al.* (1989) Treatment of infantile spasms with high dose ACTH: Efficacy and plasma levels of ACTH and cortisol. *Neurology* **39**, 1027–1030.

Sofijanov NG. (1982) Clinical Evolution and Prognosis of Childhood Epilepsies. *Epilepsia* **23**, 61–69.

Somer M, Sainio K. (1993) Epilepsy and the electroencephalogram in progressive encephalopathy with edema, hypsarrhythmia, and optic atrophy (The PEHO syndrome). *Epilepsia* **34**, 727–731.

Sorel L. (1972) 196 cases of infantile myoclonic encephalopathy with hypsarrhythmia (IEMH: West syndrome) treated with ACTH. Danger of synthetic ACTH. *Electroencephalogr Clin Neurophysiol* **32**, 576.

Sorel L. (1978) Le syndrome de West atypique ou incomplet: a propos de 80 observations. *Boll Lega It Epil* **22/23**, 181–182.

Sorel L, Dusaucy-Bauloye A. (1958) A propos de cas d'hypsarythmie; de Gibbs: son traitement spectulaire par l'ACTH. *Acta Neurol Belg* **58**, 130–141.

Sorel L, Dusaucy-Bauloye A. (1959) A propos de 21 cas d'hyparythmie de Gibbs. *Rev Neurol* **100**, 333–334.

Sperber EF, Moshé SL. (1988) Age-related differences in seizure susceptibility to flurothyl. *Dev Brain Res* **39**, 295–297.

Sperber EF, Wong BY, Wurpel JND, Moshé SL. (1987) Nigral infusions of muscimol or bicuculline facilitate seizures in developing rats. *Dev Brain Res* **37**, 243–250.

Sperber EF, Brown LL, Wurpel JND, Moshé SL. (1988) Nigral infusions of muscimol in rat pups produce local cerebral glucose utilization effects different from adult rats. *Soc Neurosci Abstr* **14**, 1296.

Sperber EF, Wurpel JND, Moshé SL (1989a): Evidence for the involvement of nigral $GABA_B$ receptors in seizures in rat pups. *Dev Brain Res* **47**, 143–146.

Sperber EF, Brown LL, Smith DM, Moshé SL. (1989b) GABA-sensitive nigral efferents mapped with ^{14}C deoxyglucose autoradiography in rat pups. *Soc Neurosci Abstr* **15**, 1033.

Sperber EF, Wurpel JND, Zhao DY, Moshé SL. (1989c) Evidence for the involvement of nigral $GABA_A$ receptors in seizures of adult rats. *Brain Res* **480**, 378–382.

Sperber EF, Haas K, Moshé SL. (1990) Mechanisms of kindling in developing animals. In: Wada JA (ed.), *Kindling*, Vol. 4. New York: Plenum Press, pp. 157–167.

Sperber EF, Pellegrini-Giampietro DE, Friedman LK, Zukin RS, Moshé SL. (1991) Maturational differences in gene expression of $GABA_A$ $\alpha 1$ receptor subunit in rat substantia nigra. *Soc Neurosci Abstr* **17**.

Sperber EF, Brown LL, Moshé SL. (1992) Functional mapping of different seizure states in the immature rat using ^{14}C-2 deoxyglucose. *Epilepsia* **33**, 44.

Spranger J, Benirschke K, Hall JG. *et al.* (1982) Errors in morphogenesis: concepts and terms. *J Pediatrics* **100**, 160–165.

Stafstrom C, Mannheim GB, Marks D, Schiffmann R, Holmes G. (1989) Hemihypsarrhythmia: presenting features, etiological factors, and outcome. (abstract) *Ann Neurol* **26**, 469.

Stafstrom CE, Patxot OF, Gilmore HE, Wisniewski KE. (1991) Seizures in children with Down syndrome: etiology, characteristics and outcome. *Dev Med Child Neuro* **33**, 191–200.

Stagno S. (1990) Cytomegalovirus. In: Remington J, Klein J. (eds), *Infectious Diseases of the Fetus and Newborn Infant*. London: W.B. Saunders.

Stamps FW, Gibbs EL, Rosenthal IM, Gibbs FA. (1959) Treatment of hypsarrhythmia with ACTH. *J Am Med Assoc* **171**, 408–411.

Stefan H, Bauer J, Feistel H. *et al.* (1990) Regional cerebral blood flow during focal seizures of temporal and frontocentral onset. *Ann Neurol* **27**, 162–166.

Stephenson JPB. (1988) A study of tuberous sclerosis seizures using visual recording techniques. Tuberous sclerosis symposium. Nottingham Sept 15–16 (Abst).

Stephenson JBP (1990) *Fits and Faints*. Clinics in Developmental Medicine No. 109, London: MacKeith Press.

Sterio M, Gebauer E, Vucicevic G. *et al.* (1990) Intravenous immunoglobulin in the treatment of malignant epilepsy in children. *Wein Klin Wochenschr* **102**, 230–233.

Stewart RM, Richman DP, Caviness VS Jr. (1975) Lissencephaly and pachygyria. An architectonic and topographical analysis. *Acta Neuropathol* **31**, 1–12.

Su TP, London ED, Jaffe JH. (1988) Steroid binding at s receptors suggests a link between endocrine, nervous, and immune systems. *Science* **240**, 219–221.

Suchy FJ, Balistreri WJ, Bucjhine JJ. (1975) Acute hepatic failure associated with the use of sodium valproate. Report of two fatal cases. *N Engl J Med* **300**, 962–964.

Sugimoto T, Yasuhara A, Ohta T. *et al.* (1992) Angelman syndrome in free siblings: characteristic epileptic seizures and EEG abnormalities. *Epilepsia* **33**, 1078–1082.

Suhren O, Bruyn GW, Tuynman JA. (1966) Hyperekplexia: a hereditary startle syndrome. *J Neurol Sci* **3**, 577–605.

Sutula T, Cascino G, Cavazos J, Parada I, Ramirez L. (1989) Mossy fiber synaptic reorganization in the epileptic human temporal lobe. *Ann Neurol* **26**, 321–330.

Swann JW, Brady RJ. (1984) Penicillin-induced epileptogenesis in immature rats CA3 hippocampal pyramidal cells. *Dev Brain Res* **12**, 243–254.

Swann JW, Smith KL, Brady R. (1990) Neural networks and synaptic transmissions in immature hippocampus. In: Ben-Ari Y. (ed.), *Excitatory Amino Acids and Neuronal Plasticity. Advances in Experimental Medicine and Biology*. New York: Putnam Press, pp. 161–171.

Swann JW, Smith KL, Brady RJ. (1991) Age-dependent alterations in the operations of hippocampal neural networks. *Ann NY Acad Sci* **627**, 264–276.

Szélies B, Herholz K, Heiss D. *et al.* (1983) Hypometabolic cortical lesion in tuberous sclerosis with epilepsy: demonstration by PET. *J Comput Assist Tomogr* **7**, 946–953.

Tacke E, Kupferschmid C, Lang D. (1983) Hypertrophic cardiomyopathy during ACTH treatment. *Klin Padiatr* **195**, 124–128.

Taft LT, Cohen HJ. Hypsarrhythmia and infantile autism: a clinical report. *J Autism Dev Disord* **1**, 327–336.

Tamaki K, Okuno T, Ito M. *et al.* (1990) MRI in relation to EEG epileptic foci in tuberous sclerosis. *Brain Dev* **12**, 316–320.

Tardieu M, Khoury Y, Navelet E, Questiaux E, Landrieu P. (1986) Un syndrome spectaculaire et bénin de convulsions néonatales. Les myoclonies du sommeil profond. *Arch Fr Pediatr* **43**, 259–260.

Tatzer E, Groh C, Nueller R, Lischka A. (1987) Carbamazepine and benzodiazepines in combination: a possibility to improve the efficacy of treatment of patients with intractable infantile spasms. *Brain Dev* **9**, 451–417.

Taylor DC, Falconer MA, Bruton CJ, Corsellis JAN. (1971) Focal dysplasia of the cerebral cortex in epilepsy. *J Neurol Neurosurg Psychiat* **34**, 369–387.

Thibault JH, Manuelidis EE. (1970) Tuberous sclerosis in a premature infant. Report of a case and review of the literature. *Neurology* **20**, 139–146.

Tibbles JAR, Barnes SE (1980) Paroxysmal dystonic choreoathetosis of Mount and Reback. *Pediatrics* **65**, 149–151.

Tjiam AT, Stefanko S, Schenk VWD, de Vlieger M. (1978) Infantile spasms associated with hemihypsarrhythmia and hemimegalencephaly. *Dev Med Child Neurol* **20**, 779–798.

Todt H. (1984) The late prognosis of epilepsy in childhood: Results of a prospective follow-up study. *Epilepsia* **25**, 137–144.

Toga M, Gambarelli D. (1982) Ultrastructural study of 3 cases of encephalopathy with hypsarrhythmia. Similarities of lesions with subacute spongiform encephalopathies. *Acta Neuropathol* **56**, 311–314.

Tominaga I, Yanai K, Kashima H, Kato Y, Sekiyama S, Yokochi A, Miura I. (1986) Observation anatomo-clinique d'une séquelle d'encéphalopathie aiguë. *Rev Neurol* **142**, 524–529.

Tortella FC, Robles L, Holaday JW. (1985) Seizure threshold studies with dynorphin (1–13) in rats: possible interactions among k-, m, and d-opioid binding sites. *Pharmacologist* **27**, 179.

Trajaborg W, Plum P. (1960) Treatment of "hypsarrhythmia" with ACTH. *Acta Paediatr Scand* **49**, 572–582.

Trottier S, Evrard B, Haul-Dupas C. (1992) Etude structurale des lesions focales dysplasiques. 1er colloque de la Société des Neurosciences. Strasbourg, A154, p. 100.

Tsao CY, Ellingson RJ. (1990) Infantile spasms in two brothers with broad thumbs syndrome. *Clin Electroencephalogr* **21**, 93–95.

Tsuboi T. (1988) Prevalence and Incidence of Epilepsy in Tokyo. *Epilepsia* **29**, 103–110.

Unerstall JR, Kuhar MJ, Niehoff DL, Palacios JM. (1981) Benzodiazepine receptors are coupled to a subpopulation of GABA receptors: Evidence from a quantitative autoradiographic study. *J Pharm Exp Ther* **218**, 797–804.

Urban I, DeWeid D. (1976) Changes in excitability of the theta generating substrate by ACTH 4-10 in the rat. *Exp Brain Res* **24**, 325–334.

Urban I, Lopes de Silva FH, Storm van Leeuwen W, DeWeid D. (1974) A frequency shift in the hippocampal theta activity: an electrical correlate of central action of ACTH analogues in the dog? *Brain Res* **69**, 361–365.

Uthman BM, Reid SA, Wilder BJ, Andriola MR, Beydoun AA. (1991) Outcome for West syndrome following surgical treatment. *Epilepsia* **32**, 668–671.

Uvebrant P, Bjure J, Hedstrom A, Ekholm S. (1991) Brain single photon emission computed tomography (SPECT) in neuropediatrics. *Neuropediatrics* **22**, 3–9.

Valk J, Knaap MS. (1989) *Magnetic Resonance of Myelin, Myelination and Myelin Disorders.* Berlin: Springer Verlag.

Vanasse M, Bedard P, Andermann F. (1976) Shuddering attacks in children: an early clinical manifestation of essential tremor. *Neurology* **26**, 1027–1030.

Van Bogaert P, Chiron C, Adamsbaum C. *et al.* (1993) Value of magnetic resonance imaging in West syndrome of unknown etiology. *Epilepsia* **34**, 701–706.

Van Delft AML, Kitay JI. (1972) Effect of ACTH on single unit activity in the diencephalcon of intact and hypophysectomized rats. *Neuroendocrinology* **9**, 188–196.

Van den Berg BJ, Yerushalmy J. (1969) Studies on convulsive disorders in young children. *Pediat Res* **3**, 298–304.

Van Rijckevorsel Harmant K, Delire M, Rucquoy Ponsar M. (1986) Treatment of idiopathic West and Lennox-Gastaut syndromes by intravenous administration of human polyvalent immuno-globulins. *Eur Arch Psychiatr Neurol Sci* **236**, 119–122.

Van Wagenen W, Herren R. (1940) Surgical division of commissural pathways in the corpus callosum: relation to spread of an epileptic attack. *Acta Neurol Psychiat*, 440–759.

Vandvik B, Sköldenberg G, Forsgren M. *et al.* (1985) Long-term persistence of intrathecal virus-specific antibody responses after herpes simplex virus encephalitis. *J Neurol* **231**, 307–312.

Vasella F, Pavlincova E, Schneider HJ, Rudin HJ, Karbowski K. (1973) Treatment of infantile spasms and Lennox-Gastaut syndrome with clonazepam. *Epilepsia* **14**, 165–175.

Vazquez HJ, Turner M. (1951) Epilepsia en flexion generalizada. *Archivos argentinos de pediatria* **35**, 111–141.

Velez A, Dulac O, Plouin P. (1990) Prognosis for seizure control in infantile spasms preceded by other seizures. *Brain Dev* **12**, 306–309.

Vesikari T, Meurman O, Mäki R. (1980) Persistent rubella-specific IgM-antibody in the cerebro-spinal fluid of a child with congenital rubella. *Arch Dis Child* **55**, 46–48.

Viani F, Beghi E, Atza MG, Gulotta MP. (1988) Classifications of epileptic syndromes: Advantages and limitations for evaluation of childhood epileptic syndromes in clinical practice. *Epilepsia* **29**, 440–445.

Vidal C, Jordan W, Zieglgansberger W. (1986) Corticosterone reduces the excitability of hippocampal pyramidal cells *in vitro. Brain Res* **383**, 54–59.

Vigevano F, Aicardi J, Lini M, Pasquinelli A. (1984) La sindrome del nevo sebaceo lineare: presentazione di una casistica multicentrica. *Boll Lega Ital Epil* **45/46**, 59–63.

Vigevano F, Di Capua M, Dalla Bernardina B. (1989a) Startle disease: an avoidable cause of sudden infant death. *Lancet* **i**, 216.

Vigevano F, Bertini E, Boldrini R. *et al.* (1989b) Hemimegalencephaly and intractable epilepsy: benefits of hemispherectomy. *Epilepsia* **30**, 833–843.

Vigevano F, Fusco L, Di Capua M, Cusmai R, Claps D. (1991a) Ictal Video/EEG recording of infantile spasms: semiology helps etiological diagnosis. (abstract) *Epilepsia* **32**, 17–18.

Vigevano F, Bertini E, Claps D. *et al.* (1991b) Emimegalencefalia: correlazione tra neuroimaging, dati neurofisiologici ed evoluzione clinica. *Boll Lega It Epil* **74**, 157–159.

Vigevano F, Fusco L, Cusmai R, Claps D, Ricci S, Milani L. (1993) The idiopathic form of West syndrome. *Epilepsia* **34**, 743–746.

Vinters HV, Fisher RS, Cornford ME. *et al.* (1992) Morphological substrates of infantile spasms: studies based on surgically resected cerebral tissue. *Child's Nerv Syst* **8**, 8–17.

Vinters HV, Armstrong DL, Babb TL. *et al.* (1993a) The neuropathology of human symptomatic epilepsy. In: J Engel Jr. (ed.) *Surgical Treatment of the Epilepsies*, 2nd edn. New York: Raven Press.

Vinters HV, De Rosa MJ, Farrell MA. (1993b) Neuropathologic study of resected cerebral tissue from patients with infantile spasms. *Epilepsia* **34**, 772–729.

Vinters HV, Wang R, Wiley CA. (1993c) Herpesviruses in chronic encephalitis associated with intractable childhood epilepsy. *Hum Pathol* **24**, 871–879.

Vles BIS, Van der Heyden AMHG, Ghils A, Troost J. (1993) Vigabatrin in the treatment of infantile spasms. *Neuropediatrics* **24**, 230–231.

Volpe JJ. (1987) *Neurology of the Newborn*. London, Philadelphia: W.B. Saunders.

Vrensen G, De Groot D, Nunes-Cardozo J. (1977) Postnatal development of neurons and synapses in the visual and motor cortex of rabbits: A quantitative light and electron microscopic study. *Brain Res Bull* **2**, 405–416.

Wada JA, Osawa T. (1976) Spontaneous recurrent seizure state induced by daily electric amygdaloid stimulation in Senegalese baboons. *Neurol* **26**, 273–286.

Wada JA, Sato M, Corcoran ME. (1974) Persistent seizure susceptibility and recurrent spontaneous seizures in kindled cats. *Epilepsia* **15**, 465–478.

Waeber C, Dietl MM, Hoyer D. *et al.* (1988) Visualization of a novel serotonergic recognition site (5-HT$_{1D}$) in the human brain by autoradiography. *Neurosci Lett* **88**, 11–16.

Waeber C, Hoyer D, Palacios JM. (1989) GR 43175: A preferential 5-HT$_{1D}$ agent in monkey and human brains as shown by autoradiography. *Synapse* **4**, 168–170.

Wamsley JK, McCabe RT, Gehlert DR. (1988) Autoradiographic localization of binding sites in several GABA and benzodiazepine receptor complexes. In: Squires RF. (ed.), *GABA and Benzodiazepine Receptors*. Florida: CRC Press, pp. 80–90.

Watanabe K, Iwase K, Hara K. (1973) The evolution of EEG features in infantile spasms: a prospective study. *Dev Med Child Neurol* **15**, 584–596.

Watanabe K, Hara K, Iwase K. (1976) The evolution of neurophysiological features in holoprosencephaly. *Neuropediatrics* **7**, 19–41.

Watanabe K, Kuroyanagi M, Hara K, Miyazaki S. (1982) Neonatal seizures and subsequent epilepsy. *Brain Dev* **4**, 341–346.

Watanabe K, Takeuchi T, Hakamada S, Hayakawa F. (1987a) Neurophysiological and neuroradiological features preceding infantile spasms. *Brain Dev* **9**, 391–398.

Watanabe K, Negoro T, Matsumoto A, Furune S. (1987b) *The Malignant Epilepsies of Childhood. Recent Advances and Prognostic Value*. Proceedings of 2nd Congress of Asian and Oceanian Association of child neurology. Jakarta: Indonesian Council on Social Welfare, pp. 18–42.

Watanabe K, Negoro T, Aso K, Matsumoto A. (1993) Reappraisal of interictal electroencephalograms in infantile spasms. *Epilepsia* **34**, 679–685.

Watson SJ, Richard CW, Barchas JD. (1978) Adrenocorticotrophin in rat brain: immunocytochemical localization in cells and axons. *Science* **200**, 1080–1082.

Wayne HS. (1954) Convulsive seizures complicating cortisone and ACTH therapy: clinical and electroencephalographic observations. *J Clin Endocrin Metab* **14**, 1039–1045.

Weinmann H-M. (1988) Lennox-Gastaut syndrome and its relationship to infantile spasms (West syndrome). In: Niedermeyer E, Degen R. (eds), *The Lennox-Gastaut Syndrome*. New York: Alan R. Liss, pp. 419–426.

Wenderowich EL, Sokolansky GG. (1934) Ueber den lissencephalischen (pachyagyrischen) Idiotismus. *Anat Anz* **78**, 129–155.

Werlin SL, D'Souza NJ, Hogan WJ. *et al.* (1980) Sandifer syndrome: an unappreciated clinical entity. *Dev Med Child Neurol* **22**, 374–378.

West WJ. (1841) On a peculiar form of infantile convulsions. *Lancet* **i**, 724–725.

Westmoreland BF. (1988) EEG experience at the Mayo Clinic. In: Gomez MR. (ed.), *Tuberous Sclerosis*. New York: Raven Press, pp. 37–49.

Westmoreland BF, Gomez MR. (1987) Infantile spasms (West syndrome). In: Lüders H, Lesser RP. (eds), *Epilepsy: Electroclinical Syndromes*. New York: Springer-Verlag, pp. 49–70.

Whitley R. (1990) Herpes simplex virus infections. In: Remington J, Klein J. (eds), *Infectious Diseases of the Fetus and Newborn Infant*. London: W.B. Saunders.

Wilkins DE, Hallet M, Wess MM. (1986) Audiogenic startle reflex of man and its relationship to startle syndromes. *Brain* **109**, 561–573.

Willemse J. (1986) Benign idiopathic dystonia with onset in the first year of life. *Dev Med Child Neurol* **28**, 356–363.

Williams RS. (1976) The cellular pathology of microgyria. A Golgi analysis. *Acta Neuropathol* **36**, 269–283.

Williams RS, Ferrante RJ, Caviness US. (1979) The isolated human cortex. A Golgi analysis of Krabbe's disease. *Arch Neurol* **36**, 134–139.

Willig RP, Lagenstein I, Iffland E. (1977) Cortisoltagesprofile unter ACTH- und Dexamethason-Therapie Frühkindlicher Anfälle (BNS- und Lennox-Syndrom). *Mschr Kinderheilk* **126**, 191–197.

Willig RP, Lagenstein I. (1980) Therapiever such mit einem ACTH-Fragment (ACTH 4-10) bei Frühkinklichen Anfällen. *Mschr Kinderheilk* **128**, 100–103.

Willig RP, Lagenstein I. (1982) Use of ACTH fragments in children with intractable seizures. *Neuropediatrics* **13**, 55–58.

Willis J, Rosman P. (1980) The Aicardi syndrome versus congenital infection: diagnostic considerations. *J Pediatr* **96**, 235–239.

Willoughby JA, Thurston DL, Holowach J. (1966) Infantile myoclonic seizures: An evaluation of ACTH and corticosteroid therapy. *J Pediatr* **69**, 1136–1138.

Willshire (1851) Spasmus nictitans, Eclampsia nutans oder der sogennante Nick-krampf- und Salaam-convulsion (Kompliementierkrampf). *Jahrbuch für Kinderheilkunde* **16**, 293.

Wilson J, Carter C. (1978) Genetics of tuberous sclerosis. *Lancet* **i**, 340.

Wisden W, Morris BJ, Darlison MG, Hunt SP, Barnard EA. (1988) Distinct $GABA_A$ receptor alpha subunit mRNAs show differential patterns of expression in bovine brain. *Neuron* **1**, 937–947.

Wisden W, McNaughton LA, Darlison MG, Hunt SP, Barnard EA. (1989a) Differential distribution of $GABA_A$ receptor mRNAs in bovine cerebellum—localization of $\alpha2$ mRNA in Bergmann glia layer. *Neurosci Lett* **106**, 7–12.

Wisden W, Morris BJ, Darlison MG, Hunt SP, Barnard EA. (1989b) Localization of $GABA_A$ receptor α-subunit mRNAs in relation to receptor subtypes. *Mol Brain Res* **5**, 305–310.

Wisden W, Laurie DJ, Monyer H, Seeburg PH. (1992) The distribution of 13 $GABA_A$ receptor subunit mRNAs in the rat brain. I. Telencephalon, diencephalon, mesencephalon. *J Neurosci* **12**, 1040–1062.

Wöhler. Zur aetiologie der bösartige Blitz- und Nickkrampfe. Dissertatio Med Göttingen 1941. (Quoted by Zellweger).

Woodbury LA. (1977) Incidence and prevalence of seizure disorders including the epilepsies in the USA, a review and analysis of the literature. In: *Plan for the Nationwide Action of Epilepsy.* Washington DC: DHEW Publications, pp. 24–77.

Wurpel JND, Tempel A, Sperber EF, Moshé SL. (1988) Age-related changes of muscimol binding in the substantia nigra. *Dev Brain Res* **43**, 305–307.

Wurpel JND, Sperber EF, Moshé SL. (1990) Baclofen inhibits amygdala kindling in immature rats. *Epilepsy Res* **5**, 1–7.

Wyllie E, Wyllie R, Cruse RP, Erenberg G, Rothner D. (1984) Pancreatitis associated with valproate therapy. *Am J Dis Child* **138**, 912–914.

Wyllie E, Luders H, Morris HH. *et al.* (1988) Subdural electrodes in the evaluation for epilepsy surgery in children and adults. *Neuropediatrics* **19**, 80–86.

Xu SG, Garant DS, Sperber EF, Moshé SL (1991a) Effects of substantia nigra γ-vinyl-GABA infusions on flurothyl seizures in adult rats. *Brain Res* **566**, 108–114.

Xu SG, Sperber EF, Moshé SL. (1991b) Is the anticonvulsant effect of substantia nigra infusion of γ-vinyl GABA (GVG) mediated by the $GABA_A$ receptor in rat pups? *Dev Brain Res* **59**, 17–21.

Xu SG, Garant DS, Sperber EF, Moshé SL. (1992) The proconvulsant effect of nigral infusion of THIP on flurothyl-induced seizures in rat pups. *Develop Brain Res* **68**, 275–7.

Yakovlev PI, Wadsworth RC. (1946) Schizencephalies. A study of the congenital clefts in the cerebral mantle. II. Clefts with hydrocephalus and lips separated. *J Neuropathol Exp Neurol* **5**, 169–206.

Yamagata T, Momoi M, Miyamoto S, Kobayashi S, Kamoshita S. (1990) Multi-institutional survey of the Aicardi syndrome in Japan. *Brain Develop* **12**, 760–765.

Yamamoto N, Watanabe K, Negoro T, Matsumoto A. *et al.* (1985) Aicardi's syndrome: report of 6 cases and a review of Japanese literature. *Brain Dev* **7**, 443–449.

Yamamoto N, Watanabe K, Negoro T. *et al.* (1987) Long-term prognosis of tuberous sclerosis with epilepsy in children. *Brain Dev* **9**, 292–295.

Yamamoto N, Watanabe K, Negoro T, Furune S. *et al.* (1988) Partial seizures evolving to infantile spasms. *Epilepsia* **29**, 34–40.

Yasujima M, Konishi Y, Kuriyamo M. *et al.* (1989) MR imaging in infantile spasms. *No to Hattatsu* **21**, 537–542.

Zellweger H. (1948) Krämpfe in kindersalter. *Helvetica Pediatrica Acta* (Suppl. 5), 1–195.

Zellweger H, Hess R. (1950) Familiare Blitz-nick und salaam krämpfe. *Helvetica Paediatrica Acta* **5**, 85–94.

Zimmerman JF, Ishak KG. (1982) Valproate induced hepatic injury: analysis of 23 fatal cases. *Hepatology* **2**, 591–607.

Index

Note: the definitions as explained on page 11 will be useful as a guide for users of the index.